KEY ASPECTS OF CARING FOR THE CHRONICALLY ILL

Sandra G. Funk, PhD, is Professor and Director of the Research Support Center (RSC) at the School of Nursing, the University of North Carolina at Chapel Hill. A faculty member of the School of Nursing for over 16 years, she served as coordinator of the graduate research sequence, teaching graduate research methods, statistics, and computer applications for 10 years, and has been Director of the RSC for the past 7 years. She has served as research and statistical advisor to nursing faculty and graduate students in several universities, and for 5 years was research advisor to the Robert Wood Johnson fellows in general pediatrics at Duke University. She has served as principal and co-investigator of numerous grants and has published in the areas of preschool development screening, research utilization, decision making, scaling, and cluster analysis.

Elizabeth M. Tornquist, MA, has been a member of the faculty of the School of Nursing at the University of North Carolina at Chapel Hill for 16 years, where she teaches scientific writing to graduate students and serves as editor in residence. Ms. Tornquist is also on the faculty of the Curriculum of Public Health Nursing at the School of Public Health, the University of North Carolina at Chapel Hill. She is a former journalist and freelance writer and is the author of *From Proposal to Publication: An Informal Guide to Writing about Nursing Research* as well as numerous articles on writing.

Mary T. Champagne, PhD, RN, is Associate Professor and Dean at the School of Nursing, Duke University; Associate Director of Nursing Services, Duke University Hospital; and Senior Fellow at the Duke University Center for Study of Aging and Human Development, Durham, North Carolina. She is co-principal investigator of a 5-year study that is testing interventions to prevent the development of acute confusion in hospitalized elderly patients. She is currently the National Nurse Advisor for Humana Heart Institute International in Louisville, Kentucky.

Ruth A. Wiese, MSN, RN, a former faculty member of the University of Nebraska College of Nursing and an in-service instructor and coordinator of staff development in a clinical setting, is currently a Research Instructor at the School of Nursing, the University of North Carolina at Chapel Hill, and Project Coordinator for "Moving New Nursing Knowledge Into Practice: A CE Program."

KEY ASPECTS OF CARING FOR THE CHRONICALLY ILL

Hospital and Home

Sandra G. Funk, PhD
Elizabeth M. Tornquist, MA
Mary T. Champagne, PhD, RN
Ruth A. Wiese, MSN, RN
Editors

Springer Publishing Company
New York

Springer Publishing Company, Inc.
536 Broadway
New York, NY 10012–3955

94 95 96 97 / 5 4 3 2

Library of Congress Cataloging-in-Publication Data

Key aspects of caring for the chronically ill: hospital and home / Sandra Funk . . . [et al.], editors.
p. cm.
Includes bibliographical references and index.
ISBN 0–8261–8080–9
1. Chronic diseases—Nursing. 2. Chronically ill—Care. 3. Long-term care of the sick. I. Funk, Sandra G.
[DNLM: 1. Home Care Services—nurses' instruction. 2. Chronic Disease-nursing. WY 115 K437 1993]
RT120.C45K48 1993
610.73—dc20
DNLM/DLC
for Library of Congress 93–19828
CIP

Printed in the United States of America

MOVING NEW NURSING KNOWLEDGE INTO PRACTICE*

ADVISORY COMMITTEE

Chair: **Carolyn A. Williams,** PhD, RN, FAAN
Professor and Dean, School of Nursing
University of Kentucky

Members: **Linda R. Cronenwett,** PhD, RN, FAAN
Director, Nursing Research and Education
Dartmouth-Hitchcock Medical Center

Cynthia M. Freund, PhD, RN, FAAN
Professor and Dean, School of Nursing
The University of North Carolina at Chapel Hill

PROJECT TEAM

Project Director: **Sandra G. Funk,** PhD
Professor and Director, Research Support Center
School of Nursing
The University of North Carolina at Chapel Hill

Co-Project Director: **Elizabeth M. Tornquist,** MA
Lecturer, School of Nursing
The University of North Carolina at Chapel Hill

Clinical Nursing Research Specialist: **Mary T. Champagne,** PhD, RN
Associate Professor and Dean, School of Nursing
Duke University, Durham, NC

Project Coordinator: **Ruth A. Wiese,** MSN, RN
Research Instructor, School of Nursing
The University of North Carolina at Chapel Hill

Administration Specialist: **Sheila P. Englebardt,** MEd, RN, CNA
Clinical Assistant Professor, School of Nursing
The University of North Carolina at Chapel Hill

General Advisor: **Laurel Archer Copp,** PhD, RN, FAAN
Professor, School of Nursing
The University of North Carolina at Chapel Hill

*The "Moving New Nursing Knowledge Into Practice" Project is funded by the Division of Nursing, DHHS, Grant # D10 NU24318.

Contents

Acknowledgments *xi*
Contributors *xiii*

Part I. Caring for the Chronically Ill: An Overview

1 Caring for the Chronically Ill: From Research to Practice 3
Sandra G. Funk, Elizabeth M. Tornquist, Mary T. Champagne, and Ruth A. Wiese

2 Managing Chronicity: The Heart of Nursing Care 8
Angela Barron McBride

3 Managing the Hospitalized Chronically Ill 21
Barbara J. Daly

4 Assisting with Transitions from Hospital to Home 30
Dorothy Brooten

5 Managing Home Care 38
Patricia A. Cloonan

6 Living with Chronic Illness: Living with Uncertainty 46
Merle H. Mishel

7 Exercise Interventions for the Chronically Ill: Review and Prospects 59
Carol C. Hogue, Sharon M. Cullinan, and Eleanor McConnell

8 Evaluating Research Findings for Practice 79
Linda R. Cronenwett

Part II. Caring for Chronically Ill Adults

9 A Special Care Unit for the Chronically Critically Ill 93
Barbara J. Daly and Ellen B. Rudy

10 Special Care Units for Persons with Alzheimer's Disease: A Successful Intervention? 112
Kathleen Coen Buckwalter, Meridean L. Maas, Elizabeth A. Swanson, and Geri Richards Hall

11 Managing Acute Exacerbations of Chronic Illness in the Elderly 132
Denise M. Kresevic, C. Seth Landefeld, Robert Palmer, and Jerome Kowal

12 Meeting the Discharge Needs of Hospitalized Elderly and Their Caregivers 142
Mary D. Naylor, Roberta L. Campbell, and Janice B. Foust

13 Effect of a Self-Help Course on Adaptation in People with Arthritis 150
Ann Mabe Newman

14 Promoting a Learned Self-Help Response to Chronic Illness 158
Carrie Jo Braden

15 Uncertainty Management for Women Receiving Treatment for Breast Cancer 170
Judith McHenry, Carol Allen, Merle H. Mishel, and Carrie Jo Braden

16 Quantitative Progressive Exercise Rehabilitation: Rehabilitation of Patients with Osteoarthritis 178
Nadine M. Fisher and David R. Pendergast

17 Exercise Testing and Training in Physically Disabled Subjects with Coronary Artery Disease 189
Barbara J. Fletcher and Lilian M. Vassallo

18 Exercise Training for Frail Rural Elderly: A Pilot Study 202
Carol C. Hogue and Sharon M. Cullinan

19 Family Caregivers of Severely Head-Injured Adults in the Community Setting 212
Joanne V. Hickey

20 Role Acquisition in Family Caregivers for Older People Who Have Been Discharged from the Hospital 219
Barbara J. Stewart, Patricia G. Archbold, Theresa A. Harvath, and Ngozi O. Nkongho

21 Chronic Sorrow: An Examination of Nursing Roles 231
Georgene G. Eakes, Mary L. Burke, Margaret A. Hainsworth, and Carolyn L. Lindgren

Part III. Caring for Chronically Ill Children

22 Nurses' and Parents' Negotiation of Caregiving Roles for Medically Fragile Infants: Barriers and Bridges 239
Margaret Shandor Miles and Annette C. Frauman

23 The Behaviors and Nursing Care of Preterm Infants with Chronic Lung Disease 250
Diane Holditch-Davis and Deborah Assad Lee

24 Cost Burden of Low Birthweight 271
Susan Gennaro, Dorothy Brooten, Audrey Klein, Marilyn Stringer, Ruth York, and Linda Brown

25 Parental Role Alterations Experienced by Mothers of Children with a Life-Threatening Chronic Illness 281
Margaret Shandor Miles, Jennifer Piersma D'Auria, Ellen M. Hart, Debra A. Sedlack, and Melody Ann Watral

26 Family Response to a Child's Chronic Illness: A Description of Major Defining Themes 290
Kathleen A. Knafl, Agatha M. Gallo, Bonnie J. Breitmayer, Linda H. Zoeller, and Lioness Ayres

27 Quality of Life and Family Relationships in Families Coping with Their Child's Chronic Illness 304
Becky J. Christian

28 Impact of Childhood Cancer on Families at Home 312
Ida M. Martinson

29 The Effects of an Asthma Education Program on Selected Health Behaviors of School-Aged Children with Asthma 319
Laurel R. Talabere

Part IV. Caring for the Chronically Ill: Implications for the Future

30 Clinical Implications of Research on Caring for Chronically Ill Adults and Children: Where Can We Go From Here? 333
Barbara Germino

Index 339

Acknowledgments

Support for this project was provided by a special projects grant (#1 D10 NU24318), "Moving New Nursing Knowledge Into Practice: A CE Program," awarded to the School of Nursing, The University of North Carolina at Chapel Hill, from the Division of Nursing, Bureau of Health Professions, Department of Health and Human Services. We are most appreciative of the support provided by the Division of Nursing for this project and of the thoughtful direction and guidance provided by our Advisory Committee: Dr. Carolyn A. Williams, Dr. Linda R. Cronenwett, and Dr. Cynthia M. Freund. For this volume and the conference it reports, Ms. Barbara J. Daly, Assistant Director of Nursing at the University Hospitals of Cleveland and Assistant Clinical Professor, Case Western Reserve University; Dr. Dorothy Brooten, Professor, University of Pennsylvania; Dr. Patricia A. Cloonan, Clinical Assistant Professor, The University of North Carolina at Chapel Hill; Dr. Merle H. Mishel, Professor, The University of North Carolina at Chapel Hill, and Dr. Carol C. Hogue, Associate Professor, The University of North Carolina at Chapel Hill, provided content expertise in the areas of managing acute exacerbations of chronic illness, assisting with transitions to home, managing home care, living with a chronic illness, and exercise interventions, respectively. We are grateful for their contributions. Heartfelt thanks are extended to our project secretary, Frances G. Hoffman, for her work on this volume, and to Brian Neelon and Michael Terry, who worked with the editors in developing conference materials and preparing this volume.

Contributors

Patricia G. Archbold, DNSc, RN, FAAN
Professor, Department of Family Nursing, School of Nursing, Oregon Health Sciences University, Portland

Carol Allen, BSN, RN
Graduate Research Assistant, College of Nursing, University of Arizona, Tucson

Lioness Ayres, MS, RN
Doctoral Candidate, Department of Nursing Sciences, College of Nursing, University of Illinois at Chicago

Carrie Jo Braden, PhD, RN
Associate Professor, College of Nursing, University of Arizona, Tucson

Bonnie J. Breitmayer, PhD, RN
Associate Professor, Psychiatric Nursing, College of Nursing, University of Illinois at Chicago

Dorothy Brooten, PhD, RN, FAAN
Professor and Chair, Health Care of Women and Childbearing, School of Nursing, University of Pennsylvania, Philadelphia

Linda Brown, PhD
Associate Professor, School of Nursing, University of Pennsylvania, Philadelphia

Kathleen Coen Buckwalter, PhD, RN, FAAN
Professor and Associate Director, Office of Nursing Research, College of Nursing, The University of Iowa, Iowa City

Mary L. Burke, DNSc, RN
Associate Professor, Department of Nursing, Rhode Island College, Providence

Roberta L. Campbell, MSN, RN, C
Research Associate, School of Nursing, University of Pennsylvania, Philadelphia

Becky J. Christian, PhD, RN
Assistant Professor, Department of Women's and Children's Health, School of Nursing, The University of North Carolina at Chapel Hill

Patricia A. Cloonan, PhD, RN
Clinical Assistant Professor, Department of Social and Administrative Systems, School of Nursing, The University of North Carolina at Chapel Hill

Linda R. Cronenwett, PhD, RN, FAAN
Director, Nursing Research and Education, Dartmouth-Hitchcock Medical Center, Hanover, New Hampshire

Sharon M. Cullinan, BSN, RN
Clinical Research Nurse, School of Nursing, The University of North Carolina at Chapel Hill

Jennifer Piersma D'Auria, PhD, RN, CPNP
Assistant Professor, Department of Women's and Children's Health, School of Nursing, The University of North Carolina at Chapel Hill

Barbara J. Daly, MSN, RN, FAAN, CCRN
Assistant Director of Nursing, University Hospitals of Cleveland, and Assistant Professor, Frances Payne Bolton School of Nursing, Case Western Reserve University, Cleveland, Ohio

Georgene G. Eakes, EdD, RN
Associate Professor, School of Nursing, East Carolina University, Greenville, North Carolina

Nadine M. Fisher, EdD
Clinical Assistant Professor, Department of Rehabilitation Medicine, School of Medicine, State University of New York at Buffalo

Barbara J. Fletcher, MN, RN
Director of Research, Department of Rehabilitation Medicine, School of Medicine, Emory University, Atlanta, Georgia

Janice B. Foust, MS, RN
Research Assistant, School of Nursing, University of Pennsylvania, Philadelphia

Annette C. Frauman, PhD, RN, FAAN
Associate Professor, Department of Women's and Children's Health, School of Nursing, The University of North Carolina at Chapel Hill

Agatha M. Gallo, PhD, RN
Associate Professor, Maternal and Child Nursing, College of Nursing, University of Illinois at Chicago

Susan Gennaro, DSN, RN, FAAN
Assistant Professor and Director Perinatal Program, School of Nursing, University of Pennsylvania, Philadelphia

Barbara B. Germino, PhD, RN, FAAN
Associate Professor and Chair, Department of Adult and Geriatric Health, School of Nursing, The University of North Carolina at Chapel Hill

Margaret A. Hainsworth, PhD, RN
Professor, Department of Nursing, Rhode Island College, Providence

Geri Richards Hall, MA, RN, CS
Gerontology Clinical Nursing Specialist, University of Iowa Hospitals and Clinics, Iowa City

Ellen M. Hart, MSN, RN
Clinical Nurse Specialist, Department of Pediatric Cardiology and Cardiac Surgery, Duke University Medical Center, Durham, North Carolina

Theresa A. Harvath, PhD, RN
Assistant Professor, Department of Family Nursing, School of Nursing, Oregon Health Sciences University, Portland

Joanne V. Hickey, PhD, RN, CNRN
Assistant Professor, School of Nursing, Duke University Medical Center, Durham, North Carolina

Carol C. Hogue, PhD, RN, FAAN
Associate Professor and Associate Dean for Graduate Studies, School of Nursing, The University of North Carolina at Chapel Hill

Diane Holditch-Davis, PhD, RN
Assistant Professor, Department of Women's and Children's Health, School of Nursing, The University of North Carolina at Chapel Hill

Audrey Klein, MSN, RN
Clinical Liaison, Paidos Health Care, Inc., Paoli, Pennsylvania

Kathleen A. Knafl, PhD
Professor and Associate Dean, College of Nursing, University of Illinois at Chicago

Jerome Kowal, MD
Professor, School of Medicine, Case Western Reserve University and University Hospitals of Cleveland, Ohio

Denise M. Kresevic, MSN, RN, CS
Clinical Nurse Specialist, University Hospitals of Cleveland, and Clinical Instructor, Frances Payne Bolton School of Nursing, Case Western Reserve University, Cleveland, Ohio

C. Seth Landefeld, MD
Associate Professor, Department of Internal Medicine, Case Western Reserve University and University Hospitals of Cleveland, Ohio

Deborah Assad Lee, MSN, RN
Research Assistant, Department of Women's and Children's Health, School of Nursing, The University of North Carolina at Chapel Hill

Carolyn L. Lindgren, PhD, RN
Assistant Professor, College of Nursing, Wayne State University, Detroit, Michigan

Meridean L. Maas, PhD, RN, FAAN
Associate Professor and Chair, Department of Organizations and Systems, College of Nursing, The University of Iowa, Iowa City

Ida M. Martinson, PhD, RN, FAAN
Professor, Department of Family Health Care Nursing, School of Nursing, University of California, San Francisco

Angela Barron McBride, PhD, RN, FAAN
Distinguished Professor and University Dean, School of Nursing, Indiana University, Indianapolis

Eleanor McConnell, MSN, RN
Clinical Nurse Specialist, Department of Veterans' Affairs Medical Center, Durham, North Carolina

Judith McHenry, BSN, RN
Research Nurse, College of Nursing, University of Arizona, Tucson

Margaret Shandor Miles, PhD, RN
Professor and Chair, Department of Women's and Children's Health, School of Nursing, The University of North Carolina at Chapel Hill

Merle H. Mishel, PhD, RN, FAAN
Professor, Department of Adult and Geriatric Health, School of Nursing, The University of North Carolina at Chapel Hill

Mary D. Naylor, PhD, RN, FAAN
Associate Dean and Director of Undergraduate Studies, School of Nursing, University of Pennsylvania, Philadelphia

Ann Mabe Newman, DSN, RN, C
Assistant Professor, College of Nursing, and Adjunct Assistant Professor of Women's Studies, The University of North Carolina at Charlotte

Ngozi O. Nkongho, PhD, RN
Postdoctoral Fellow, School of Nursing, Oregon Health Sciences University, Portland

Robert Palmer, MPH, MD
Associate Professor, School of Medicine, Case Western Reserve University, and Medical Director, ACE Unit, University Hospitals of Cleveland, Ohio

David R. Pendergast, EdD
Professor, Department of Physiology, School of Medicine, State University of New York at Buffalo

Ellen B. Rudy, PhD, RN, FAAN
Professor and Dean, School of Nursing, University of Pittsburgh, Pennsylvania

Debra A. Sedlack, MSN, RN
Nurse Clinician, Department of Pediatrics, Division of Allergy and Immunology, Duke University Medical Center, Durham, North Carolina

Barbara J. Stewart, PhD
Professor, Department of Family Nursing, School of Nursing, Oregon Health Sciences University, Portland

Marilyn Stringer, MSN, RN
Clinical Specialist, School of Nursing, University of Pennsylvania, Philadelphia

Elizabeth A. Swanson, PhD, RN
Associate Professor and Chair, Department of Theory and Health Promotion, College of Nursing, The University of Iowa, Iowa City

Laurel R. Talabere, PhD, RNC, CPNP
Professor, School of Nursing, Capital University, Columbus, Ohio

Lilian M. Vassallo, MD
Medical Assistant, Coronary Care Unit, Department of Cardiology, Guillermo Almenara Hospital, Lima, Peru

Melody Ann Watral, MSN, RN
Head Nurse, Pediatric Surgery Unit, University of North Carolina Children's Hospital, Chapel Hill

Ruth York, PhD, RN, FAAN
Associate Professor and Director of Health Care of Women, School of Nursing, University of Pennsylvania, Philadelphia

Linda H. Zoeller, MPH, RN
Assistant Professor, Department of Public Health Nursing, University of Illinois at Chicago, and Lecturer, School of Nursing, Indiana University at South Bend

Part I

CARING FOR THE CHRONICALLY ILL: AN OVERVIEW

[1]

Caring for the Chronically Ill: From Research to Practice

Sandra G. Funk, Elizabeth M. Tornquist, Mary T. Champagne, and Ruth A. Wiese

Arthritis, cancer, diabetes, stroke, heart disease, respiratory illness, neuromuscular disorders, dementia, and AIDS are but a few of the major chronic illnesses facing us today. Over half of the American population have one or more chronic illnesses, and almost 30% of these individuals have sufficient disability to limit their normal daily activities (Lambert & Lambert, 1987). Further, 31% of children under the age of 18 years are estimated to be affected by chronic illnesses or chronic conditions such as respiratory allergies, repeated ear infections, and asthma; for over a third of these children, the severity of the condition results in limitation of activity (Newacheck & Taylor, 1992). With the graying of our population, the prevalence of chronic conditions will continue to increase.

Chronic illnesses are caused by pathological changes in the body that are non-reversible, permanent, or leave residual disability; they may be characterized by periods of recurrence and remission, and they generally require extended periods of supervision, observation, care, and rehabilitation (Commission on Chronic Illness, 1956; Kerson & Kerson, 1985). Chronic illnesses have a major impact on all aspects of a person's life—physical, psychological, familial, social, vocational, and economic (Lubkin, 1990; Falvo, 1991). They may result in impaired functioning, limitations in self-care and activities of daily living, loss of independence, pain and discomfort, problems with sleep and rest, changes in mood and affect, and disruption of family and social life (Lubkin, 1990; Kerson & Kerson, 1985). Chronic illnesses are by definition beyond the realm of traditional medical science, which has focused on "cure." They are at the heart of nursing, whose focus is on "care."

Nurses in hospitals, long-term care, community settings, and home health play key roles in caring for the chronically ill—from neonates to the elderly—and in helping these patients and their families maintain quality of life. Nurses deal with acute episodes, ease transitions between hospital and community, and promote functional independence. They also assist patients and families to deal with high-tech home care, manage complex regimens, and live with persistent problems.

Research can offer guidance to the nurse who is caring for the chronically ill. It can provide the data to help nurses better understand the life situation of the chronically ill and their caregivers—their experiences, their needs, and their capabilities; it can provide interventions to meet those needs and maximize those capabilities—to enhance function, promote self-care, and reduce symptoms; and it can show us ways to adapt the environment to the special needs of the chronically ill, or it can teach them and their caregivers to better navigate environments that cannot be changed. While much about caring for the chronically ill remains to be studied, important studies are available to guide clinicians. Unfortunately, in this area, as in many other areas of nursing, there is a sizable gap between research and practice (Kirchhoff, 1982; Brett, 1987). The purpose of this volume is to share the latest nursing research on key aspects of caring for the chronically ill with practicing nurses—to move the ideas and findings of the research into the practice setting.

This book is one part of our multifaceted approach to improving the dissemination of nursing research and, ultimately, the use of research in nursing practice. There are four major components to the approach:

1. carefully structured topic-focused conferences present nursing research findings that are ready for practice in a form that is easy to understand and that emphasizes usefulness in the clinical setting;
2. pre- and post-conference workshops assist clinicians and administrators in selecting research-based innovations appropriate for use in their settings and assist them in identifying suitable implementation strategies;
3. carefully edited books, based on the conference research presentations and discussions, are published to ensure that the research is broadly disseminated; and
4. an information center and newsletter provide consultation and a communication mechanism for clinicians and administrators during the implementation of the innovations. (See Funk, Tornquist, & Champagne, 1989a, for a fuller explanation of this approach.)

Topics for the conferences are selected based on their importance to the practice of nursing, their applicability to a broad range of settings, the availability of ongoing research in the area, the ability of nurses to control interventions, and the perceived gap between knowledge and practice. Researchers are invited through a national call to submit their research for presentation at the conference, and submissions are reviewed by a panel of individuals with practice and research expertise in the topic area, or with methodological or statistical expertise. Papers are selected based on scientific merit, significance, and readiness for practice. The conference is structured to include information on the current bases for practice, the selected research papers, discussions by clinicians and researchers that focus on moving the research into practice, discussion of strategies for implementation, and demonstration sessions. Extensive consultation is provided to researchers to assist them with the preparation of research presentations that are scientifically sound, clearly presented, and practice oriented.

Three previous conferences using this approach to dissemination of nursing research focused on comfort—management of pain, fatigue, and nausea; recovery—improving nutrition, rest, and mobility; and elder care—managing falls, incontinence, and cognitive impairment. These conferences were attended by hundreds of nurses from many countries, the majority of whom were employed in clinical settings. Evaluations of the conferences conveyed the participants' excitement and enthusiasm for improving their practice based on the research they had heard (Funk, Tornquist, & Champagne, 1989b). Springer Publishing Company has published the books emanating from the conferences (Funk, Tornquist, Champagne, Copp, & Wiese, 1989, 1990; and Funk, Tornquist, Champagne, & Wiese, 1992); all have received *American Journal of Nursing* Book of the Year awards.

The fourth conference was equally successful. Held in April of 1992, it focused on key aspects of caring for the chronically ill. This volume stems from the conference. Its purpose is to provide a wider audience of practicing nurses with the most current research on caring for the chronically ill—research that describes new ways to manage acute exacerbations of chronic illness and new types of hospital units designed to meet the special needs of the chronically ill; research that evaluates new exercise programs that enhance the mobility, strength, and endurance of the chronically ill; research that tests interventions to promote self-help, reduce uncertainty, and enhance independence; and research that describes the psychological, social, and economic impact of chronic illness on families and caregivers. Since the purpose of the volume is to present the latest in nursing research, the selected papers necessarily reflect the scope and focus of research today. Negative findings are included when they are felt to illustrate an important point. Replicated findings were preferred, but unreplicated research is also included if aspects of the findings are ready for informal use or clinical trials, point to important factors that should be considered in practice, or alert the reader to important future research in a new area. Collectively, these works provide the clinician with the knowledge and means to enhance practice and improve patient care.

Each paper has been edited extensively with the clinical audience in mind. Each study is presented as a full research report, but technical language is minimized, only directly relevant literature is cited, research methods are presented directly and simply, results sections focus on describing the major findings rather than the statistics, and discussion sections detail implications for practice. Introductory papers describe strategies for using the research in practice and the current bases for nursing practice with regard to managing the hospitalized chronically ill, assisting with transitions from hospital to home, managing home care, and living with chronic illness. New research studies follow. A discussion of this new research, emphasizing implications for practice and directions for further research, concludes the volume.

This book represents an effort to effectively communicate research findings that are relevant and ready for use, in a form that is understandable to practicing nurses, with suggestions for implementation and further clinical evaluation. The book is only one—though we think crucial—step in the process of moving from the conduct of research to its use in practice. As outlined in the chapter on improving practice through research utilization, it is hoped that the clinician reading this book will take note of particularly relevant findings and begin to use the new knowledge in practice—whether informally through viewing chronically ill patients in a new light or formally through making changes in patient care. Always, the clinician should evaluate the impact of such changes.

Nurses are the key players in caring for the chronically ill; it is essential that they build on the research presented here and take the lead in further developing and testing cost-effective interventions to promote independence, assist the chronically ill to maintain or recover function, and enhance quality of life. In particular, interventions are needed to enhance aerobic capacity, mobility, strength and endurance; provide new ways to maximize available function to allow performance of ADLs and IADLs; reduce the magnitude and interference of symptoms such as pain, fatigue and nausea; improve rest and sleep; decrease the psychological sequelae of chronic illness; and teach patients how to care for themselves, caregivers how to provide care, and both how to access needed services. Special attention needs to be given to underserved populations such as the rural and poor chronically ill. And adaptations of environments, including acute care settings, long-term care settings, and the home, are needed.

Care of the chronically ill is the task of the future. It is nurses who will take the lead in making it a caring future, one in which the ill and disabled and those facing death are not simply "maintained" but are nurtured, supported, and encouraged to live life fully.

REFERENCES

Brett, J. L. (1987). Use of nursing practice research findings. *Nursing Research, 36*, 344–349.

Commission on Chronic Illness. (1956). *Chronic illness in the United States: Vol II: Care of the long-term patient*. Cambridge, MA: Harvard University Press.

Falvo, D. R. (1991). *Medical and psychosocial aspects of chronic illness and disability.* Gaithersburg, MD: Aspen Publishers, Inc.

Funk, S. G., Tornquist, E. M., & Champagne, M. T. (1989a). A model for improving the dissemination of nursing research. *Western Journal of Nursing Research, 11*, 359–365.

Funk, S. G., Tornquist, E. M., & Champagne, M. T. (1989b). Application and evaluation of the dissemination model. *Western Journal of Nursing Research, 11*, 486–491.

Funk, S. G., Tornquist, E. M., Champagne, M. T., Copp, L. A., & Wiese, R. A. (Eds.). (1989). *Key aspects of comfort: Management of pain, fatigue, and nausea*. New York: Springer Publishing Co.

Funk, S. G., Tornquist, E. M., Champagne, M. T., Copp, L. A., & Wiese, R. A. (Eds.). (1990). *Key aspects of recovery: Improving nutrition, rest, and mobility.* New York: Springer Publishing Co.

Funk, S. G., Tornquist, E. M., Champagne, M. T., & Wiese, R. A. (Eds.). (1992). *Key aspects of elder care: Managing falls, incontinence, and cognitive impairment*. New York: Springer Publishing Co.

Kerson, T. S., & Kerson, L. A. (1985). *Understanding chronic illness: The medical and psychosocial dimensions of nine diseases*. New York: Free Press.

Kirchhoff, K. T. (1982). A diffusion survey of coronary precautions. *Nursing Research, 31*, 196–201.

Lambert, V. A., & Lambert, C. E., Jr. (1987). Psychosocial impacts created by chronic illness. *Nursing Clinics of North America, 22*, 527–533.

Lubkin, I. M. (1990). *Chronic illness: Impact and interventions*. Boston: Jones & Bartlett Publishers.

Newacheck, P. W., & Taylor, W. R. (1992). Childhood chronic illness: Prevalence, severity, and impact. *American Journal of Public Health, 82*, 364–371.

[2]

Managing Chronicity: The Heart of Nursing Care

Angela Barron McBride

Our health care system has been so oriented towards acuity in its efforts both to extinguish diseases (e.g., smallpox, tetanus, diphtheria, polio) and to provide intensive care in medical emergencies (e.g., trauma, myocardial infarction, hemorrhage, septicemia) that chronic illness has historically not been considered particularly worthy of high-profile attention. Yet managing chronicity needs to be at the heart of nursing care. Chronic illness should not be perceived primarily in passive terms as a failure of technology (e.g., the problems that develop when one-pound babies survive) or as a failure of health prevention (e.g., the life experience of a paraplegic after a motorcycle accident), but in active terms, as central to the mission of the nursing profession.

Mortality rather than morbidity has traditionally been the primary concern of health care providers—to some extent because morbidity may seem a morbid (in the sense of darkly dull) topic; but we must change that. If we see nursing as responsible for limiting morbidity, we must take seriously the role we can play in the development of "successful aging" programs aimed at compressing morbidity (i.e., forestalling the onset of chronic health problems and delaying the appearance of signs and symptoms). Managing chronicity also opens up opportunities not just to minimize the effects of the disease process, but to take the lead in helping patients address their dis-eases, that is, the disequilibriums occasioned by diminished health.

Soon after the establishment of the National Center for Nursing Research, Representative Edward R. Madigan (R-Illinois) wrote this about the promise of nursing research in helping individuals deal effectively with chronic problems:

> The government's concern for quality health care in the face of cost-cutting measures; the limitation of acute, hospital-based care in a society that now has chronic—rather than infectious—disease as its most pressing health problem; and the graying of our population, with its corresponding long-term care needs, are just a few of the trends that must be addressed. I believe that nursing research can provide much of the needed data to enhance the provision of high quality effective and efficient care. (1986, p. 3)

His view is—and ours must be—that nursing has a solemn responsibility to find answers to the questions that increasingly concern members of the general public as they recognize the limits of medical treatment and cure. In meeting that responsibility, I would argue, we will finally get the full recognition our field has sought from other disciplines, influential people in government, and consumers of our services. We are being asked to take the lead in managing chronicity, and instead of grumbling about the fact that we get asked to do what no one else wants to do (as we sometimes have), we must assume that leadership with flair and regard it as further evidence that our domain is in the ascendancy. As a psychiatric nurse I have seen us shy away from chronic care, yet the need is great and the public wants us to provide services, both in and out of institutions.

Few of us were socialized to think of managing chronic illness as an exciting challenge, but I am going to describe some areas that excite me about an emphasis on chronicity. My selection is not meant to be exhaustive, but merely illustrative of the opportunities before us. The word "chronic" derives from *chronicus* in Latin and *chronikos* in Greek, and primarily means *for the time*—referring, in some sense, to health problems that are constant, recurring, tedious, habitual, or lasting. Thus the emphasis in managing chronicity is not on that which is sudden or intense, but on the sense of burden, strain, and irritation that accumulates over time. Interestingly, there is a convergence in the "over time" component of chronic health problems and the "over time" component of nursing's mission to provide 24-hour care, and we need to build on this. One of the most comforting promises we can make to the public is that *our profession will be there over time for the health problems that persist*. Let me elaborate further on the overlap between nursing's values and the needs of the chronically ill.

EMPHASIS ON FUNCTIONAL ABILITY

The historical emphasis in nursing on putting patients in the best condition for nature to act on them (Nightingale) or helping them do what they would do unaided if they had the necessary strength, will, or knowledge (Henderson) presupposes an abiding commitment on our part to the restoration of maximal function in our patients. Nurses deal with medical diagnoses per se far less than they address the effectiveness of an individual's responses to actual or potential health problems. When the American Nurses' Association (1980, p. 10) put together a list of human responses that might be the focus for nursing interventions, many items reflected the concerns of the chronically ill: impaired functioning, self-care limitations, pain and discomfort, emotional problems related to illness and treatment, and self-image changes brought about by health status.

Because our profession has responsibility for what happens to individuals around the clock, assessing functional ability is crucial in order to plan both staffing ratios and patient care; a key method of assessing function is examining how the individual handles the activities of daily living (ADL). Activities of daily living have been subdivided into (1) basic ADL—bathing, dressing, toileting; (2) household ADL—meal preparation, shopping, housework; and (3) advanced ADL—managing money, using the telephone (Wolinsky, Callahan, Fitzgerald, & Johnson, 1992). Another method of assessing function distinguishes between lower body limitations and upper body limitations as a way of determining level of impairment (Nagi, 1976), because the former can be useful in predicting the likelihood of needing a nursing home, while the latter are predictive of subsequent death. Psychiatric nurses working with the persistently mentally ill are interested in adaptive functioning (Mezzich, Evanczuk, Mathias, & Coffman, 1984) or self-care functioning (Morrison, Fisher, Wilson, & Underwood, 1985), because these encompass a range of biopsychosocial behaviors the field is concerned about facilitating (Stuart, 1986).

The reason that functional ability is emphasized when dealing with chronic conditions is that a particular medical diagnosis may come to belong to a patient for life, but that does not in and of itself give any meaningful estimate of functioning. It is possible to have a serious disability or disease—for example, be deaf or have multiple sclerosis, yet function well within the constraints imposed by the condition. Two children can have chronic illnesses that are equally life threatening and comparably invisible to the eye—epilepsy versus asthma, say, and have differences in adjustment (Austin, 1988, 1989). It is this range of possibilities with which the nurse works.

In my own research, I have collaborated with a number of colleagues (1991) to develop the Indiana Nursing Assessment of Functioning (INAF), which has been found useful in evaluating both chronic and acute psychiatric patients. Table 2.1 gives the ten areas assessed by that instrument. The measure was developed because psychiatric diagnosis was such a poor way of determining which patients had similar capabilities and because a means was needed to monitor relatively small, but clinically important shifts in functioning.

TABLE 2.1. Indiana Nursing Assessment of Functioning

Item	Sample function descriptors
Body self-care	Ability to engage in self-care activities, including maintaining diet, grooming, dressing, and personal activities, and/or to handle toileting activities.
Balance in rest/activity	Ability to balance rest and activity, to understand bodily needs, and/or to maintain regular patterns of sleep, rest, and physical activity.
Care of environment	Ability to maintain safe and sanitary living quarters (this includes disposal of garbage and waste, keeping possessions in working order, eliminating fire and health hazards, and proper handling of food).
Dealing with emotions	Ability to understand and manage feelings, handle impulses, express feelings (including sexual feelings), and/or feel good about self.
Cognitive functioning	Ability to understand what is going on, think clearly, communicate ideas, make judgments, pay attention to things, learn from experience, remember information, and/or identify beliefs and values.
Presentation of self	Ability to present self to advantage, dress for the occasion, handle one's body appropriately, adapt one's behavior to the situation, and/or know what is proper and what is not.
Coping/adaptation	Ability to think before acting, assess own strengths and weaknesses, make use of what is available, and/or deal with problems.
Social/interpersonal skills	Ability to develop and maintain relationships with others, accept others' ideas, take an active interest in others, and/or meet the needs of others.
Use of time	Ability to use time constructively, set realistic work/leisure goals, select activities that promote self-expression and/or satisfaction, and/or carry out projects successfully.
Family relationships	Ability to relate to family, initiate open and honest communication with family members, keep up relationships, and/or promote shared understanding with family.

Each item is rated on a 35-point scale. For each item, the rater first chooses one of seven score ranges for that category of behavior [grossly impaired (1–5), very poor (6–10), poor (11–15), fair (16–20), good (21–25), very good (26–30), and superior (31–35)]. Then the rater fine tunes that judgment by selecting a number within the 5-point score range, bearing in mind the person's lowest level of functioning in that area in the last week.

In and of itself, an emphasis on functional ability can have a positive effect on patients because it makes the locus of control not invasive agents or pathology but the behavior of the individual with the problem. Since responses to similar pathology vary so widely, the individual is encouraged to focus on her/his functioning and what affects it—which puts the person into the posture of being a detective taking advantage of helpful clues, rather than a victim. This purposeful self-scrutiny, which Price (1989) has termed "body listening," has the potential for transforming passivity into constructive activity because it presupposes that the affected individual is in the best position to monitor implementation of a medical regimen and other therapeutic strategies. For example, the person managing bipolar illness is urged to become sensitive to how rest/activity cycles, stress, and colds/flu affect coping and the effectiveness of lithium treatment. The complex problem-solving that patients with chronic health conditions must undertake requires careful coaching in order to transform suggestions into health-enhancing habits. For example, the elderly patient with diminished endurance may have to experiment under the tutelage of the nurse to figure out how to maintain important activities while being mindful of limitations.

QUALITY OF LIFE

Quality of life is related to functioning, but is a still larger concept. The fact that so many components—physical, psychological, and social—shape a person's quality of life makes these components of great importance in managing chronicity. For example, quality of life involves not only physical functioning, energy/stamina, self-care ability, absence of pain, and control of symptoms, but also includes coping ability, life satisfaction, adjustment to illness, role functioning, and usefulness to others (Grant, Padilla, Ferrell, & Rhiner, 1990; Jalowiec, 1990). This multidimensional construct is intriguing to clinicians because the determinants of quality of life can be independent of disease categories and age. For example, one study of the perceptions of elderly patients with the five most common chronic diseases found that quality of life was largely based on their perception of their health, interpersonal relationships, and finances; interestingly, patients generally saw themselves as more advantaged than did their physicians, who presumably saw them more in terms of their diseases (Pearlman & Uhlmann, 1988).

Quality of life is important to nurses managing chronicity for at least three major reasons. First, the concept reflects our field's holistic perspective that seeks to view individuals as much more than their disease status. Second, the range of variables considered under quality of life serves to remind patients and nurses alike that more things are important in life than falling or not falling into a diagnostic category—for example, the degree to which individuals succeed in accomplishing what they wish despite constraints imposed by a health problem (Gerson, 1976). The focus is on patients defining for themselves what makes for quality of life, confirming nursing's emphasis on taking seriously the lived experience and proceeding from the perspective of the patient. Third, researchers welcome the use of multiple indicators within the umbrella term quality of life, because it affords them new measures of effectiveness when evaluating treatment outcomes (Goodinson & Singleton, 1989; Revicki, 1989). This is significant because many nursing interventions are not likely to eliminate untoward situations but, rather, may help patients feel better *despite* their problems. Quality of life deals with two separate but related sets of needs: (1) the need to avoid, diminish, and/or adjust to distressing life experiences; *and* (2) the need to develop and sustain life satisfaction by increasing competence and mastery over the environment (Holmes, 1989). To put it another way, there's living and then there's *how* you live (Burckhardt, Woods, Schultz, & Ziebarth, 1989).

THE PERSON-ENVIRONMENT FIT

One of the major values of nursing that is also of importance in managing chronicity is the fit between person and environment. Nursing's metatheory has traditionally been concerned about what the nurse can do to promote health for the person embedded in a particular environment (Fawcett, 1984). Yet most change strategies focus on what the individual can or should do rather than on environmental interventions. Managing chronicity must involve behavioral change not only at the level of individuals and their families but at the macro level of the community (Flynn & Rider, 1991).

The leading causes of death in the United States are heart disease, cancer, cerebrovascular accident, accidents, and lung disease. All five of these conditions have life-style correlates associated with morbidity—alcohol/drug usage, exposure to sun, cigarette smoking, poor diet, failure to use seat belts, lack of exercise, stress, etc. These personal habits/behaviors are themselves affected by whether the environment makes healthy choices the easy choices. The question is whether the larger social conditions make it possible for individuals to perform the activities of daily living in a way that maximizes their sense of well-being.

Indiana University School of Nursing's Institute of Action Research for Community Health has recently been designated by the World Health Organization as the first WHO Collaborating Center in Healthy Cities (Flynn, Rider, & Ray, 1991). The emphasis on healthy cities recognizes the extent to which the health of individuals is shaped by environmental cues and by larger community policies. The Institute is following in the footsteps of Lillian Wald and Margaret Sanger, whose work in the tenements of New York City concerned both the needs of individuals and the social conditions that contributed to personal tragedies. Nursing at its best has always considered the individual and her/his health as embedded in a series of interlocking contexts (familial, cultural, social, political, etc.), and this is especially the case when helping individuals deal with chronic problems. For example, managing alcoholism as a chronic health problem requires understanding genetic predisposition, the link with depression/anxiety, co-morbidity factors, and the effects on families, while also developing employee assistance programs in the work place, responsible beverage service training for restaurant personnel, and enforcement programs to reduce the illegal sale of alcohol to minors.

Based on Stokols' thinking about a social ecology of health promotion (1992), Table 2.2 illustrates how various components of health can be played out in the person and the environment of a woman managing the dietary restrictions imposed by diabetes. Her adherence to a health-promoting dietary regimen will be influenced by how attractive supermarkets make healthy choices and by whether nutritious foods cost more than those full of sugar and fat. Her sense of personal competence and control may be enhanced by media coverage of all that Mary Tyler Moore has accomplished while living with diabetes.

Recognition of the importance of the person-environment fit to managing chronicity has at least two major consequences for nursing. First, being sensitive to the person-environment fit means that nursing has to be concerned with the interface between the behavioral and biomedical sciences; moreover, health behavior must be conceptualized both in terms of micro level and macro level changes possible. The second consequence follows

TABLE 2.2 Health and the Person-Environment Fit

Health	Person	Environment
Physical	Health-promoting dietary regimen adopted because of changes in pancreatic functioning	Supermarkets make health choices easy and appealing
Emotional/Mental	Sense of personal competence and control encouraged	Role models provided of individuals living full lives despite chronic health problems
Socio-Economic	"Soul food" preferences are not full of sugar and fat, and personal income allows for food variety	Healthy choices do not cost more; family does not force woman to prepare sweets that she cannot eat

from the first: nursing care must include *facilitating* coping by the individual and her/his family, organizing effective systems of care, and managing the individual's connections to other caregivers and to the various components of the health and human services system. In effect, being a case manager is as important as providing care yourself as a nurse.

CHRONICITY AS A FEMINIST ISSUE

Because women tend to live longer than men and thus are more likely to have to deal with the consequences of aging (Cassel & Neugarten, 1988; Kandrack, Grant, & Segall, 1991; Seely, 1990), chronicity may be considered a feminist issue. The consequences of aging include greater likelihood of both suffering from chronic conditions (e.g., Alzheimer's disease, lupus, multiple sclerosis, osteoporosis, diabetes, urinary incontinence, arthritis) and suffering from outliving one's peers—the latter means that women are more likely to be cared for in nursing homes than men (Grau, 1987; Lewis, 1985; Older Women's League, 1988). Also, because women make less money throughout their lives than men, they have fewer economic resources—social security benefits, insurance, and pensions—for dealing with the health problems of aging, which limits their choices as they struggle with chronic conditions. Indeed, medicine provides better coverage for services used more by men (acute care) than for those used more by women (outpatient services and long-term care) (Sofaer & Abel, 1990).

It is also women who provide the bulk of family care to aging relatives with chronic conditions (Brody & Schoonover, 1986; Faulkner & Micchelli, 1988; Horowitz, 1985; Houser & Berkman, 1985):

> Of the eight million Americans who provide some level of care to an elderly relative or friend, most are daughters; their average age is 46. One in three of the 1.2 million who provide care for the severely disabled works outside the home full time and many others hold part-time jobs. While they can be found in all occupations, caregivers are most likely to be blue collar and clerical workers. (Bernardy, 1987, p. 4)

The costs to the caregiver are many (Baum & Gallagher, 1985-1986; George & Gwyther, 1986; Goodman, 1986; Newald, 1986). Responsibilities may cripple a climb up the career ladder, while the burden of care (21-28 hours per week) can lead to financial hardship, strained personal relationships, emotional collapse, and declines in physical health (Brody, 1985; Cantor, 1983; Stone, Cafferata, & Sangl, 1986). As a result, the caregiver herself may develop chronic health problems.

RESURGENCE OF THE CASE STUDY METHOD

Benner's *From Novice to Expert* (1984) has reminded us in recent years of the importance of expert clinical judgment, and nowhere is this more true than in dealing with chronic health problems. The gifted clinician has to know how to address multiple health problems concurrently without losing sight of the fact that they co-exist in one person with hopes and dreams, all the while appreciating that the person is embarking on a journey in which her or his perceptions about life will be fundamentally changed by the condition and will, in turn, help to shape manifestations of that condition. Since the purpose of clinical practice is to improve the well-being of individuals (Gerhardt, 1990), case by case analysis is essential, and this means the resurgence of care based on case-related evidence. Such an approach becomes particularly important when one patient has multiple health problems (e.g., arthritis, hypertension, and cancer) and a complicated treatment regimen.

Qualitative approaches to understanding the patient's situation—whether grounded theory (Strauss & Glaser, 1984; Strauss, Glaser, & Quint, 1964), ethnomethodologic techniques in narrative analysis (Voysey, 1975; Williams, 1984), or biographical research (Robinson, 1986) have in common an emphasis on the meaning attached to the situation by the affected individual(s). They also are concerned about the stages that a person and his/her family go through in coming to terms with the condition and any stigma attached to a medical diagnosis. This process of reconstitution—associated with consideration of what might now be expected of everyday life—calls forth the best in nursing: helping patients modify their behaviors appropriately while understanding that their personal goals can continue to be realized, and helping individuals deal with the inevitable task of aging that calls for substituting wisdom-based values for physique-based values.

SUSTAINING OPTIMISM

The final issue I want to consider as essential to managing chronicity—sustaining optimism—has been alluded to in passing but deserves elaboration. Health problems that are never likely to be cured leave the individual vulnerable to depression because there seems no escape from the unwanted condition. Ruminating over the body's failure (or the individual's failure to avoid health problems) can activate a storehouse of negative memories that interfere with coping. But in most situations, how one thinks about setbacks and health problems matters more than whether one experiences setbacks and health problems. For example, there is evidence to suggest that "perceived" health is linked to longevity more than so-called objective health status (Kaplan & Camacho, 1983; Mossey & Shapiro, 1982). Optimism shapes health because it acts on key intervening variables—goal setting, problem solving, stress management, perseverance, and immune competence (Peterson & Bossio, 1991).

The conceptual development and measurement of hardiness as a factor in adaptation continue to be debated (Hull, Van Treuren, & Propsom, 1988; Pollock, 1989; Wagnild & Young, 1991): Is hardiness a unitary construct or a concept with three dimensions—control, commitment, and challenge? No matter what the final decision in that debate, it seems to me that nurses need to examine further the extent to which certain mind sets can have positive consequences, that is, seeing oneself as influential in the face of life's contingencies, perceiving change as likely to be ultimately beneficial rather than as a threat to security, and being deeply involved in various activities of life (Kobasa, 1979). Moreover, how can we encourage these ways of thinking so that perceived ineffectuality does not fuel depression? Individuals who think that whatever they do will not make a difference are likely to become increasingly passive and oblivious to opportunities, eventually making their hopelessness a self-fulfilling prophecy. Frankly, emphasis on sustaining optimism is also important to the caregiver, because commitment to health-related activities, believing one can exert control, and reframing problems as challenges are all essential to professional success. Both patients and caregivers need to be reminded not to overgeneralize less successful days and to use humor to handle tension-filled situations. Managing chronicity is, in many ways, a test of the possibilities of the human spirit, and that can be a mind-expanding perspective.

CONCLUSION

I hope that you believe, as I do, that managing chronicity can be exciting—even chic. It has appeal because there is such a synergistic overlap between nursing's time-honored values and the needs of the chronically ill. There is even more overlap between the health promotion values of nursing and the growing interest in compressing morbidity. The issues I have discussed (and they are by no means the only ones) will be some of the cutting-edge concerns of the 21st century:

- Facilitating functioning when cure is not possible.
- Measuring outcome effectiveness in terms of quality of life.
- Promoting health by being sensitive to the person-environment fit.
- Recognizing that chronicity disproportionately affects women's lives.
- Re-establishing the case study method as the technique of choice in addressing multiple problems in one person.

- Developing teaching strategies for sustaining optimism despite setbacks.
- Expanding our theoretical understanding of what is meant by functioning, quality of life, body listening, normalization, reconstitution, hardiness, etc.

These challenges are the agenda we must adopt as we greet a future committed to postponing the age of onset of chronic infirmity (Fries, 1990). These are the challenges our profession has been prepared to address for so long, though only now are we being asked to take the lead. And make no mistake, we are being asked by consumers, physicians, and legislators to take the lead!

REFERENCES

American Nurses' Association. (1980). *Nursing. A social policy statement.* Kansas City, MO: Author.

Austin, J. K. (1988). Childhood epilepsy: Child adaptation and family resources. *Journal of Child and Adolescent Psychiatric and Mental Health Nursing, 1,* 18–24.

Austin, J. K. (1989). Comparison of child adaptation to epilepsy and asthma. *Journal of Child and Adolescent Psychiatric and Mental Health Nursing, 2,* 119–144.

Baum, D., & Gallagher, D. (1985-1986). Case studies of psychotherapy with depressed caregivers. *Clinical Gerontologist, 4*(2), 19–29.

Benner, P. (1984). *From novice to expert: Excellence and power in clinical nursing practice.* Menlo Park, CA: Addison-Wesley.

Bernardy, R. (1987, Spring). An important new family issue. *Gray Panther Network* (pp. 4–5, 11).

Brody, E. M. (1985). Parent care as a normative family stress. *The Gerontologist, 25,* 19–29.

Brody, E. M., & Schoonover, C. B. (1986). Patterns of parent-care when adult daughters work and when they do not. *The Gerontologist, 26,* 372–382.

Burckhardt, C. S., Woods, S. L., Schultz, A. A., & Ziebarth, D. M. (1989). Quality of life of adults with chronic illness: A psychometric study. *Research in Nursing and Health, 12,* 347–354.

Cantor, M. H. (1983). Strain among caregivers: A study of experience in the United States. *The Gerontologist, 23,* 597–604.

Cassel, C., & Neugarten, B. L. (1988). A forecast of women's health and longevity. Implications for an aging America. *Western Journal of Medicine, 149,* 712–717.

Faulkner, A. O., & Micchelli, M. (1988). The aging, the aged, and the very old: Women the policy makers forgot. *Women & Health, 14*(3/4), 5–19.

Fawcett, J. (1984). The metaparadigm of nursing. Current status and future refinements. *Image: Journal of Nursing Scholarship, 16,* 84–87.

Flynn, B. C., & Rider, M. S. (1991). Notes from the field. Healthy cities Indiana: Mainstreaming community health in the United States. *American Journal of Public Health, 81,* 510–511.

Flynn, B. C., Rider, M., & Ray, D. W. (1991). Healthy cities: The Indiana model of community development in public health. *Health Education Quarterly, 18,* 331–347.

Fries, J. F. (1990). The compression of morbidity: Near or far? *The Millbank Quarterly, 67*, 208–232.

George, L. K., & Gwyther, L. P. (1986). Caregiver well-being: A multidimensional examination of family caregivers of demented adults. *The Gerontologist, 26*, 253–259.

Gerhardt, U. (1990). Qualitative research on chronic illness: The issue and the story. *Social Science and Medicine, 30*, 1149–1159.

Gerson, E. M. (1976). On "Quality of life." *American Sociological Review, 41*, 793-806.

Goodinson, S. M., & Singleton, J. (1989). Quality of life: A critical review of current concepts, measures and their clinical implications. *International Journal of Nursing Studies, 26*, 327–341.

Goodman, C. (1986). Research on the informal career: A selected literature review. *Journal of Advanced Nursing, 11*, 705–712.

Grant, M., Padilla, G. V., Ferrell, B. R., & Rhiner, M. (1990). Assessment of quality of life with a single instrument. *Seminars in Oncology Nursing, 6*, 260–270.

Grau, L. (1987). Illness-engendered poverty among the elderly. *Women & Health, 12*(3/4), 103–118.

Holmes, C. A. (1989). Health care and the quality of life: A review. *Journal of Advanced Nursing, 14*, 833–839.

Horowitz, A. (1985). Sons and daughters as caregivers to older parents: Differences in role performances. *The Gerontologist, 25*, 612.

Houser, B. B., & Berkman, S. L. (1985). Sex and birth order differences in filial behavior. *Sex Roles, 13*, 641–651.

Hull, J. G., Van Treuren, R. R., & Propsom, P. M. (1988). Attributional style and the components of hardiness. *Personality and Social Psychology Bulletin, 14*, 505–513.

Jalowiec, A. (1990). Issues in using multiple measures of quality of life. *Seminars in Oncology Nursing, 6*, 271–277.

Kandrack, M-A., Grant, K. R., & Segall, A. (1991). Gender differences in health related behavior: Some unanswered questions. *Social Science and Medicine, 32*, 579–590.

Kaplan, G. A., & Camacho, T. (1983). Perceived health and mortality: A nine-year follow-up of the human population laboratory cohort. *American Journal of Epidemiology, 117*, 292–304.

Kobasa, S. C. (1979). Stressful life events, personality, and health: An inquiry into hardiness. *Journal of Personality and Social Psychology, 37*, 1–11.

Lewis, M. (1985). Older women and health: An overview. *Women & Health, 10*(2/3), 1–16.

Madigan, E. R. (1986). Nursing research to take its rightful place. Editorial in *Nursing and Health Care, 7*, 3.

McBride, A. B., Austin, J. K., Chesnut, E., Keeter, E., Main, S., Mishler, S., Moody, S., Richards, B., & Roy, B. (1991, October). *Clinical assessment of the INAF.* Paper presented at the biennial meeting of the Council of Nurse Researchers, Los Angeles, CA.

Mezzich, J. E., Evanczuk, K. J., Mathias, R. J., & Coffman, G. A. (1984). Admission decisions and multiaxial diagnosis. *Archives of General Psychiatry, 41*, 1001–1004.

Morrison, E., Fisher, L. Y., Wilson, H. S., & Underwood, P. (1985). NSGAE. Nursing adaptation evaluation. *Journal of Psychosocial Nursing, 23*(8), 10–13.

Mossey, J. M., & Shapiro, E. (1982). Self-rated health: A predictor of mortality among the elderly. *American Journal of Public Health, 72*, 800–808.

Nagi, S. Z. (1976). An epidemiology of disability among adults in the United States. *Milbank Memorial Fund Quarterly, 54*, 439–468.
Newald, J. (1986). Women as care givers face crisis at home. *Hospitals, 60*, 106.
Older Women's League. (1988). The picture of health for midlife and older women in America. *Women & Health, 14*(3/4), 53–74.
Pearlman, R. A., & Uhlmann, R. F. (1988). Quality of life in chronic diseases: Perceptions of elderly patients. *Journal of Gerontology, 43*, M25–M30.
Peterson, C., & Bossio, L. M. (1991). *Health and optimism*. New York: Free Press.
Pollock, S. E. (1989). The hardiness characteristic: A motivating factor in adaptation. *Advances in Nursing Science, ll*(2), 53–62.
Price, M. J. (1989). Perceived uncertainty associated with the management trajectory of a chronic illness—diabetes mellitus. *Dissertation Abstracts International* (University Microfilms, No. 49–9).
Revicki, D. A. (1989). Health-related quality of life in the evaluation of medical therapy for chronic illness. *Journal of Family Practice, 29*, 377–380.
Robinson, I. (1986). *Multiple sclerosis*. London: Tavistock.
Seely, S. (1990). The gender gap: Why do women live longer than men? *International Journal of Cardiology, 29*, 113–119.
Sofaer, S., & Abel, E. (1990). Older women's health and financial vulnerability: Implications of the Medicare benefit structure. *Women & Health, 16*(3/4), 47-67.
Stokols, D. (1992). Establishing and maintaining healthy environments. Toward a social ecology of health promotion. *American Psychologist, 47*, 6–22.
Stone, R., Cafferata, G. L., & Sangl, J. (1986). *Caregivers of the frail elderly: A national profile*. Rockville, MD: National Center for Health Services Research and Health Care Technology Assessment.
Strauss, A., & Glaser, B. (1984). *Chronic illness and the quality of life* (2nd ed.). St. Louis: Mosby.
Strauss, A., Glaser, B., & Quint, J. (1964). The non-accountability of terminal care. *Hospitals, 36*, 73–87.
Stuart, G. W. (1986). NSGAE update. Nursing adaptation evaluation. *Journal of Psychosocial Nursing, 24*(2), 31–33.
Voysey, M. S. (1975). *A constant burden: The reconstitution of family life*. London: Routledge & Paul.
Wagnild, G., & Young, H. M. (1991). Another look at hardiness. *Image: Journal of Nursing Scholarship, 23*, 257–259.
Williams, G. (1984). The genesis of chronic illness: Narrative reconstruction. *Sociology in Health and Illness, 6*, 175.
Wolinsky, F. D., Callahan, C. M., Fitzgerald, J. F., & Johnson, R. J. (1992). The risk of nursing home placement and subsequent death among older adults. *Journal of Gerontology, 47*, S173–S182.

[3]

Managing the Hospitalized Chronically Ill

Barbara J. Daly

Almost no research has been done on caring for hospitalized chronically ill patients. There are very few studies which have directly measured or described the response of chronically ill patients to hospitalization, none which have compared chronically ill with acutely ill patients, and almost none which have tested nursing interventions designed specifically for the hospitalized chronically ill. So the first message concerning the state of the art is that our understanding of issues in the care of hospitalized persons who are chronically ill is primarily derived by transferring, combining, and attempting to apply what we know about the characteristics of chronically ill persons to the context of modern hospitals.

In the discussion that follows we will see that the predominant characteristics of the hospital environment work against meeting patient needs that are related to chronic illness. In some ways, despite the astonishing accomplishments of hospitals in managing patients with acute conditions, when it comes to caring for patients with chronic conditions, we seem to be perilously close to losing sight of Florence Nightingale's 1863 message: "The first requirement of a hospital is that it should do the sick no harm" (quoted in Mitchell, 1989, p. 3).

To make the point in another way, I'd like to quote from an article in the *Journal of the American Medical Association*:

> The large number of chronically ill persons in general hospitals who require long-term care represents a serious problem to hospital administrators. The general hospital as at present constituted is often unsuited to the care of long-term patients since it is geared primarily to the therapeutic and general requirements of the acutely ill. It may lack adequate departments for physical

> therapy, occupational therapy, and rehabilitation, as well as . . . [lacking] an understanding of the social and psychologic needs of the chronically ill. (American Hospital Association, American Public Welfare Association, American Public Health Association, & American Medical Association, 1947, p. 345)

The interesting thing about the quote is that it is accurate today though it comes from a 1947 issue of *JAMA*, suggesting, I think, that we still have not come to grips with the problem of caring for chronically ill patients in an environment designed for acute, short-term illnesses.

With this as an introduction, let me now discuss some facts and findings I believe have direct applicability to chronically ill hospital patients. We need to first define the population. In 1950 a multidisciplinary group, The Commission on Chronic Illness, was formed, composed of representatives from the American Medical Association, the American Hospital Association, the American Public Health Association, and the American Public Welfare Association. Concerned about the growing population of chronically ill in the U. S., the representatives from these organizations proposed a definition that is still used today:

> Chronic diseases are all impairments or deviations from normal which have one or more of the following characteristics: permanency, leave residual damage, caused by non-reversible pathology, require specialized training of the patient for rehabilitation, and/or require a long period of supervised care. (Commission on Chronic Illness, 1954, p. 7)

At the time of the Commission's initial work, in 1950, an estimated 28 million persons in the U. S. had one or more chronic diseases; 5.3 million of these people were further classified as disabled in that they could not independently perform at the usual level of activity or carry out activities of daily living (Commission on Chronic Illness, 1954). Fifty percent of the 28 million were under the age of 45. As communicable diseases have decreased and technologic ability to prolong the life of the chronically ill has increased, the numbers of chronically ill have also significantly increased. By 1967, there were 95 million persons with one or more chronic illnesses, 22 million of whom were disabled (Strauss & Glaser, 1975). By 1986, this figure had grown to 110 million persons with at least one chronic illness, and 32.4 million disabled. That means that roughly one of every two persons in the U. S. has at least one chronic illness (Lambert & Lambert, 1987).

The diseases contributing to these numbers have changed somewhat over the years. In the early 1950's, chronic illnesses included, in order of frequency, heart disease, nervous or mental disorders, TB, arthritis, diabetes, asthma, and cancer (American Hospital Association et al., 1947). Today, heart disease and cancer are still among the most common, along with arthritis, diabetes, COPD, chronic pain disorders, and neuromuscular disorders such as MS. Most recently, researchers have added AIDS to the list.

In order to set the stage for understanding the dilemmas posed by having chronically ill persons in an environment oriented towards acute care, let me briefly review some hospital statistics. At the time of the article from *JAMA* quoted above, the predominant pattern of care for persons with chronic illnesses who required institutional care was the use of free-standing facilities specializing in chronic care. There was a notable blurring of definitions among conditions of chronic illness, disability, and long-term care. Today we recognize that not all persons who are chronically ill are disabled, many disabled persons do not require any significant amounts of health care, and many chronic illnesses do not require long-term care in an institution. However, in the 1940's and 1950's, when there were few treatment modalities available, anyone who needed long-term care received it in chronic disease hospitals. The emphasis of these facilities was on long-term placement, custodial care, and rehabilitation. Patients were not expected to require acute care. To illustrate this, a survey of these facilities in 1950 revealed that while 63% of them had libraries for patients, only 40% of them had ECG services available and only 53% could perform diagnostic x-rays (Commission on Chronic Illness, 1956).

As treatment modalities expanded, it became increasingly difficult to care for these persons with less than the full range of services available in conventional acute care hospitals, and chronic disease institutions began to close. In 1950 there were 406 long-term or chronic disease hospitals (Commission on Chronic Illness, 1956). Today there are 135 such institutions (American Hospital Association, 1991).

Unfortunately, the trends in modern hospital care have exacerbated problems which have always been present. In 1950 the Commission recognized several shortcomings of general hospitals as places of care for the chronically ill. These included operating at a "tempo" unsuited to the needs of the long-term patient, inability or unwillingness to assume responsibility for aggressive discharge planning, and failing in the concept and practice of rehabilitation. If this was true in 1950, consider the effect of cost containment and reduced reimbursement. We have seen the average length of stay in acute care hospitals decrease from 10.6 days in 1952 (Commission on Chronic Illness, 1956) to 7.2 in the average community hospital (American Hospital Association, 1991), and there is continuing demand to further reduce length of stay in order to reduce unreimbursed costs. Yet we know that the presence of chronic disease superimposed on an acute condition inevitably results in a longer stay. For example, the average length of stay for cholecystectomy patients in 1985 was 7.6 days; in the presence of multiple diagnoses, the length of stay increased to 11.8 days (Commission on Professional and Hospital Activities, 1986).

The need to reduce costs has also led to a reduction in the number and variety of support services available. Hospitals of less than 300 beds represent 81% of all acute care hospitals; only 33% of these facilities have occupational therapy services, which are among the most frequently needed services for the chronically ill, who must learn to adjust their life-style to the limitations of their illness (American Hospital Association, 1991).

This is just a preliminary look at what sets up the problem of lack of fit between the needs of the chronically ill and the trends in acute care facilities. Now let's take a look at some of what we have learned over the past few decades about chronic illness. Much of this is from nursing research, but a great deal of important information comes from other disciplines, and I don't want to ignore those findings.

In fact, two of the best known researchers on chronic illness are Anselm Strauss and Barney Glaser, sociologists from the University of California, who began their work in the 1960s. Strauss and Glaser have conducted numerous studies, have specifically looked at the characteristics of chronic illness, and have considered the conflicts which occur when these patients enter an acute care hospital (Strauss & Glaser, 1975). They found several common problems of daily living among persons with chronic illness:

1. prevention of medical crises and management of crises that do occur;
2. carrying out of prescribed regimens and management of problems associated with the prescribed regimen;
3. control of symptoms;
4. prevention of and living with the social isolation caused by lessened contact with others;
5. adjustment to changes in the course of the illness;
6. attempts to normalize life and interaction; and
7. funding—managing with loss of employment and the cost of care.

Strauss and Glaser found that in order to handle these problems, patients and families develop basic strategies, establish relationships with helpers, and develop organizational patterns for managing the disease and its crises. I mention these here to point out one of the first issues in hospitalization. The chronically ill person differs significantly from the acutely ill person in that he or she has been shouldering the responsibility for management of illness. While the acutely ill person has no pattern of managing this new illness, no organization of family and personal resources, the chronically ill person's very existence has depended on his ability to manage.

The management of illness that chronically ill persons have learned is far from a passive following of medical prescriptions. Regimens are learned, then modified, juggled, and coordinated around multiple illnesses and the demands of maintaining a normal life-style. The COPD patient, for example, develops a pattern of spacing activities in order to avoid dyspnea episodes (Shekleton, 1987). Yet, what happens when the patient is admitted into the acute care setting? The caregivers take control, imposing their schedule as if the specific condition precipitating hospitalization were the only focus of concern.

Strauss and Glaser note that usual patterns of health care reflect a home-facility dichotomy. Home is the patient's domain, meaning that whatever happens there is his business. The corollary is that whatever happens in the hospital is mostly the staff's business. The consequence of this is not only mismanagement of the chronic disease regimen, but disruption of the precarious balance the patient has achieved and damage to the patient's identity as a competent manager of his condition.

The importance of control over one's response to illness and ability to perform self-help behaviors was supported in a study by Braden in 1990. She looked at 396 patients with arthritis, using a Self-Help Model, and found that as levels of uncertainty and dependency in illness increased, the level of enabling skills, or perceived ability to manage adversity decreased. Similarly, as enabling skills increased, the level of self-help, or the ability to carry out usual adult roles increased. As we would expect, as self-help increased, the patient's overall quality of life also increased. While there has been no demonstration that caregivers' assumption of total control of activities and management of chronic conditions directly leads to reduced enabling skills, this seems a reasonable hypothesis.

This leads to the question of what could be done differently. Four areas have been examined by researchers: issues of control, education, the psychosocial aspects of chronic disease, and alterations in the environment.

Regarding control, some fairly obvious and very practical recommendations stemming from the work of Strauss and Glaser might include letting patients manage their own schedules of treatment, and letting them keep and take their own medications. Dennis (1990) looked at the types of activities in the hospital which contributed to patients' sense of control. Patients found control through being informed, through being involved in decision making, and through directing interpersonal and environmental interactions. Importantly, these were not major issues or significant aspects of their medical care, but often included such simple things as controlling the temperature of their room. They also gained a sense of control by being able to fulfill the patient role. What this study indicates is that for patients, control does not mean taking over all the decisions or self-treating. In fact, it includes being compliant and cooperative with hospital staff's efforts to treat the acute problem. Thus this study suggests that there is reason to believe that we can contribute to the patient's sense of control by making very minor adjustments to our usual functioning. It also points to the importance of negotiating with patients who have chronic illness when they are admitted, making explicit our expectations of them, and offering them a clear opportunity to participate in managing routines.

Another aspect of the patient's involvement in his or her care is education. Although much of the research about educational interventions for the chronically ill has involved patients at home, there are a few studies that emphasize how important education is in the course of hospitalization, not just in outpatient care. First, education about one's illness is positively related to control, as mentioned above. In addition, in Lipman's study of 30 newly diagnosed diabetic children, matched for acuity of illness and socioeconomic status, the presence of a clinical nurse specialist as diabetes educator actually decreased the length of hospitalization by 1.8 days (Lipman, 1987).

Education has been consistently shown to be related to effective disease management, particularly with diabetic persons. O'Connell and associates found that patients who had accurate information on the relation between specific symptoms and low blood glucose levels—termed "accuracy of symptom beliefs"— were in better metabolic control (O'Connell, Hamera, Schorfheide, & Guthrie, 1990). Similarly, in a large study conducted in Indianapolis, researchers found that the combination of patient and physician education resulted in significant improvements in diabetic patients' physiologic health outcomes (Vinicor et al., 1987). Yet when Moriarty and Stephens (1988) interviewed staff nurses, they found that diabetic teaching was often not done because of lack of time and inadequate teaching skills. Most worrisome, provision of an 8-hour workshop on diabetes did not change these perceptions. These researchers concluded that a better approach may be to recognize the environmental limits on nurses' time and provide educational services by a specialist. Obviously this has cost implications, but in view of the research demonstrating the potential of education to shorten length of stay and achieve better metabolic control, this seems to be an intervention which needs to be pursued.

A third focus of much of the research on chronically ill patients is on psychosocial factors and patterns. Chronic illness obviously imposes additional stress and requires additional coping, and attempts have been made to describe these. The goal, of course, is to gain a better understanding of the patterns associated with this kind of illness in order to plan interventions appropriate to the patient's needs. Several investigators have documented a higher than average incidence of depression among COPD patients, suggesting that patients with this diagnosis should be specifically assessed for this complication (Shekleton, 1987). Nickel, Brown, and Smith (1990) also found that one-third of over 1,000 patients with chronic heart disease reported symptoms of emotional distress and one-fourth were taking anti-anxiety medication. It seems reasonable to suggest that, given the additional stress of hospitalization, it might be wise to routinely involve psychiatric nurse clinicians in the care of patients with these diagnoses rather than waiting for a crisis to occur. This is another intervention that needs to be tested to determine efficacy.

In planning interventions to support coping during exacerbations of illness, we would do well to remember that chronically ill persons are accustomed to managing their own illness and have developed their own patterns of coping. Rather than assuming that help should come from caregivers, we might more appropriately focus on facilitating or strengthening the patient's usual methods. Primomo, Yeates, and Woods (1990) studied the sources of social support for 125 chronically ill women and, not surprisingly, found the women perceived more support from their spouse or partner than any other source. Yet what do we routinely do as part of hospital routines? Limit visiting. While the attitudes of staff members regarding strict visiting policies have loosened considerably lately, is it not the exception rather than the rule to allow spouses to stay overnight, or to arrange for a meal to be delivered for the spouse so that he or she can eat with the patient? Again, these are very simple alterations in hospital routine, yet they have at least the potential for significantly aiding the patient's recovery.

Thus far we have been discussing specific aspects of chronic illness and specific interventions which might be used by hospital staff. Another approach is to focus on the whole environment of care, and several researchers have begun work in this area. Ironically, this is the approach recommended by clinicians in 1947 (American Hospital Association et al., 1947), who suggested that special care units be set up to meet the unique needs of the chronically ill. The early work on hospice care, which demonstrated the effectiveness of creating alternative environments of care for patients with needs significantly different from those of the acutely ill, set the stage for this approach (Greer et al., 1986). Current efforts to test such special care units are reported in later chapters; Kathleen Buckwalter discusses the work at the University of Iowa with a unit designed for Alzheimer's patients; Denise Kresevic discusses an acute care unit for the elderly, designed to reduce the detrimental effects of hospitalization on the elderly, many of whom have coexisting chronic diseases; and I discuss a special care unit for the chronically critically ill which has shown encouraging results in reducing the cost of care, mortality rates, and some complications.

These approaches—essentially redesigning care around the needs of the chronically ill—reflect what is probably the greatest need in hospital care of the chronically ill. That is, we need to reconceptualize both our view of the recipients of care and our responsibilities to these very vulnerable patients. The predominant paradigm for acute care is still the traditional biomedical model in which the patient's illness is conceived of primarily in terms of physical pathology, isolated from social experience and accessible only through technologic interventions. Appropriate behaviors on the part of both caretakers and patients are fairly rigidly defined in terms of orientation towards the primary goal of disease eradication. In the presence of conditions which are poorly defined, which are incurable, and in which social adaptation is a major component of health, our traditional approaches are unlikely to produce good results. Stewart and Sullivan (1982), studying doctor-patient relationships and illness behaviors among patients with chronic diseases, noted that when physicians have difficulty diagnosing and treating an illness, such as occurs with many chronic diseases, the situation is less normatively controlled, leading to disharmony and lack of consensus. Plough (1981) illustrated the same phenomenon with renal failure patients and commented on the tension and uncertainties generated by our attempts to use traditional technologies with inadequate attention to the lived experience of the chronically ill.

It may be tempting for us to think that allegiance to the biomedical model is primarily a characteristic of physicians and that, as nurses, we are much more able to approach the chronically ill person as an individual. However, Brillhart, Jay, and Wyers (1990) reported a disturbing study in which they interviewed disabled persons, nursing faculty, beginning students, graduating students, and registered nurses about their attitudes towards people with disabilities. The disabled persons themselves, as might be expected, had the most positive attitudes. What is disturbing is that faculty members had the least positive attitudes, followed closely by the graduating students. In other words, it appeared that the relatively positive attitudes of beginning students were changed by their faculty members, who held negative stereotypes of the disabled. In another study of chronic pain, despite the importance of pain as a clinical phenomenon, nurses perceived pain as less intense when the patient had no overt signs of pathology and when the duration of the pain was long term (Taylor, Skelton, & Butcher, 1984).

Both of these studies should serve as cautions to us that registered nurses, as well as other caregivers, may be prone to bias and misunderstanding regarding the needs of the chronically ill. Clearly more research needs to be done in this area, but the studies to date suggest that we also need to reconsider the paradigm under which we perform our work. I suspect when we take a new look, from a different angle, we will make some surprising discoveries.

REFERENCES

American Hospital Association. (1991). *AHA hospital statistics, 1990.* Chicago: Author.

American Hospital Association, American Public Welfare Association, American Public Health Association, & American Medical Association. (1947). Planning for the chronically ill. *Journal of the American Medical Association, 135,* 343–347.

Braden, C. J. (1990). A test of the self-help model: Learned response to chronic illness experience. *Nursing Research, 39*, 42–46.

Brillhart, B. A., Jay, H., & Wyers, M. E. (1990). Attitudes toward people with disabilities. *Rehabilitation Nursing, 15*, 80–82.

Commission on Chronic Illness. (1954). *Care of the long-term patient*. Washington DC: United States Department of Health, Education, & Welfare, Public Health Service Publication No. 344.

Commission on Chronic Illness. (1956). *Chronic illness in the United States: Vol. II: Care of the long-term patient*. Cambridge, MA: Harvard University Press.

Commission on Professional and Hospital Activities. (1986). Lengths of stay: Geriatric length of stay by diagnosis and operation, U.S., 1985. Ann Arbor, MI: Commission of Professional and Hospital Activities.

Dennis, K. E. (1990). Patients' control and the information imperative: Clarification and confirmation. *Nursing Research, 39*, 162–166.

Greer, D. S., Mor, V., Morris, I. N., Sherwood, S., Kidder, D., & Birnbaum, H. (1986). An alternative in terminal care: Results of the national hospice study. *Journal of Chronic Diseases, 39*, 9–26.

Lambert, C. E., & Lambert, V. A. (1987). Psychosocial impacts created by chronic illness. *Nursing Clinics of North America, 22*, 527–533.

Lipman, T. H. (1987). Length of hospitalization of children with diabetes: Effect of a clinical nurse specialist. *The Diabetes Educator, 14*, 41–43.

Mitchell, M. K. (1989). *Indices of quality in long-term care* (p. 3). New York: National League for Nursing.

Moriarty, D. R., & Stephens, L. C. (1988). Factors that influence diabetes patient teaching performed by hospital staff nurses. *The Diabetes Educator, 16*, 31–35.

Nickel, J. T., Brown, K. J, & Smith, B. A. (1990). Depression and anxiety among chronically ill heart patients: Age differences in risk and predictors. *Research in Nursing and Health, 13*, 87–97.

O'Connell, K. A., Hamera, E. K., Schorfheide, A., & Guthrie, D. (1990). Symptom beliefs and actual glucose in Type II diabetes. *Research in Nursing and Health, 13*, 145–151.

Plough, A. L. (1981). Medical technology and the crisis of experience: The costs of clinical legitimation. *Social Science and Medicine, 15F*, 89–101.

Primomo, J., Yeates, B. C., & Woods, M. F. (1990). Social support for women during chronic illness: The relationship among sources and types to adjustment. *Research in Nursing and Health, 13*, 153–161.

Shekleton, M. E. (1987). Coping with chronic respiratory difficulty. *Nursing Clinics of North America, 22*, 569–81.

Stewart, D. C., & Sullivan, T. J. (1982). Illness behavior and the sick role in chronic disease. *Social Science and Medicine, 16*, 1397—1404.

Strauss, A. L., & Glaser, B. G. (1975). *Chronic illness and the quality of life*. St. Louis, MO: C. V. Mosby.

Taylor, A. G., Skelton, J. A., & Butcher, J. (1984). Duration of pain condition and physical pathology as determinants of nurses' assessments of patients in pain. *Nursing Research, 33*, 4–8.

Vinicor, F., Cohen, S., Mazzuca, S. A., Moorman, N., Wheeler, M., Kuebler, T., Swanson, S., Ours, P., Fineberg, S. E., Gordon, E. E., Duckworth, W., Norton, J. A., Fineberg, N., & Clark, C. M., Jr. (1987). DIABEDS: A randomized trial of the effects of physician and/or patient education on diabetes patient outcomes. *Journal of Chronic Diseases, 40*(4), 345–354.

[4]

Assisting with Transitions from Hospital to Home

Dorothy Brooten

The nursing science on transitions from hospital to home is extremely thin. There is little empirical data; most of what we know is opinion. This chapter, therefore, first focuses on the overriding issues that have arisen from the literature on transitional care; second, briefly mentions the major current and emerging models of transitional care reported in the literature; and third, presents the model of transitional care developed and used by our research team for over a decade.

TRANSITIONAL CARE—WHAT IS IT?

In response to earlier discharge, there has been a tremendous growth in various types of "transitional care services." These services are defined differently and implemented differently; seldom have they had sound evaluations of the outcomes of care. Most commonly, transitional care refers to care and services required for the transfer of patients from the hospital to home or from one level of care to another (Goldson, 1981; Ritz & Walker, 1989; Smith & Marien, 1989). The term has also been used in reference to the transfer of patients from the home back to the hospital or the transfer of patients from one facility to another, as in the care of the elderly or the disabled. Key features of transitional care include discharge planning, coordination of needed post-discharge services, provision of in-home services over the short run, and continued health care follow-up.

ISSUES IN TRANSITIONAL CARE

In examining transitional care services, several issues arise. They include the nature of the service, the length of the service, and questions about who requires the service, who should be the providers, and what are the costs.

Nature of the Service

In regards to the nature of the services, we know that transition implies an in-between period. These services, therefore, are not long-term, but temporary short-term services, which are quite different from, and not to be confused with, long-term home care (Ritz & Walker, 1989).

Length of the Service—Beginning and End

Transitional care services begin with discharge planning—which should begin on the day of the patient's admission. This is essential in this time of very short hospital stays and increased patient acuity, for only thus can services be projected and referrals made (Morrow-Howell, Proctor, & Mui, 1991). However, this appears to be an ideal. A recent panel of experts in the care of the elderly, for example, rated the quality of current planning for care after discharge as very poor. A study of over 900 Medicare-certified hospitals revealed that only 9% of elderly patients were discharged with plans for further care, and of that 9%, only half actually received the care (GAO, 1987).

The selection of patients who require discharge planning and transitional care remains very haphazard. In one study, the presence or absence of a family member was often used to determine the need for follow-up care. Living with someone frequently excludes the patient from receiving essential posthospital services. A study of hospitalized elderly who had experienced a hip fracture, for example, reported that 94% of patients who lived alone were visited by a discharge planner while only 40% of those who lived with someone else received a similar visit. One of the patients not visited was an 89-year-old woman who accurately reported that she lived with someone—her 91- and 93-year-old sisters, who clearly were not capable of her post-discharge care (Furstenberg & Mezy, 1987).

Transitional services ideally end with normal functioning and recovery, or stabilization of the patient's condition. The length of the service should vary with the specific needs of the patient or group of patients. We do not, however, have data indicating the most effective and cost efficient endpoint for receipt of these services by specific patient groups or subgroups. Realistically, in today's era of health care cost containment, the services end with as much home care or service as is reimbursable.

Who Requires the Service?

There is widespread agreement that vulnerable groups such as the elderly, the technologically dependent, the disabled, and some high-risk infants and children should receive transitional services (Berk & Berstein, 1985). Yet, as many researchers have noted, not everyone within these groups may need the full complement of services or services over the same length of time, or services at the same level and type of provider.

For example, the data to date suggest that not all hospitalized elderly are at risk for poor post-discharge outcomes. Many elderly and their families who receive effective preparation while in the hospital do quite well after discharge and do not require transitional care services. Naylor (1990) and Kennedy, Neidlinger, and Scroggins (1987) have demonstrated this. Some research findings have helped to identify those patients who will require transitional care services. The group includes elderly with major mental and functional deficits, those without people who are able or willing to help them, and those with complex medical problems.

Who Should Be the Providers?

The providers of transitional care are as varied as the programs and services (Brooten et al., 1986; Schwartz, Blumenfield, & Perlman Simon, 1990). Those providing daily direct care range from individuals with little health care training to master's prepared nurses plus a variety of providers who offer specialized services such as respiratory therapy, physical therapy, occupational therapy, etc. What is clear is that success is possible only with a multidisciplinary approach, from the multidisciplinary team in the hospital to the many community agencies and resources needed by the patient and family. However, some member of the multidisciplinary team must coordinate the care.

What are the Costs of the Services?

The direct costs of services can be calculated. The data we do not have are on indirect costs, such as prevention of re-hospitalization, acute care visits, decreased employment, and burden on family caregivers. These data are important in examining the overall cost benefit or cost effectiveness of such services.

CURRENT AND EMERGING MODELS

Current and emerging models of transitional care include the following:

- Multidisciplinary discharge planning teams with referral to a variety of community agencies. These models use a main discharge planner or case manager (MacAdam et al., 1989).
- Hospital-based home care services (Floyd & Buckle, 1987; Schwartz et al., 1990).
- Community agencies with hospital liaison personnel. Some of these models include a community health nurse who makes rounds with the hospital team and discharge planner (Edelstein & Lang, 1991).
- Community-based groups with services such as the famous Block Nurse Program, developed in Minnesota by Ida Martinson ("Award Recognizes," 1986).
- Entrepreneurial groups serving specific groups of patients, including high-risk infants and those who are technologically dependent. These groups provide a variety of services and give care mainly to patients with private insurance.
- Transitional units in hospitals. Here family caregivers spend time in the units learning to care for the patient. Following discharge, they have continued telephone access to providers and are linked with community services (Goldson, 1981).

Although all of the models attempt to improve continuity of care and the transition to the home and more normal functioning, there has been relatively little research on the outcomes of these many programs. What is needed are comparisons of the patient outcomes of these services and evaluation of which type and level of provider result in improved outcomes, what mix of services is necessary for which vulnerable group, and which services are most cost effective.

QUALITY-COST MODEL OF NURSE SPECIALIST TRANSITIONAL CARE

The model of quality-cost transitional follow-up care by nurse specialists was developed in 1981 and tested with very low birthweight (VLBW) infants beginning in 1982. The model has been refined and modified and is now being applied to a variety of patient groups including the elderly, women post-hysterectomy surgery, women with unplanned cesarean birth, women with high-risk pregnancies, and children with perinatal AIDS and their families.

The quality-cost model is designed for use in both research and care delivery for any patient population. It provides a well-developed framework for examining both quality of care as reflected in patient outcomes and cost of care in providing transitional follow-up services at home to specific patient groups. Its comprehensiveness, with discharge planning early in the hospital stay, coordination of needed post-discharge services, in-home direct care provided by nurse specialists, and continued health care follow-up, allows for thorough documentation of interventions (Brooten, Brown, et al., 1988).

The model can be used to compare quality and cost outcomes of routine care and early discharge with transitional care using a nurse specialist who has advanced practice skills. The model can also be used to compare home care using a nurse specialist with advanced practice skills and a myriad of other levels and types of health care providers.

The Model and VLBW Infants

The model was first developed for use with VLBW infants in 1981. The impetus came from the movement toward earlier hospital discharge for vulnerable groups despite a lack of postdischarge outcome data, the lack of community home follow-up services by nurses in Philadelphia for VLBW infants due to budget cuts, concern for the women who deliver VLBW infants at the University of Pennsylvania hospital since they are poor women with few resources in the home to care for high risk infants, and increasing Federal efforts to reduce social programs, which placed families functioning on the margin in an even more precarious position.

The study was designed as a randomized clinical trial with one group of infants and families receiving usual routine care, while a second group received early infant discharge and nurse specialist home follow-up for 18 months postdischarge (Brooten et al., 1986). For the early discharge group, the transition from the hospital to the home began following the birth of a VLBW infant. The discharge planning protocol included assessment of the parents' perception of the infant; teaching of care-taking skills to the parents or caretakers; a return demonstration of care-taking skills to the nurse specialist; assessment of the home environment and coordination of needed postdischarge services, including home monitoring services; follow-up health care services; and provision of utility services, including heating and telephone services.

Actual discharge criteria were developed by the physicians and nurse specialists with input from primary nurses and a variety of other members of the care team. The aim was to achieve infant readiness for discharge, family readiness, and an environment adequate to support the infant's basic needs. The infant was discharged upon agreement of the team, mainly the physician, nurse specialist, and primary nurse.

Following discharge, home visits were made during the first 2 weeks post-discharge and then at 1, 9, 12, and 18 months. In addition, the nurse specialist made a series of telephone calls to the family, and the family had 7-day-a-week telephone access to the nurse specialist. Whenever possible the nurse specialist also met with the family at the infant's routinely scheduled clinic or physician office visits. All of these interventions focused on continuity of care for the infant and family and continued follow-up care.

The study results indicated that the early discharge group followed by a nurse specialist was able to be discharged a mean of 11 days earlier, a mean of 200 grams less in weight, and 2 weeks younger than the control group, with no significant differences in rehospitalizations, acute care visits, or growth and development. Hospital charges were reduced a mean of 27% and physician charges a mean of 22% for the early discharge group (Brooten et al., 1986). The study's secondary findings were almost as important as the primary findings. They demonstrated the following:

- Despite the many telephone calls made to families, the parents still had major concerns and need for access to a nurse who was familiar with the infant's health care needs. Parents made over 300 telephone calls to the nurse specialists. Seventy-four percent of the calls were made within the first 6 months post-infant discharge. The number and type of telephone calls did not differ according to type of medical insurance held by parents (Butts et al., 1988).
- Ninety-five percent of rehospitalizations occurred within the first year following infant discharge, with 79% occurring within the first 6 months. Major diagnoses were respiratory problems, surgery, infections, and gastrointestinal problems. These data are important for discharge and follow-up teaching (Termini, Brooten, Brown, Gennaro, & York, 1990).
- Maternal anxiety was high the week after birth and the week the infant went home. Multiparas and mothers with infants who had shorter hospital stays were more depressed at the time of infant discharge (Brooten, Gennaro, et al., 1988).
- The study resulted in significant savings in ancillary costs (Finkler, Brooten, & Brown, 1988).
- Major teaching needs were in the areas of infant feeding, both breast and bottle, and helping parents manage the complex system of health care services (Brooten, Gennaro, Knapp, Brown, & York, 1989).
- Parental visiting and telephoning while the infant was hospitalized were mainly the responsibility of the mother, and the pattern was not linked to infant health outcomes (Brown, Gennaro, York, Swinkles, & Brooten, 1991; Brown, York, Jacobsen, Gennaro, & Brooten, 1989).
- Sociodemographic data documented the lack of resources of this group to provide complex home care for these vulnerable infants (Brown, Brooten, et al., 1989).

These findings provided much useful data on the transitional care services needed by this group of vulnerable infants. The model was then refined and tested with women who had hysterectomies, high-risk pregnancies, and unplanned cesarean births. Results of the work with these groups are currently being analyzed. In addition, Dr. Mary Naylor is testing the model with the elderly, and Drs. Deatrick and Thurber are applying it to HIV-positive infants. Doctoral student efforts include a follow-up of the original VLBW infant group and their families to examine infant and family outcomes some 10 years later; classification of the functions of the nurse specialist with the various groups followed; and examination of treatment adherence, help seeking, and outcomes of patients followed by the nurse specialist and the control groups.

In summary, assisting with the transition from hospital to home is critical in this time of shortened hospital length of stay. What is needed is quality discharge planning, coordination of needed postdischarge services, provision of in-home services over the short run, and continued health care follow-up or retention of patients in the health care system.

REFERENCES

Award recognizes block program for cost efficient nursing care. (1986, Nov/Dec). *American Nurse, 18*(10), 9.

Berk, M., & Berstein, A. (1985). Home health services: Some findings from the national medical care expenditure survey. *Home Health Care Services Quarterly, 6*, 13–23.

Brooten, D., Brown, L., Munro, B., York, R., Cohen, S., Roncoli, M., & Hollingsworth, A. (1988). Early discharge and specialist transitional care. *Image: The Journal of Nursing Scholarship, 20*, 64–68.

Brooten, D., Gennaro, S., Brown, L., Butts, P., Gibbons, A., Bakewell-Sachs, S., & Kumar, S. (1988). Maternal anxiety, depression and hostility in mothers of preterm infants. *Nursing Research, 37*, 213–216.

Brooten, D., Gennaro, S., Knapp, H., Brown, L., & York, R. (1989). Clinical specialist pre and post discharge teaching of parents of very low birthweight infants. *Journal of Obstetric, Gynecologic and Neonatal Nursing, 18*, 316–22.

Brooten, D., Kumar, S., Brown, L., Butts, P., Finkler, S., Bakewell-Sachs, S., Gibbons, A., and Delivoria-Papadopoulos, M. (1986). A randomized clinical trial of early discharge and home follow-up of very low birthweight infants. *The New England Journal of Medicine, 315*, 934–939.

Brown, L., Brooten, D., Kumar, S., Butts, P., Finkler, S., Bakewell-Sachs, S., Gibbons, A., and Delivoria-Papadopoulos, M. (1989). Families of very low birthweight infants: A sociodemographic profile of 72 families. *Western Journal of Nursing Research, 11*, 520–532.

Brown, L., Gennaro, S., York, R., Swinkles, K., & Brooten, D. (1991). VLBW infants: Association between visiting and telephoning and maternal and infant outcome measures. *The Journal of Perinatal & Neonatal Nursing, 4*(4), 39–46.

Brown, L., York, R., Jacobsen, B., Gennaro, S., & Brooten, D. (1989). Very low birthweight infants: Parental visiting and telephoning during initial infant hospitalization. *Nursing Research, 38*, 233–236.

Butts, P., Brooten, D., Brown, L., Bakewell-Sachs, S., Gibbons, A., & Kumar, S. (1988). Concerns of parents of low birthweight infants following hospital discharge: A report of parent initiated telephone calls. *Neonatal Network, 7*(2), 37–42.

Edelstein, H., & Lang, A. (1991). Posthospital care for older people: A collaborative solution. *The Gerontologist, 31*, 267–270.

Finkler, S., Brooten, D., & Brown, L. (1988). Utilization of inpatient services under shortened lengths of stay: A neonatal care example. *Inquiry, 25*, 271–280.

Floyd, J., & Buckle, J. (1987). Nursing care of the elderly. *Journal of Gerontological Nursing, 13*(2), 20–25.

Furstenberg, A., & Mezy, M. (1987). Mental impairment of elderly hospitalized hip fracture patients. *Comprehensive Gerontology, 1*, 80–86.

Goldson, E. (1981). The family care center. *Children Today, 10*(4), 15–20.

Kennedy, L., Neidlinger, S., & Scroggins, K. (1987). Effective comprehensive discharge planning for hospitalized elderly. *The Gerontologist, 27*, 577–80.

MacAdam, M., Capitman, J., Yee, D., Prottas, J., Leutz, W., & Westwater, D. (1989). Case management for frail elders: The Robert Wood Johnson Foundation's program for hospital initiatives in long-term care. *The Gerontologist, 29*, 737–744.

Morrow-Howell, N., Proctor, E., & Mui, A. (1991). Efficacy of discharge plans for elderly patients. *Social Work Research & Abstracts, 27*, 6–13.

Naylor, M. (1990). Comprehensive discharge planning for hospitalized elderly: A pilot study. *Nursing Research, 39*, 156–161.

Post-hospital care: Discharge planners report increasing difficulty in planning for Medicare patients. (1987, January). *GAO/PMED-87-5-BR*.

Ritz, L., & Walker, M. (1989). Transitional care services and chronicity: Oncology as a case in point. *The Hospice Journal, 5*(2), 55–66.

Schwartz, P., Blumenfield, S., & Perlman Simon, E. (1990). The interim homecare program: An innovative discharge planning alternative. *Health and Social Work, 15*, 152–160.

Smith, C., & Marien, L. (1989). Transitional care of adults dependent on technological care at home. *The Kansas Nurse*, pp. 1–2.

Termini, L., Brooten, D., Brown, L., Gennaro, S., & York, R. (1990). Reasons for acute care visits and rehospitalizations in very low birthweight infants. *Neonatal Network, 8*(5), 23–25.

[5]

Managing Home Care

Patricia A. Cloonan

Home health research is still embryonic. The focus of the chapter, then, will be on the state of our system of home health care delivery—where we are, where we've been, where we're going—and how we might use research to get there. It is also my hope to stimulate research in this exciting arena.

I'd like to start with a story about a home care nurse and her patient (this is an actual case history that is part of the public record). The story captures in an especially poignant way what "managing home care" is all about in today's environment. This is the story of Harvy Simms, age 72, who lives in northeastern Pennsylvania in a tiny, sparsely furnished single room. Mr. Simms has congenital hearing loss, is mildly retarded, and is legally blind because of congenital cataracts. In 1986 he developed cancer of the larynx. Following his laryngectomy, Mr. Simms was discharged to home care for treatment of his stoma and for instruction on how to manage his own care, including suctioning his trachea. With great patience and skill, the home care nurse taught Mr. Simms self-care. Slowly he gained strength and regained his independence. He learned to suction his trachea and do his own stoma care. Mr. Simms, however, was denied Medicare coverage for the home care he received; he was declared not homebound because he was able to go to the hospital for radiation therapy.

The home care nurse was outraged. Joining with other Pennsylvania nurses who had had similar experiences with Medicare, they went to Washington, DC, and they enlisted the concern of the late Senator John Heinz, who subsequently made a home visit to Mr. Simms. With shaky but deliberate hands, Mr. Simms proudly demonstrated his newly learned self-care skills. Not surprisingly he made his way into Senator Heinz's heart and eventually into the Congressional Record. In the 1987 Omnibus Reconciliation Act (OBRA), Congress added the provision that homebound patients may make trips for medical treatment without forfeiting their right to home care services (Pera & Gould, 1989). This story reflects nurses' understanding that providing home health care often means putting forth extraordinary effort for patients. Home health nurses do this every day—they call landlords when the heat is off, they arrange needed medications and supplies, and they help patients and families navigate a very complex and fragmented health care system.

Since the trend in health care is away from the hospital and toward the community, this is a wonderful time to be in home health nursing. The potential seems limitless; but to take hold of the opportunities before us, we need to reflect on where we've been, to analyze where we are today, and to create a vision of where we might go. This chapter begins that journey.

Caring for the chronically ill at home is not new; health care has been delivered at home, primarily by women, for centuries (home care is reported in the Bible). However, the first organized program for providing care to the sick at home was established at the Boston Dispensary in 1796 (Cary, 1989). A century later, in 1892, the first organized home nursing service, the Visiting Nurse Service of New York, was established (Spiegel, 1987). These visiting nurses assumed responsibility for a broad spectrum of health and social services. They provided home nursing services, including coordination of health and social services, and they served as patient advocates to improve housing, workplaces and neighborhoods. They also were responsible for school health. Indeed, this sounds like the first case management program! What is important to note is that these nurses understood the links between social and environmental influences and health status. They also understood that to improve health, environmental issues that have an impact on health must be addressed. The nursing model developed by these early visiting nurse programs was holistic, blending clinical care with political activism—like the nursing care provided to Mr. Simms nearly a century later.

In today's environment the cost of such care would be of concern; at the turn of the century, however, there was a combination of public welfare and philanthropic support for this kind of health care (Rose, 1989). Concern for the sick, especially the sick poor, was widespread among communities and citizens. There was a sense of stewardship, a belief that responsibility for the good of the individual rested with the community.

Home remained the central location for care delivery until the 1940s when advances in scientific medicine and surgery—disease could now actually be cured—combined with technological developments to shift care delivery from homes into hospitals. The Hill-Burton Act funded construction of hospitals, and insurance companies reimbursed the care delivered in them; hospitals reigned supreme in the health care delivery system. The scientific paradigm was empiricism, with its accompanying objectivity and detachment. Medicine came into its own, claiming status, power, and authority (Jecker & Self, 1991). And as a society we began a love affair with the biggest, the brightest and slickest, and the most technologically sophisticated hospitals that money could buy.

During the 1940s and 1950s home health care remained primarily within the purview of visiting nurse associations and health departments. Their scope narrowed from the model developed by the Visiting Nurse Service of New York, however, and became more specialized; yet home and public health nursing practice continued to be dictated by patient need.

During the 1950s and 1960s the cost of health care began a dramatic escalation, but the nation's social conscience was alive and well, and as a society we became concerned about access to care for those in need. By 1964, the climate was right for addressing the health needs of at least two segments of the population—the poor and the elderly. In 1965, through an amendment to the Social Security Act, Medicare and Medicaid were established. Because home care was thought to be a cost-effective alternative to hospital care, it was reimbursed under both (Kent & Hanley, 1991). However, this federal involvement in home care precipitated a radical shift in the scope and authority of home care services. Physicians were designated as the gatekeepers to home care, and a medical diagnosis, rather than a health or social need, was required for care to be delivered and reimbursed. The result was a shift from comprehensive health care for people of all ages to short-term care for the acutely ill, primarily the elderly. The implementation of Medicare and Medicaid thus marked the shift from a nursing model of comprehensive home care delivery to a medical model that limited services to acute care for the ill (Wood & Estes, 1988). It is important to note that nursing and medicine need not be dichotomized, with one viewed as good and the other as bad. Rather, we need to acknowledge the two models of care delivery that have become known as the medical model and the nursing model. The medical model, with its attention to technology, objectivity, and scientific rationality, was more consistent with the societal values and the financial and political agendas of the 1970s and 1980s. As a result, it became the dominant model of care delivery. Home nursing care began to be defined by the medical model, and for the first time, influences other than patient need determined the type and amount of nursing care delivered.

Medicare and Medicaid were only the first of the forces that have shaped the current environment for home care delivery. Costs continued to escalate, and legislative and regulatory bodies continued to try to contain them. In 1981 OBRA was passed. This law expanded the benefits for Medicare recipients of home care and eliminated the state licensure requirements for proprietary agencies (Kent & Hanley, 1991). The result was a 98% increase in the number of agencies delivering care, from 3,012 agencies in 1981 to 5,953 in 1987 (Harrington, 1988). A concomitant increase occurred in the number of different types of agencies delivering home care. In 1982, Congress passed the Tax Equity and Fiscal Responsibility Act (TEFRA), which established a prospective payment system for the hospital care of Medicare patients and essentially changed the financial incentives for health care (Cowart, 1985). One ripple effect was that a growing number of frail and sick elderly began to receive care in the community (Phillips & Cloonan, 1987). Societal values and technical advances made this shift possible. But is the home care system, with its now deeply entrenched medical model, able to meet the needs of this population?

Home care has been defined by the World Health Organization as the provision of comprehensive services to patients and families in their place of residence to promote, maintain, and restore health; maximize independence; or support a peaceful death. The services typically provided include skilled nursing, rehabilitation therapy, social services, supplies and equipment, and such technologically advanced care as continuous infusion and continuous ventilation.

Patients who receive home care today are typically acutely ill; however, the needs of the chronically ill, not generally reimbursed by third parties, are becoming more pressing as the population ages and the number of chronically ill increases (Gould, 1989). It is these chronic patients that home care agencies report being unable to serve because of poor reimbursement for their care (Gould, 1989; Rinke, 1989; Rose, 1989). It is especially ironic that the home care delivery system has the capability to provide the care needed, but the limits of reimbursement make this care difficult to access.

The needs of chronic illness care are primarily integrative, with the goal for care being constructive integration of the patient's illness into daily life, thus mitigating the limitations of the chronic condition. Although many of us identify these as skilled needs, they do not fit the narrowly prescribed definition of skilled care required for Medicare reimbursement. Unfortunately, home care is increasingly becoming known by this narrowly prescribed definition: One must have a medical diagnosis, be homebound, and require part-time skilled nursing. This definition virtually eliminates those whose care needs are primarily for nonprofessional assistance with ADLs.

So who provides the needed care to the chronically ill at home? The informal system, often referred to as the silent arm of the health care delivery system, carries much of the burden of chronic illness care (O'Neill & Sorensen, 1991). Family responsibility for care is not a new concept; indeed, it is deeply embedded in our culture, with 95% of personal care delivered by informal caregivers (Folden, 1989). Of the 2.2 million unpaid caregivers, 72% are women (Gaynor, 1990), making this clearly a woman's issue. Women provide this care without, for the most part, financial rewards or resources and often without sufficient information (Anderson, 1990). Studies of caregivers suggest a cycle of neglect: many caregivers are in poor health themselves, suffering from sleep deprivation, chronic fatigue, and depression; they experience an increased incidence of stress-related disorders such as hypertension and heart disease, and they have an increased number of physician's visits, take more medications, and use more sick days (Gaynor, 1990; Given & Given, 1991). Many report that caregiving can be a positive experience, but all report needing support, respite, affirmation, and knowledge. The formal system has an important role in designing strategies that support informal caregivers and promote wellness and integration of care for chronic conditions into daily life (Noelker & Bass, 1989; Schirm, 1990). This role needs to be developed, valued, and funded.

Clearly the medical model, with its individualistic and reductionistic thinking, and the home care system that has fashioned itself on this model, have limitations for chronic illness care. The basic premises of the medical model are that patients are biological organisms and disease is an external threat to be cured (Roth & Harrison, 1991). While this model might be appropriate within the context of acute illness, it is not useful for the management of chronic illness. Indeed, it is inconsistent with the needs of a society with many aged, chronically ill, and frail members who need supportive services to maintain independence. The nursing model incorporates aspects of the medical model, but it is broader and more integrative. Nurses' values and expertise can provide unique insights into the human experience of health and illness.

We need to work together with our colleagues in other disciplines to develop a comprehensive model that addresses the economic, social, and environmental factors associated with chronic illness—a model that integrates the psyche and the body, health and illness, patients and families, and that defines quality broadly and values care as well as cure. How do we get there? Research is a way of reclaiming home care from the existing model that is so incompatible with chronic illness. Yet although home care is probably the oldest nursing specialty, the research in this area is in its infancy. Like society, nursing research in general and home care research in particular have embraced the scientific paradigm and have not been enamored of low tech, chronic illness care. Our research has adopted the concerns of the medical model; we have defined outcomes in pragmatic, medically oriented ways (Barkauskas, 1990; Green, 1989, 1990). Let me point out, however, that the home health field is growing so quickly and is so competitive that answers to important questions of effectiveness and cost are needed quickly. Therefore, studies have been primarily cost and mortality comparisons between home care and institutional options. Thus, most of what we know about home care is related to cost effectiveness and efficacy. For example, studies have demonstrated that for some patients, home care is a cost-effective alternative to acute inpatient care (Brickner et al., 1976; Hughes et al., 1992; Zimmer, Groth-Juncker, & McCusker, 1985); it reduces hospital and nursing home length of stay (Gaumer et al., 1986); a variety of treatment and care regimes can be provided safely at home by patients and caregivers (Barrera, Cunningham, & Rosenbaum, 1986; Brooten et al., 1986); and home care is a more acceptable way of care delivery for many patients (Bull, 1992; Hughes et al., 1992).

However, problems with design and methods make even these findings suspect. For example, two well-controlled studies have produced contradictory findings about the cost-effectiveness of home care services; one found that the cost of home care was higher than the cost of inpatient care (Hughes, Cordray, & Spiker, 1984; Hughes, Manheim, Edelman, & Conrad, 1987), while the other found cost savings in home care (Zimmer et al., 1985). Home care research is often conducted in a single agency, with participants who are selected because of their ability to participate in self-care; thus the findings cannot be generalized. Further, research reports in the literature often only loosely define variables, so replication is difficult. For example, nursing interventions are usually broadly defined as home visits or telephone calls, telling us little about the components and dynamics of home-based nursing interventions. Many home care agencies are small and rural, with few opportunities for professional contact and collaboration. Research is not well disseminated to these agencies. Finally, much home care nursing research lacks a theoretical basis. Some of the chapters in this book, especially those reporting on work with chronically ill infants and children, are important first steps in advancing the field.

We need a diverse, multidimensional research agenda. First, we need to define our terms (Storfjell, 1989; Martin, 1988). We have not even defined what we mean by home care quality and effectiveness from a nursing perspective. Is effectiveness the same as quality? Is effectiveness demonstrated by lower mortality rates? Is quality care defined by the consumer or the government? It is clear that definitions are vital to any progress. If we do not know what it is we want, how can we achieve it? Once we have identified the outcomes that need to be measured, we need to develop specific, reliable, and valid tools to adequately measure achievement of these outcomes. We need some measurable index to indicate success or failure. Our research also needs a more holistic array of outcomes. In Chapter 2, McBride speaks of functional level and quality of life as clear domains for nursing inquiry. Ware (1987) suggests five domains that should be measured to determine changes in total health status: physical health, mental health, social functioning, role functioning, and general well-being. These foci will perhaps help us move beyond considerations of cost, mortality, and morbidity. In addition, there are other important questions that may not easily be answered by empirical methodologies. For example, the meaning of life with chronic illness, the establishment of supportive health care environments in which chronically ill persons can construct meaningful lives, and the integration of family caregivers into coordinated networks of health and social services are legitimate areas of inquiry for nursing and of major importance to an aging society facing increasing chronic illness and functional disability.

As a profession we have both private and public concerns. Our private concerns are rooted in the interests and rights of individual patients; our public duty involves serving the public as a whole in areas such as policy, resource allocation, and the protection of human rights (Roth & Harrison, 1991). We need to use our research not only to advance our private concerns but also to articulate our public voice. The policy arena is how we got here; we need to make the links between the concerns of nurses caring for patients and our concern for the way health care is delivered in this country, in much the same way that Mr. Simms' home care nurse did. Major policy decisions are being made based on research that has serious deficits.

To orchestrate social change in chronic illness care, nurses must be creative, politically astute, and willing to move against the current of existing societal norms and toward a new vision of health (Roth & Harrison, 1991). Although we cannot go home again, I believe that we can revisit our roots and learn again from the rich traditions of home care nursing practice. That is the message of this stanza from T. S. Eliot's *Four Quartets*:

> What we call the beginning is often the end
> And to make an end is to make a beginning
> The end is where we start from.

REFERENCES

Anderson, J. (1990). Home care management in chronic illness and the self-care movement: An analysis of ideologies and economic processes influencing policy decisions. *Advances in Nursing Science, 12*, 71–83.

Barkauskas, V. (1990). Home health care. *Annual Review of Nursing Research, 8*, 103–132.

Barrera, M., Cunningham, C., & Rosenbaum, P. (1986). Low birth weight and home intervention strategies: Preterm infants. *Journal of Developmental and Behavioral Pediatrics, 7*, 361–366.

Brickner, P., Janeski, J., Rich, G., Duque, T., Starita, L., LaRoccom, R., Flannery, T., & Werlin, S. (1976). Home maintenance for the home-bound aged. *The Gerontologist, 16*, 25–29.

Brooten, D., Kumar, S., Brown, L., Butts, P., Finkler, S., Bakewell-Sachs, G. S., Gibbons, A., & Delivoria-Papadopoulos, M. (1986). A randomized clinical trial of early hospital discharge and home follow-up of very low birth weight infants. *New England Journal of Medicine, 315*, 934–939.

Bull, M. (1992). Managing the transition from hospital to home. *Qualitative Health Research, 2*(1), 27–41.

Cary, A. (1989). Home health care. In C. Lambert & V. Lambert (Eds.), *Perspectives in nursing: The impacts on the nurse, the consumer, and society* (pp. 379-402). Norwalk, CT: Appleton & Lange.

Cowart, M. (1985). Policy issues: Financial reimbursement for home care. *Family and Community Health, 8*(2), 1–10.

Folden, S. (1989). Caring for older homebound adults: A chronic illness perspective. *Journal of Home Health Care Practice, 2*(1), 57–62.

Gaumer, G., Birnbaum, H., Pratter, F., Burke, R., Franklin, S., & Ellingson-Otto, K. (1986). Impact of the New York Long-Term Care Program. *Medical Care, 24*, 641–653.

Gaynor, S. (1990). The long haul: The effects of home care on caregivers. *Image: Journal of Nursing Scholarship, 22*, 208–212.

Given, B., & Given, C. (1991). Family caregiving for the elderly. *Annual Review of Nursing Research*, 77–101.

Gould, E. (1989). Home care nursing: Professional and political issues. *Journal of the New York State Nurses' Association, 20*(1), 4–7.

Green, J. (1989). Indices of quality in long-term care: Research and practice. *Long-term home care research* (pp. 125-143). New York: National League for Nursing.

Green, J. (1990). Long-term home care research. *Nursing and Health Care, 10*, 139–144.

Harrington, C. (1988). Quality, access, and costs: Public policy and home health care. *Nursing Outlook, 36*(4), 164–166.

Hughes, S., Cordray, D., & Spiker, V. (1984). Evaluation of a long term home care program. *Medical Care, 22*, 460–475.

Hughes, S., Manheim, L., Edelman, P., & Conrad, K. (1987). Impact of long term home care on hospital and nursing home use and cost. *Health Services Research, 22*, 19–47.

Hughes, S., Cummings, J., Weaver, F., Manheim, L., Braun, B., & Conrad, K. (1992). A randomized trial of the cost-effectiveness of VA hospital-based home care for the terminally ill. *Health Services Research, 26*, 817.

Jecker, N., & Self, D. (1991). Separating care and cure: An analysis of historical and contemporary images of nursing and medicine. *Journal of Medicine and Philosophy, 16*, 285–306.

Kent, V., & Hanley, B. (1991). Home health care. *Nursing and Health Care, 11*, 234–240.

Martin, K. (1988). Research in home care. *Nursing Clinics of North America, 23*, 373–385.

Noelker, L., & Bass, D. (1989). Home care for elderly persons: Linkages between formal and informal caregivers. *Journal of Gerontology, 44*, 563–570.

O'Neill, C., & Sorensen, E. (1991). Home care of the elderly: A family perspective. *Advances in Nursing Science, 13*(4), 28–37.

Pera, M., & Gould, E. (1989). Home care nursing: Integration of politics and nursing. *Holistic Nursing Practice, 3*(2), 9–17.

Phillips, E., & Cloonan, P. (1987). DRG ripple effects on community health nursing. *Public Health Nursing, 4*(2), 84–88.

Rinke, L. (1989). Replacing a failing old paradigm with a vital new paradigm: Home care. *Nursing and Health Care, 8*, 330–333.

Roth, P., & Harrison, J. (1991). Orchestrating social change: An imperative in care of the chronically ill. *Journal of Medicine and Philosophy, 16*, 343–359.

Rose, M. (1989). Home care nursing: The new frontier. *Holistic Nursing Practice, 3*(2), 1–8.

Schirm, V. (1990). Shared caregiving responsibilities for chronically ill elders. *Holistic Nursing Practice, 5*(1), 54–61.
Spiegel, A. (1987). *Home health care.* Owing Mills, MD: Rynd Communications.
Storfjell, J. (1989). A response to home health care: Caregivers and quality (pp. 145–154). *Long-term home care research.* New York: National League for Nursing.
Ware, J. (1987). The science of quality of life. *Journal of Chronic Diseases, 40,* 459-463.
Wood, J., & Estes, C. (1988). Medicalization of community services for the elderly. *Health and Social Work,* 35–42.
Zimmer, J., Groth-Juncker, A., & McCusker, J. (1985). A randomized controlled study of a home health care team. *American Journal of Public Health, 75,* 134–141.

[6]

Living with Chronic Illness: Living with Uncertainty

Merle H. Mishel

Conrad (1987) has identified five recurring themes in the literature on living with chronic illness. These are, in order of importance: uncertainty, stigma, loss of self, managing regimens, and family relations. This chapter focuses on uncertainty. Chronic illness has been described by Wiener (1975) as an experience of living with chronic uncertainty. According to Viney and Westbrook (1982), uncertainty has been reported in patients in the early stages of illness and when new treatments are introduced. Uncertainty regarding the duration of an illness or its outcome has been reported as the greatest single psychological stressor for the patient with a life-threatening illness (Koocher, 1984). Uncertainty does not represent the total experience of chronic illness, yet it is a constant part of the illness from the earliest symptoms through immediate treatment and into the long process of learning how to manage life. This chapter discusses situations promoting uncertainty and methods to manage the uncertainty. The situations promoting uncertainty in chronic illness may be divided into the categories of symptom uncertainty, medical uncertainty, and daily living uncertainty. Methods to manage the uncertainty include managing symptom/ medical uncertainty and managing daily living uncertainty.

UNCERTAINTY IN ILLNESS

Uncertainty in illness may be defined as the inability to determine the meaning of illness-related events. It is the cognitive state created when the person cannot adequately structure or categorize an event because of lack of sufficient cues. Uncertainty occurs in a situation in which the decision maker is unable to assign definite value to objects or events and/or is unable to accurately predict outcomes (Mishel, 1988).

Uncertainty in illness has been referred to by Koocher (1984) as the "Damocles Syndrome," after the Greek myth about a courier who was forced to sit through a banquet under a sword suspended overhead by a single horsehair. This analogy highlights the stressful nature of uncertainty—not knowing when tragedy, difficulty, untoward events, or whatever else will occur; not knowing what form it will take; not knowing what to do about it; not knowing how to manage or survive it.

Why should we place such emphasis on uncertainty? Why is it important? Probably the major reason is that most people consider the experience of uncertainty as emotionally painful. The common phrase is "an agony of uncertainty." Studies by Mishel, Hostetter, King, and Graham (1984) conducted on women with gynecological cancer, by Hilton (1988) on women with breast cancer, and by Webster and Christman (1988) and Richardson and colleagues (1987) on persons undergoing radiotherapy, all found that uncertainty led to anxiety and depression. These findings were replicated in Wineman's (1990) study of uncertainty in persons with multiple sclerosis.

When the uncertainty centers upon an event that will have a definite answer in the immediate future, uncertainty causes anxiety until an answer is available; examples include a diagnostic workup such as HIV testing, cardiac catheterization, or exploratory surgery to determine presence of cancer, or the waiting period for obtaining organ transplant. Although the outcome may not be the desired choice, the decision removes the uncertainty. People often remark that any outcome is preferable to crippling uncertainty. With an outcome, action can be undertaken. With uncertainty, people report that they are immobilized.

Although uncertainty may be a factor in maintaining hope, uncertainty commonly undermines quality of life. In their study of quality of life after heart transplantation, Murdaugh and Mishel (1991) found that uncertainty was related to emotional distress and lower levels of life satisfaction. Uncertainty sabotages adjustments in the major areas of family, work, and recreation because the family's day-to-day living becomes ill-defined and indeterminate (Mishel et al., 1984). Problems in family relationships have been reported as resulting from uncertainty (Mishel et al., 1984; Rowat & Knafl, 1985). Among women receiving treatment for breast cancer, uncertainty weakens the sense of mastery over a situation (Mishel, Padilla, Grant, & Sorenson, 1991; Mishel & Sorenson, 1991). Uncertainty has a similar impact on other related variables such as locus of control and learned resourcefulness. Among patients living with a heart transplant, uncertainty weakens internal locus of control (Murdaugh & Mishel, 1991). Braden (1990) reported that among persons with rheumatoid arthritis, uncertainty reduced their sense of learned resourcefulness, which then lessened their ability to help themselves. In the research on cancer and cardiac disease and on rheumatoid arthritis, uncertainty has consistently been shown to increase a person's sense of threat and danger.

In some situations, however, uncertainty is not strongly related to negative outcome. In fact, there is support for viewing uncertainty as a positive experience in persons with a chronic illness. Among patients receiving kidney dialysis, higher levels of uncertainty were found related to compliance, while lower levels of uncertainty were related to non-compliance (Mishel, 1988). Persons with lupus have reported that the longer they lived with the illness, the more positive was their evaluation of uncertainty (Mishel, 1988). Also, among care providers for persons with Alzheimer's disease, uncertainty was found to be related to lower catecholamine and cortisol levels (Pergrin, Mishel, & Murdaugh, 1987). Mishel and Murdaugh (1987) found that spouses of heart transplant candidates viewed the uncertainty surrounding heart transplantation as a second chance at life.

Symptom Uncertainty

A major type of uncertainty in chronic illness is uncertainty about symptoms. This occurs when the person cannot determine a pattern to his/her symptoms. In chronic illness, symptom uncertainty is part of living with the illness. Many chronic illnesses are characterized by their fluctuating nature. Examples include epilepsy, rheumatoid arthritis, lupus, Crohn's disease, multiple sclerosis, and AIDS. A major characteristic of many of these illnesses is not that they are curable or incurable, but that their manifestations and trajectory are unpredictable and the success of management methods is uncertain. A primary task of persons with these chronic illnesses is to control the physical attack.

Weitz (1989) notes that AIDS, like many chronic illnesses, causes unpredictable flare-ups and remissions. Similar illness characteristics have been reported by Wiener (1975) as a major aspect of rheumatoid arthritis. Rheumatoid arthritis, lupus, and multiple sclerosis are diseases that do not follow a strictly downhill course. Flare-ups occur suddenly and, in some cases, they can also be suddenly arrested. These diseases can be quite calm for a long time, only to burst out again.

Not only is there uncertainty present in the flare-up of symptoms and their remission, but the areas of involvement vary. Persons complain that they do not know where symptoms will be located (place of body involvement), what type of symptoms will occur (pain, swelling, stiffness, or numbness), how severe they will be, or how long they will last. Weitz (1989) reports that persons with AIDS never know from one day to the next how sick they will be. She quotes one man as saying:

> Probably the hardest thing is not knowing when you're well what's going to happen tomorrow because when you're well, all you're thinking about is, "What's the next infection I'm going to have to put up with?" (Weitz, 1989, p. 275)

King and Mishel (1986) found that for persons with lupus, it was the lack of a pattern of symptoms that caused them the greatest uncertainty prior to diagnosis. Patients with diseases characterized by symptom variability, such as immunological conditions, lupus, and rheumatoid arthritis, have higher levels of uncertainty than do persons with illnesses characterized by symptom consistency (Mishel, 1988). Rowat and Knafl (1985) also report that spouses of patients with chronic pain complain about uncertainty concerning the persistence of pain. Spousal caregivers are stressed by their uncertainty about how to manage their partner's pain, their inability to effect any change in the pain, and their uncertainty about how to make their partner more comfortable.

Medical Uncertainty

Medical uncertainty can also be termed diagnostic uncertainty because difficulty in achieving a diagnosis is the pivotal feature of this area of uncertainty. Cohen and Martinson (1988) describe the attempt to reduce diagnostic uncertainty as a trip through a diagnostic funnel—or a progressive narrowing of possible alternatives in examining a specific set of symptoms. When a person brings ambiguous symptoms to the physician, the person hopes for a quick conclusion with a label of a specific diagnosis.

However, seeing a physician does not necessarily end the uncertainty. Weitz (1989), for example, reports that physicians may not consider the diagnosis of AIDS unless they know their clients well. Some physicians, even knowing the client is at risk for HIV, are reluctant or refuse to conduct HIV testing because the doctor cannot deal with the possibility of a positive result from testing. This leaves the person wallowing in uncertainty about the nature of the symptoms.

In the case of illnesses such as lupus or multiple sclerosis, the process of achieving a diagnosis can be harrowing. Patients report that it can take a number of years to achieve an accurate diagnosis. According to Stewart and Sullivan (1982), 60 persons with multiple sclerosis reported the number of physicians they contacted as 227, for a total of 420 diagnostic tests and treatments.

A variety of diagnoses have been given to persons with lupus, multiple sclerosis, and other vague collagen-related conditions. With each of these diagnoses goes an array of treatments. With each diagnosis, the person's uncertainty decreases, and then, with each failed treatment and return to the diagnostic funnel, the uncertainty increases again. Belief in any initial explanation erodes, leaving the person in an amorphous situation: symptoms of illness and no certainty about what they mean. This leads to increased urgency to obtain a diagnosis or at least to get someone with credibility to recognize the seriousness of the observations. As one patient told me:

> I look back on my medical history. I lost my teeth and lost my gall bladder. One thing after another. It was diagnosed different things, lupus was never in there. I complained for years about fatigue. I'd walk upstairs, lie down, tears would roll down my cheeks. The doctor would say, slow down, you're doing too much; you have family problems, go to a psychiatrist, go to a psychologist. I went to the chaplain. I'm 43 now; this started when I was 24 years old, and then all those operations. It feels good to know what it is. I was doing things that went against me, but how would I know that if someone didn't tell me.

Another result of the lack of diagnosis is erosion of faith in the physician's judgment. Once this occurs, persons are less likely to consider any diagnosis credible. This leaves them in the difficult position of defining themselves or their children as sick, but not being socially defined as ill. Stewart and Sullivan (1982) report that this in turn heightens diagnostic uncertainty.

Lack of trust and confidence in the physician results in high levels of uncertainty. In a number of studies, the physician has been found to have a greater influence on levels of uncertainty than other social and person factors (Mishel & Braden, 1988; Mishel, 1988). In fact, trust/confidence in the physician has been shown to explain about 35% of the variance in uncertainty (Mishel, 1988). The relationship with the physician is important in reducing uncertainty because the physician is a source of information about causes and consequences of symptoms. The physician confirms that symptoms indicate a diagnostic category. The more credible the physician, the less the uncertainty.

Trust and confidence in the physician are a major means of preventing uncertainty. However, although physicians have a powerful impact on the degree of uncertainty experienced by patients, physicians themselves experience uncertainty in their practices. Doctors complain that they never expected the degree of uncertainty involved in medicine when they chose it as a career and poorly tolerate the stress the uncertainty exerts. A person, who eventually was diagnosed with lupus, said to me:

> It is such an indecisive thing. I went to the doctor, he gave me a blood test, and all these different tests, and said "you may have it, or you may not." Then I went to another doctor who said "you probably have it but not bad enough to put you on any medication." I said to heck with it and just sort of regulate myself according to how I feel.

Daily Living Uncertainty

Charmaz (1983) suggests that when symptom uncertainty exists and illness is characterized by an unpredictable course, the unpredictability causes some persons to voluntarily restrict their lives more than need be. Because of the unpredictability of their condition, patients suffer disruptions of their lives and selves that go far beyond the experience of physical discomfort. Such disruptions include the felt necessity to quit work, limit social engagements, and avoid activity. These actions are taken to protect the person's life, but they are done at a great cost to self-image.

Persons living with unpredictability attempt to manage the condition by finding something that they can correlate with remissions so that they bring the physical instability under control. This effort can lead people to try various types of remedies and to structure life according to various protocols or beliefs. If self-help can be initiated, often some symptom stability can be achieved, only to be disrupted again. The person swings through hope and disappointment, both fueled by uncertainty.

Loveys (1990) describes the "at-risk role" as a state of being neither sick nor well in which all the patterns of preillness life are gradually resumed but modified in various ways. At-risk status is based on the uncertainty of recurrence and/or disease extension in persons who may look and feel well or stabilized.

In the at-risk role, persons may function in a near normal world, aware of the potential of illness only at uncertainty stress points. Hilton (1988), for example, describes situations that increase uncertainty about outcomes of breast cancer in women who have terminated treatment. Certain events activate concern about an unknown outcome. These events include returning for checkups, hearing of others diagnosed or dying from breast cancer, hearing of treatment controversies, and experiencing new symptoms or further recurrence (Hilton, 1988).

Koocher (1985), who studied cancer in children, refers to the at-risk period as survivorship—one characterized by the uncertainty of outcome. Like Hilton, Koocher identifies uncertainty stress points as reminders of the original risk. For children, such reminders include anniversary phenomena. If cancer was diagnosed at the beginning of a school year, then uncertainty may recur as September draws closer. Other important transition points in life, such as birthdays and school graduations, may remind the child that he might not live long enough to achieve future goals. Just as with women with breast cancer, uncertainty about security or vulnerability is produced in children by learning of another's illness or by seeing media presentations about the illness.

The survivorship experience described by Koocher for children with cancer can also be applied to their parents. Brett and Davies (1988) report that parents of children with leukemia live with constant uncertainty, questioning every bruise and every cold, always wondering if the illness has returned. Cohen and Martinson (1988) report that parents show a heightened sensitivity to any sign of threat to the child's health. Yet the parents' ability to distinguish between normal variations in their child and those due to illness becomes impaired. The first response to any deviation from usual or normal is to ask, "Is this it again?" No behavior is considered benign or irrelevant (Cohen & Martinson, 1988). This extreme vigilance and the inability to distinguish pathology from normal are also transferred to parents' appraisal of siblings' health. Parents guard against being surprised again.

MANAGING SYMPTOM AND MEDICAL UNCERTAINTY

Four major methods of managing symptom and medical uncertainty have been identified in the literature: forming illness schemas and constructing a normative framework; formulating timetables, and using benchmarks; managing unpredictability; and maintaining hope.

Forming illness schemas and constructing a normative framework are techniques for constructing some cognitive meaning for illness experiences. An illness schema or normative framework is the person's representation of the illness—whether the person has it, why or how he got it, how it will progress, and how he will recover. It is the subjectively formed cognitive meaning; it is not necessarily factually accurate. When it is constructed, the person has a personally logical explanation for his situation.

Constructing a personal explanation of illness events is facilitated by uncertainty. Because an uncertain situation is vague, unstructured, and ill-defined, it allows the viewer to superimpose a structure on the events and setting that fits the desired view. This is one of the advantages of uncertainty. An amorphous structure allows a person to interpret a situation any way he desires. The vague and amorphous nature of an uncertain situation allows it to be reformed by the person, just like putty, to make a more positive situation.

One method used to form a cognitive schema when initial symptoms appear, but prior to a diagnosis, is to minimize one's susceptibility to the potential illness. This involves generating reasons why one is not at risk for the illness. It includes identifying characteristics of people with the illness and then reasoning how those with the illness are different from oneself. Differences can be based upon age, gender, race, etc. Parents may argue that children do not get such serious diseases, or that cardiac problems are diseases of old people, or that only men have cardiac problems, not women. Location may also be the basis for the rationale. As Weitz (1989) reports, "One Phoenix resident explained that he and his friends did not practice safe sex because they believed that 'there's only nine people in Arizona who have AIDS, four of them are dead and two of them live in Tucson, so what are our chances of getting it?'" (p. 273).

Another approach to developing an illness schema and normative framework is gathering information. Information is sought from other ill persons who are doing well, maintaining a good level of health, and surviving. This information is usually consistent with the desires of the seeker and solidifies the belief structure about what will occur.

Hilton (1988) reports that seeking information from reading and talking with others, both personal friends and professionals, is a common way for women with breast cancer to make sense of their situation. Seeking information is a very frequent method of modifying uncertainty. But the information must be personally relevant to the individual. Programmed information is often not useful because it is not directed toward the specific source of uncertainty.

Another approach to developing normative frameworks is taking self-care actions that the person believes will prevent illness or cure illness. Such self-care actions include changes in dietary patterns and changes in attitudes toward life—for example, reducing life stress and altering lifestyle. These methods are seen as a way to control the person's world. These self-care activities form a belief system that reduces uncertainty by allowing the person to redefine the situation as one that he can manage.

Formulating timetables/benchmarks is a second approach to managing symptom/medical uncertainty. This involves setting personally defined timelines for a variety of illness events. For example, a person receiving radiation may set a timeline of 2 months for resolution of treatment-induced fatigue. These timelines may have no basis in fact, but they help the person structure the future. Benchmarks have a similar purpose. Patients use these to gauge recovery. Benchmarks are particular activities that, when they can be accomplished, signify progression in recovery. Walking a certain distance, lifting certain objects, and carrying out certain activities are all benchmarks that indicate progress and remove ambiguity and vagueness from the treatment/recovery phase. It is crucial to recognize the importance of these timelines and benchmarks and to respect the purpose they serve. It does not matter whether they fit so-called "reality."

Unpredictability management, a third approach to managing symptom/medical uncertainty involves a series of methods used to reduce uncertainty/unpredictability. These techniques have been observed in family members waiting for the patient to receive an organ transplant. The techniques include containing investment, setting limits, filtering information, and monitoring. These are strategies used to decrease uncertainty during the waiting period and after transplantation (Mishel & Murdaugh, 1987). Containing investment involves the removal of stakes in the future and a strengthened focus on the present. Affect is absent from future plans, if they are made. Any future plans are described in a factual tone; excitement is tempered. Emotion is not invested in future events because there is too much uncertainty about whether they will occur.

A second method, called setting limits, involves generating rules for avoiding events that could threaten the patient's stability, such as infection. When to use protective devices such as masks and what type of mask to wear are important decisions. As one spouse of a transplant candidate said, "If people cough on you, what can you do about it? If you have a mask, that might protect you. How can we protect our husbands in restaurants or the supermarket? They must have a mask on at all times."

Filtering information is a third method of managing uncertainty/unpredictability. Information is filtered so that only supportive information is acknowledged. Information that is certain and non-conflictual is allowed. Information that raises uncertainty about the present or future is omitted from awareness. Family problems such as finances and family illnesses are not shared. Information on other patients who died or who are not progressing well is withheld.

Monitoring the patient for any type of treatment regimen indiscretion is another method of managing uncertainty. Keeping a close watch on any inattention to the regimen can provide the patient or family member with an early cue to the onset of complications. This reduces the unpredictability of the onset and the uncertainty of the course of recovery.

Maintaining hope involves a group of methods to manage medical/symptom uncertainty. These techniques include blaming the victim, making downward comparisons, seeing the situation as temporary, believing in powerful others, and avoiding painful material. With these techniques, the uncertainty is used to generate a positive view of the outcome. The techniques are not geared to reducing uncertainty or avoiding the arousal of uncertainty, but instead, they use the uncertainty to reformulate what is occurring in a more positive light. Mishel and Murdaugh (1987) observed these methods among spouses of patients awaiting organ transplantation.

Blaming the victim is a method of maintaining hope by finding some reason to blame a complication that occurred to another patient upon that patient. If another patient does not do well, then poor performance after treatment is blamed on some personal characteristic that is not present in the evaluator. For example: "She didn't watch what she ate, so of course she would have a rejection and get sick. Since she didn't follow her diet, this is an example of a wasted heart."

Downward comparison has the same purpose as blaming the victim. The patient's situation is elevated and seen as preferable to that of others, who are viewed as in worse situations. For example, two spouses of heart transplant candidates said that having a heart transplant was not so bad and compared themselves to people waiting for a heart and lung transplant. Another aspect of downward comparison is emphasizing the positive benefits of the situation. As one spouse said, "When I talk to women my age, I am so much stronger than they are and I don't get upset about the trivial things that seem to bother them."

Seeing the situation as temporary is a method in which all events are viewed as of short duration. The present situation is seen as not continuing. When patients take a turn for the worse, this is also viewed as short lived. As one spouse of a heart transplant patient said, "They can surprise you. People can make a sudden change and can turn right around. Look at how sick F. was; he came right out of it."

Belief in powerful others involves faith, religion, or viewing the physician as a source of power. When this method is used, the patient adopts the attitude that the problem will be handled by the powerful other.

Avoiding painful material involves selective attending so that the spouse and/or patient is not exposed to negative information. Articles that contain information about problems after treatment are not read or circulated. Patients who are doing poorly are not visited. This keeps the belief in a positive outcome alive.

MANAGING DAILY LIVING UNCERTAINTY

There are five major approaches to managing the uncertainty associated with daily life in chronic illness: constructing normative frameworks, focusing on the positive, specifying controllable circumstances, carrying out ritualistic behavior, and incorporating uncertainty.

Constructing a normative framework differs somewhat in the phase of living with chronic illness and the phase of symptom and medical treatment. In the phase of living with uncertainty, this approach includes three strategies. The first, self-advocacy, may be defined as believing in one's own judgment concerning health care, planning one's own health care, modifying prescribed care, and seeing oneself as the health professional. An example is this statement from a person with lupus: "You've got to learn what goes for you, what goes against you; you assume the kind of position where you're the watchdog for yourself. I think I know more about my body than any physician. You have to do most of your care on your own" (King & Mishel, 1986, p. 15).

Among women with cancer, buffering the situation is a second method used to develop a normative structure. This includes controlling the meaning of the problem by minimizing, avoiding, or denying it. Hilton (1988) reported that many women, post-treatment for breast cancer, talked about not worrying about it, while others reported that they tried not to think about it. Others generated only positive thoughts about the future. Koocher (1985) found that some survivors of childhood cancer developed the belief that their prior cancer treatments provided them with immunity against a recurrence or second tumor.

Another strategy is redefining the situation. One way to do this is to redefine what one wants out of the situation. A situation is more positive if a person's expectations do not exceed the likely outcomes. If a person moves away from prior goals, then uncertainty about reaching them becomes less important.

Focusing on the positive involves another series of strategies. One is forgetting the negative—putting negative aspects of the situation out of one's mind, or simply blanking it out. This is not easy to do, but some people are able to accomplish it.

Another method is to find side benefits. Traumatic, overwhelming situations can have side benefits such as bringing families together, eliciting caring from neighbors and friends, and making one aware of other values in life.

Transforming a negative to a positive involves using the uncertainty or unpredictability of a situation to generate the possibility of a positive outcome. When a situation changes unpredictably, the probability of a desirable outcome may be equal to the probability of an undesirable outcome. Persons with lupus, for example, talk about the unpredictability of the disease as a chance to get better. As long as the disease has its ups and downs, they know that they may feel better tomorrow.

Specifying controllable circumstances—a third approach to managing daily life with uncertainty in chronic illness, involves determining what one can and cannot control. After making this distinction, emphasis is placed upon what *can* be controlled. Another way to control the situation is for the patient to find his/her good days and use them fully. Persons with lupus say that they cram all they can into their good days. They learn that they cannot do everything so they find their own way to reciprocate or participate. As one person said, "I've planned my career according to something I can do from a wheelchair in case I get worse."

Rituals are used by some persons to contain disease. These rituals take on the quality of magic because people begin to believe that if they are enacted consistently, the disease will be kept at bay. A variety of methods are used by cancer patients, for example, to increase the chances of early detection of recurrence and to increase general health. As these are enacted like a liturgy, they take on a ritualistic protection against the uncertainties of disease progression.

Incorporating the uncertainty is a final approach to living with uncertainty. It involves a change in the patient's and family's perspective on life, away from an orientation to control and predictability toward an acceptance of unpredictability and uncertainty as normal. Uncertainty ultimately is accepted as the normal rhythm of life. The expectation of certainty is abandoned as a part of reality. The new view of life involves probabilistic and conditional thinking. This method of managing uncertainty has been discussed elsewhere (Mishel, 1990).

All these methods for managing uncertainty can be used in practice. Because the existence of uncertainty can be measured, it is easy to identify in clinical populations. Once identified, these management methods can be taught to patients or supported where they are already being used.

REFERENCES

Braden, C. J. (1990). A test of the self-help model: Learned response to chronic illness experience. *Nursing Research, 39,* 42–47.

Brett, K. M., & Davies, E. M. B. (1988). "What does it mean?": Sibling and parental appraisals of childhood leukemia. *Cancer Nursing, 11,* 329–338.

Charmaz, K. (1983). Loss of self: A fundamental form of suffering in the chronically ill. *Sociology of Health and Illness, 5,* 168–195.

Cohen, M. H., & Martinson, I. M. (1988). Chronic uncertainty: Its effect on parental appraisal of a child's health. *Journal of Pediatric Nursing, 3,* 89–96.

Conrad, P. (1987). The experience of illness: Recent and new directions. *Research in the Sociology of Health Care, 6,* 1–31.

Hilton, B. A. (1988). The phenomenon of uncertainty in women with breast cancer. *Issues in Mental Health Nursing, 9,* 217–238.

King, B., & Mishel, M. H. (1986, May). *Uncertainty appraisal and management in chronic illness.* Paper presented at the Nineteenth Communicating Nursing Research Conference, Western Society for Research in Nursing, Portland, OR.

Koocher, G. P. (1984). Terminal care and survivorship in pediatric chronic illness. *Clinical Psychology Review, 4*, 571–583.

Koocher, G. P. (1985). Psychosocial care of the child cured of cancer. *Journal of Pediatric Nursing, 4*, 91–93.

Loveys, B. (1990). Transitions in chronic illness: The at-risk role. *Holistic Nursing Practice, 4*, 56–64.

Mishel, M. H. (1988). Uncertainty in illness. *Image: Journal of Nursing Scholarship, 20*, 225–232.

Mishel, M. H. (1990). Reconceptualization of the uncertainty in illness theory. *Image: Journal of Nursing Scholarship, 22*, 256–262.

Mishel, M., & Braden, C. (1988). Finding meaning: Antecedents of uncertainty in illness. *Nursing Research, 37*, 98–103.

Mishel, M. H., Hostetter, T., King, B., & Graham, V. (1984). Predictors of psychosocial adjustment in patients newly diagnosed with gynecological cancer. *Cancer Nursing, 7*, 291–299.

Mishel, M. H., & Murdaugh, C. L. (1987). Family adjustment to heart transplantation: Redesigning the dream. *Nursing Research, 36*, 332–338.

Mishel, M. H., Padilla, G., Grant, M., & Sorenson, D. S. (1991). Uncertainty in illness theory: A replication of the mediating effects of mastery and coping. *Nursing Research, 40*, 236–240.

Mishel, M. H., & Sorenson, D. S. (1991). Uncertainty in gynecological cancer: A test of the mediating functions of mastery and coping. *Nursing Research, 40*, 167–171.

Murdaugh, C. L., & Mishel, M. H. (1991, November). *Predictors of quality of life in patients who undergo heart transplantation*. Paper presented at the American Heart Association Meeting, Anaheim, CA.

Pergrin, J., Mishel, M. H., & Murdaugh, C. (1987, May). *Impact of uncertainty and social support on stress in caregivers*. Paper presented at the Twentieth Communicating Nursing Research Conference, Western Society for Research in Nursing, Phoenix, AZ.

Richardson, J. L., Marks, G., Johnson, C. A., Graham, J. W., Chan, K. K., Selser, J. N., Kishbaugh, C., Barranday, Y., & Levine, A. M. (1987). Path model of compliance with cancer therapy. *Health Psychology, 6*, 183–207.

Rowat, K. M., & Knafl, K. A. (1985). Living with chronic pain: The spouse's perspective. *Pain, 23*, 259–271.

Stewart, D. C., & Sullivan, T. J. (1982). Illness behavior and the sick role in chronic illness. *Social Science and Medicine, 16*, 1397–1404.

Viney, L. L., & Westbrook, M. T. (1982). Patients' psychological reactions to chronic illness: Are they associated with rehabilitation. *Journal of Applied Rehabilitation Counseling, 13*, 38–44.

Webster, K. K., & Christman, N. J. (1988). Perceived uncertainty and coping post myocardial infarction. *Western Journal of Nursing Research, 10*, 384–400.

Weitz, R. (1989). Uncertainty and the lives of persons with AIDS. *Journal of Health and Human Behavior, 30*, 270–281.

Wiener, C. L. (1975). The burden of rheumatoid arthritis: Tolerating the uncertainty. *Social Science and Medicine, 9*, 97–104.

Wineman, N. M. (1990). Adaptation to multiple sclerosis: The role of social support, functional disability and perceived uncertainty. *Nursing Research, 39*, 294–299.

[7]

Exercise Interventions for the Chronically Ill: Review and Prospects

Carol C. Hogue, Sharon Cullinan, and Eleanor McConnell

We know little about the etiology and less about the cure for most chronic illnesses, yet typically chronic illness is long-lasting and it is usually accompanied by substantial burden to those with the illness and to their families and society (McCorkle & Given, 1991). The prevalence of chronic illness is higher in late life (U.S. Senate Special Committee on Aging, 1986), so biological declines of aging may further diminish the functional ability of large numbers of individuals. Inactivity is a particular problem as the effects of inactivity combine with the effects of chronic illness, compounding the potential harm. Helping those with chronic illness manage symptoms in ways that promote function and well-being is paramount. Because of unwanted side effects of drugs to manage chronic disease, nonpharmacologic therapies such as weight loss, biofeedback, relaxation, and exercise are especially attractive. This chapter reviews research on the health benefits and risks of exercise for adults with chronic illness, briefly summarizing selected findings about exercise for persons with coronary artery disease, hypertension, arthritis, diabetes, cancer, chronic obstructive pulmonary disease (COPD), and mental health and illness.

The review is limited to adults, except for a few observations about adolescents. Further, the focus is on interventions for persons who already have chronic illness, even though there is a large body of literature on primary prevention of chronic illness. We consider illness conditions one at a time, though it is well known that many adults have more than one chronic condition. Because we have somewhat greater experience with and knowledge of the literature about diabetes and arthritis, we devote more attention to them than to the large literature on cardiac rehabilitation and hypertension or to the small literature on COPD and cancer. Mental health considerations cut across chronic illnesses. Mental illness, not necessarily the reciprocal of mental health, is included because of the potential for exercise in an almost unstudied area, dementia. Finally, we have generally limited our review to papers published since 1980. We make no claim to comprehensiveness or representativeness though the conclusions we draw from the studies reviewed tend to concur with several published reviews (Bouchard, Shephard, Stephens, Sutton, & McPherson, 1990; Buchner, Beresford, Larson, LaCroix, & Wagner, 1992; Pollack & Wilmore, 1990; Skinner, 1987).

EXERCISE

Physical activity is any bodily movement produced by skeletal muscles resulting in energy expenditure. Exercise, also known as training, is a systematic, planned, structured, repetitive type of physical activity. Physical fitness is a set of attributes one has or achieves; fitness requires training (Caspersen, Powell, & Christenson, 1985). Physical fitness, the ability to perform muscular work satisfactorily, includes cardiorespiratory endurance or aerobic capacity, muscle strength and endurance, and flexibility (World Health Organization, 1978). Physiologic fitness indicators that appear to be influenced by exercise include blood pressure, glucose tolerance, insulin sensitivity, blood lipid levels, lipoprotein profile, body composition and fat distribution, and stress tolerance. Aerobic capacity is the ability of the body to produce energy by using oxygen. Aerobic capacity can be measured directly by measuring maximal oxygen consumption (VO_2 max), or it can be estimated. Cardiorespiratory endurance is usually expressed relative to body weight, ml/kg/minute, or as metabolic equivalents (METS), with 1 MET = the rate of oxygen consumption at rest, or about 3.5 ml/kg/minute (Pollock & Wilmore, 1990). Cardiorespiratory endurance depends on the functional condition of the cardiorespiratory system and the skeletal muscle system.

Muscle strength is the maximal force that can be generated by a particular muscle or muscle group. Strength depends on the condition of the muscle and the neurological system. Strength can be measured as the maximum weight lifted (isotonic), as the maximum force exerted against a fixed object (isometric), or as the peak rotational force (torque) produced at a given speed of muscular contraction (isokinetic strength). Muscle endurance is the ability of a muscle group to perform repeated contractions over a period of time (de Lateur & Lehmann, 1986). Flexibility refers to the ability to move a joint through a range of motion; it is dependent on a number of factors.

Frequency, intensity, and duration of exercise are all important if a conditioning effect is to be achieved. The American College of Sports Medicine (ACSM) recommends exercise 3–5 times/week, 20–60 minutes each time, at moderate or high intensity for fitness training for healthy adults. However, there are no standards for persons with chronic illness. ACSM describes moderate intensity as 40%–60% of VO_2 max, efforts that are within an individual's current capacity, and efforts that can be sustained for a prolonged period such as 20–60 minutes (American College of Sports Medicine, 1990). In general, the lower the intensity, the longer the duration must be for an effect to occur. It was previously thought that to reap cardiovascular benefits, moderate or high-intensity exercise was necessary; however, our review has identified research that shows that low-intensity exercise may be even more beneficial in some illness conditions.

The potential benefits of exercise for persons with chronic illness include improvement on fitness tests and improvement in the illness—at least the illness becomes more manageable. Self-management of exercise requires deliberate behavioral strategies, as does self-management of chronic illness. People who are most fit tend to exercise more and need less help than those who are less fit and do not exercise.

Coronary Artery Disease

There is extensive literature on the effect of exercise interventions after acute myocardial infarction (AMI). Although exercise has been shown to have strong and significant effects in preventing first coronary events (Caspersen, 1987; Paffenbarger, Hyde, Hsieh & Wing, 1986; Paffenbarger, Hyde, Wing & Steinmetz, 1984; Peters, Cady, Bischoff, Bernstein & Pike, 1983), no reduction of reinfarction has been consistently demonstrated with exercise after AMI (Rechnitzer et al., 1983; Shaw, 1981). The large number of subjects needed and the difficulty of careful long-term follow-up have precluded definitive randomized controlled trials of cardiac rehabilitation. Additionally, it is difficult to separate the effects of exercise from other aspects of cardiac rehabilitation. Patient dropout from cardiac rehabilitation has been another limiting problem. Andrew and colleagues (1981) studied 639 dropouts and continuing participants in the Ontario Exercise Heart Collaborative Study to understand the reasons for dropout. Three main factors were associated with high dropout rate: convenience aspects of the exercise center, perceptions of the exercise program, and family/lifestyle factors. Oldridge, Guyatt, Fisher, and Rimm (1988) conducted a meta-analysis of 10 randomized controlled trials of exercise after myocardial infarction; the pooled data included 4,347 patients, about half of them controls, half cardiac rehabilitation intervention subjects. The intervention was primarily aerobic exercise. A 25% reduction in cardiovascular death was found in the exercise group, but quality of life outcomes were not reported.

There is no convincing evidence that exercise interventions after AMI lead to earlier return to work (Froelicher, 1990). There is only modest evidence that work capacity, defined as symptoms of dyspnea or pain with walking and other exertion, improves with exercise training after AMI (Carson et al., 1982).

However, exercise appears to have positive effects on well-being. Ditchey and his colleagues (1981) found subjective improvement and a 2-MET increase in aerobic capacity in 14 coronary patients who completed 3–14 months of supervised arm and leg exercises. Gulanick (1991) showed increases in self-efficacy and in performance of physical activity early in the recovery phase after myocardial infarction (MI) or cardiac surgery, but the increases were not statistically significant, possibly because the sample was very small.

Although intensity of exercise makes a difference in disease-free adults, in cardiac patients intensity seems to make little difference. Men randomly assigned to high (65%–75%) maximum oxygen consumption rate or low intensity (<45%) achieved similar cardiorespiratory benefits after 3 months of training (Blumenthal et al., 1988).

Research explaining why persons with coronary artery disease should be expected to benefit from exercise has been reviewed by Rechnitzer (1990). Elevation of the ischemic threshold is an important and likely mechanism of effect of exercise in cardiac rehabilitation. There is longstanding, strong evidence in animal models and humans with exercise-induced myocardial ischemia that, after exercise training, subjects can do more work before evidence of ischemia appears. The practical consequence of this is that after exercise training, the person with stable angina can function at a higher level in daily activities without evidence of ischemia. The effect is similar to beta blockade; that is, a lower heart rate is required for a given amount of work (Froelicher, 1990).

The effect of exercise on myocardial contractility is less certain. The persuasive evidence that contractility improves with exercise demonstrated in animal models has not been reported in humans (Froelicher, 1990).

Effect on atherogenesis has also been shown in animal studies. In young monkeys fed an atherogenic diet, regular exercise reduced the development of atherosclerotic lesions (Kramsch, Aspen, Abramowitz, Kreimendahl, & Hood, 1981).

Rechnitzer (1990) notes that although exercise in coronary artery disease does not have the power that penicillin does for pneumococcal pneumonia, it is important, perhaps most of all as evidence of potential within the individual's contol, a symbol of hope. "The realization by the patient that his or her endurance or anginal threshold has improved through his or her own effort involving self-discipline . . . is of immense and likely incalculable benefit" (1990, p. 452).

In summary, exercise decreases cardiac symptoms and lessens cardiovascular mortality. Psychosocial function may be improved; earlier return to work has not been demonstrated. Finally, our review indicates that exercise is as safe and effective as other means of secondary prevention of coronary artery disease. The excellent American Heart Association document, *Exercise Standards: A Statement for Health Professionals* (1991), provides background and guidelines for safety for exercise for cardiac patients.

Hypertension

The cardiovascular consequences of untreated hypertension have been known since the 1970s (Veterans' Administration Cooperative Study Group on Antihypertensive Agents, 1972). The benefits of drug therapy are clear for those with blood pressures greater than 160/105, but for those whose pressures are in the range of 140/90 to 160/105, the risk of side effects has fueled debate about the wisdom of drug therapy (Veterans' Administration Cooperative Study Group on Antihypertensive Agents, 1967). For those receiving drug therapy, as well as those with mild hypertension—the group for whom the risk-benefit of drug therapy may not be favorable, the use of nonpharmacologic means to lower blood pressure is attractive. Research has demonstrated that a person with blood pressure kept low by drug therapy still is at greater risk than an individual who has the same blood pressure but is without drug treatment (Kaplan, 1986).

Dozens of clinical studies on humans have been published, but findings should be viewed cautiously as only five were randomized controlled trials, though another eight to ten at least had nonexercising hypertensive control groups and careful recording of blood pressures. This research has been reviewed by Hagberg (1990), Seals and Hagberg (1984), and Tran, Weltman, Glass, and Mood (1983). We summarize some of their findings below and review some newer studies, particularly two recent randomized controlled trials (Blumenthal, Siegel, & Appelbaum, 1991; Martin, Dubbert, & Cushman, 1990). Subjects in 27 studies ranged in age from 10 to 70 years, sample size ranged from 4 to 99 subjects, and the length of the training varied from 4 to 52 weeks. In more than half the studies, only males were included in the sample, and even when women were included, rarely were data for female subjects reported separately. The studies generally found that endurance exercise training lowered both systolic and diastolic blood pressure by about 10 mm Hg in persons with essential hypertension. Blood pressures tended to be reduced but not returned to normal, and some studies did not show any reduction. Hagberg (1990) concluded that women, persons with higher initial diastolic pressure, and persons with lower initial body weight appear to benefit most from endurance exercise.

Regimens have included endurance (Cade et al., 1984; Duncan et al., 1985; Martin, Dubbert, & Cushman, 1990), strength training (Blumenthal, Siegel, & Applebaum, 1991; Harris & Holly, 1987) , and isometric exercise (Kiveloff & Huber, 1971) with different intensities and durations. Endurance exercise has usually been the type of exercise chosen to reduce blood pressure, perhaps because of the pressor response that accompanies static muscle contractions. The pressor response increases both systolic blood pressure (SBP) and diastolic blood pressure (DBP), and may place excessive demand on the myocardium, a problem for persons with compromised left-ventricular function. However, Hagberg et al. (1984) found that adolescents with mild hypertension who first lowered their SBP with endurance exercise maintained or improved those reductions with 5 months of weight training.

It appears that exercise training at 40%–60% of VO_2 max may be as (or even more) efficacious in reducing blood pressure as higher intensity training (Roman, Camuzzi, Villalon, & Klenner, 1981). It is not clear how long it takes for endurance training to lead to lower blood pressures, nor is it clear whether long-term training is better than short-term training in lowering blood pressure.

If drug therapy is aggressive, greater reductions in blood pressure, in cardiovascular mortality, in myocardial infarction, and in cerebrovascular events are achieved by drug therapy than by exercise training (Amery et al., 1985; Hypertension Detection and Follow-up Program Cooperative Group, 1979). However, given the concerns about the side effects of antihypertensive drug therapy, it is useful to compare exercise to other nonpharmacologic means of reducing hypertension. Several well-controlled studies of weight-reduction, biofeedback, and relaxation therapy have been reported. Kaplan (1986), reviewing 11 weight reduction studies, found that systolic and diastolic blood pressures were reduced 15 and 10 mmHg, respectively, after an average of 9.8 kg weight loss. Thus, substantial weight loss is likely to be accompanied by more blood pressure reduction than is exercise. However, we are aware of no controlled studies of endurance exercise training in markedly overweight persons. Several older studies found that biofeedback reduced systolic and diastolic blood pressure by 12 and 5 mmHg, respectively (Shapiro, Schwartz, Ferguson, Redmond, & Weiss, 1977). Reductions of 18 and 11 mmHg were shown in studies of relaxation therapy (Shapiro et al., 1977). In more recent well-controlled studies, only small effects on hypertension have been demonstrated with single and combined behavioral therapies (Glasgow, Gardner,

& Engel, 1982; Luborsky et al., 1982). For both biofeedback and relaxation, the studies reviewed tended to report single sessions and not long-term training or long-term effects.

Potential mechanisms for the antihypertensive effects of aerobic exercise include reduction of cardiac output and reduction of total peripheral resistance. The role of the sympathetic nervous system is not yet clear. Blumenthal et al. (1991) found that all subjects—those receiving endurance training, those receiving strength and flexibility training, and those in the waiting list control group—achieved significant reductions in systolic and diastolic blood pressure. Weight and body fat are possible confounders. A meta-analysis reported by Hagberg (1990) showed no relationship between weight change and decrease in systolic or diastolic blood pressure after endurance exercise training.

We conclude that the blood-pressure lowering effect of endurance exercise training in persons with essential hypertension compares favorably with other nonpharmacological therapies and with drug therapy, and is safe. More research, however, is needed to investigate the possibility of interactions between therapies and to shed more light on the mechanism of blood pressure reduction by exercise.

Arthritis

Controlled studies of exercise for persons with arthritis have only recently been done. Until 1991, The American College of Sports Medicine (1986) identified arthritis of any type as a relative contraindication for excercise. Arthritis is a generic term for many diseases characterized by inflammation and joint involvement. Osteoarthritis (OA) and rheumatoid arthritis (RA), the two most common types of arthritis, are also the most common causes of functional limitation and dependence in the United States. Osteoarthritis, a degenerative continuous disorder confined to affected joints, is characterized by deterioration of weight-bearing cartilage surfaces of joints, hardening of subchondral bone, and overgrowth of new bone at joint margins. Rheumatoid arthritis is episodic, a systemic disease with inflammation in the synovial lining of the joints that results in cartilage and bone destruction. Both OA and RA are associated with joint pain, loss of motion, muscle weakness, and reduced aerobic capacity (Danneskiold-Samsoe & Grimby, 1986; Gerberich et al., 1989). The disease directly restricts activity, and the therapy, which has traditionally emphasized rest and nonstress exercise, has indirectly limited physical activity (Ike, Lampman, & Castor, 1989). Psychosocial features of arthritis such as depression, helplessness, and social isolation have been shown to be correlated with restricted activity (Parker et al., 1988; Yelin, Meenan, Nevit, & Epstein, 1980).

A number of studies of exercise interventions have included patients with osteoarthritis (Fisher, Pendergast, Gresham, & Calkins, 1991; Kovar et al., 1992), or patients with rheumatoid arthritis (Danneskiold-Samsoe, Lyngberg, Risum, & Telling, 1987; Harkcom, Lampman, Banwell, & Castor, 1985; Perlman et al., 1990), or both (Beals et al., 1985; Minor, Hewitt, Webel, Anderson, & Kay, 1989). Physical training programs studied have lasted 6–16 weeks, with sessions 2 or 3 times a week. Either low- or moderate-intensity training has been offered, with the goal of improving aerobic capacity, or strength and endurance of muscles, or flexibility, or a combination of those. Approaches have included bike ergometry, walking, aerobic dance, or aquatic aerobics.

Half a dozen recent intervention studies have demonstrated that persons with arthritis can be safely tested and trained, and they show improvements in aerobic capacity (Harkcom et al., 1985), muscle strength (Fisher, Pendergast, Gresham, & Calkins, 1991), flexibility (Minor et al., 1989), and overall physical activity (Kovar et al., 1992; Minor et al., 1989; Perlman et al., 1990). Depression and anxiety were studied by two groups of researchers (Minor et al., 1989, Perlman et al., 1990), and both studies found substantial decreases in depression; one study also found a decrease in anxiety (Minor et al., 1989). Kovar et al. (1992), Harkcom et al. (1985), Minor et al. (1989), and Perlman et al. (1990) all studied the effect of exercise interventions on pain and (except for the Kovar group) on joint involvement; all of them except the Harkcom group found significantly less pain and less joint involvement (number or severity of painful or swollen joints) after the intervention than before. Fisher et al. (1991), Minor et al. (1989), and Perlman et al. (1990) found that timed walk improved; the Kovar group (1992) found an increase in walking distance in a 6-minute walk. All the exercise interventions for persons with arthritis we reviewed were tailored to those patients' particular needs. In an excellent review paper, Minor (1991) lists arthritis-specific exercise needs and modifications—important clinical considerations that are beyond the scope of this chapter.

The rationale for the positive effects of weight-bearing exercise on arthritis is that active motion and periods of compression and decompression, both of which are supplied by weight-bearing exercise, help maintain healthy cartilage. Healthy cartilage, elasticity and tone of tendons and ligaments, and muscle strength and muscle endurance are all necessary for the stability and alignment of joints and for the management of impact and compressive forces (Bland, 1988; Brandt, 1988).

We conclude that persons with arthritis can safely participate in exercise testing and training programs designed for them. Benefits include improved aerobic capacity, strength and flexibility, less pain and joint involvement, less depression and less anxiety.

Diabetes Mellitus

The importance of exercise for patients with Type I (insulin dependent) diabetes mellitus (IDDM) and Type II (noninsulin dependent) diabetes mellitus (NIDDM) diabetes has been reexamined in recent years. Research findings indicate that diabetics who exercise regularly may derive benefits related to glucoregulation as well as prevention of cardiovascular complications.

Metabolic Response to Exercise in IDDM. Increased blood flow to muscles during exercise provides insulin receptors greater exposure to insulin and results in an increased rate of glucose utilization by working muscle (Berger, Hagg, & Rudderman, 1975). Additionally, in insulin-treated diabetics, plasma insulin concentrations do not decrease during exercise (as they do in nondiabetic individuals). The resulting sustained insulin levels enhance peripheral glucose uptake and inhibit hepatic glucose production (Zinman et al., 1977).

Glucoregulatory Effects of Exercise. Several recent studies have explored the long-term glucoregulatory effect of physical training in IDDM. McCarger, Tauton, and Pare (1991) examined 12 IDDM men in a 12-week walking/jogging program. Subjects exercised moderately (60%–70% of estimated maximum heart rate) either 3 or 5 days per week for 1 hour and experienced minimal side effects. Changes in fasting serum glucose and blood lipid values were not observed, although subjects did report improved well-being and they showed improved exercise capacity. Wallberg-Henriksson and colleagues (1982) studied 9 men with IDDM who attended a training program for 1 hour two–three times a week for 16 weeks. The men showed a decrease in total cholesterol, an increase in high-density lipoproteins (HDL), and increased peripheral insulin sensitivity. No change, however, was observed in glycosylated hemoglobin, the measure of long-term glucose control. Zinman and colleagues reported similar findings (1984). Blood glucose values dropped sharply following exercise, but fasting blood glucose and glycosylated hemoglobin values remained unchanged after a 12-week program of cycling. In both studies, the lack of improvement was attributed to an increased intake of 300-400 calories on exercising days. The researchers concluded that physical training by itself does not improve blood glucose in individuals with IDDM, though other benefits may be realized.

Individuals who wish to exercise should be informed that the glucose lowering effect of training is influenced greatly by variables such as dietary intake, serum insulin levels, and length and intensity of exercise. These determine a diabetic's response to exercise and underlie many of the inconsistencies found in the literature.

Caron, Poussier, and Marliss (1982) reported that the majority of individuals who exercised moderately (30 minutes of stationary cycling) after a meal showed improved blood glucose concentrations that persisted until the next meal. However metabolic rates remained elevated after completion of exercise, and late-onset hypoglycemia is a risk for diabetics. MacDonald (1987) found that late-onset hypoglycemia occurred in 48 of 300 subjects over a 2-year period; hypoglycemia was most common 6-15 hours after vigorous or prolonged exercise and following a period of inactivity.

Hyperglycemic responses are seen when exercise is undertaken in the presence of severe insulin deficiency. Glucose utilization by working muscles is impaired, so lipolysis and hepatic glucose production are stimulated. The result is a further increase in blood glucose concentration that may result in ketosis (Kemmer et al., 1979). In light of these facts, vigorous physical activity should be postponed if blood glucose is >250 mg/dl and ketones are present in urine or blood. The individual should take supplemental insulin to reestablish good metabolic control. If blood glucose is < 100 mg/dl and the individual has taken insulin within 60-90 minutes, supplemental feedings should be taken before and during exercise.

Metabolic Response to Exercise in NIDDM. Noninsulin dependent diabetes mellitus is characterized by insulin resistance and impaired insulin secretion. In contrast to IDDM, improvements in glycemic control and glucose tolerance do occur following exercise, as a result of decreased insulin resistance. Although the mechanism remains unclear, the improvement in insulin control appears to result from an increase in insulin receptor affinity during each episode of exercise and an increase in receptor numbers over time with regular exercise (Horton, 1988). Lilloja's finding (1987) that capillary density is directly related to insulin sensitivity suggests that increased capillary density resulting from exercise may also be related to the decrease in insulin resistance.

Clinical Evidence of Glucoregulatory Effects. Bjorntorp, De Joung, and Sjostrom (1973) found that plasma insulin levels dropped in obese men after exercise and this effect was not associated with body composition. Although a change in overall glucose control was not demonstrated in this study, a decrease in glycosylated hemoglobin as a result of exercise has been documented in several recent studies. Schneider and colleagues (1984) demonstrated a 12% reduction in glycosylated hemoglobin in 20 sedentary men after 6 weeks of aerobic training. The Schneider group subsequently observed that improvement in glucose tolerance occurred rapidly, within 7 days, but the improvement ceased to be significant 18 hours after the last exercise session. These findings indicate that the cumulative effects of single exercise bouts are responsible for improvements in overall measures of glucose control. Wing and associates (1988), in a related study, demonstrated that the benefits of a combination of diet and moderate exercise exceed the benefits of either treatment by itself. All the individuals in their study were able to reduce the amount of medication they were taking.

Participation in regular exercise has also been effective in reducing risk factors associated with NIDDM. In a 6-week conditioning program of moderate intensity (65% VO_2 max), for 7 female subjects, DeFronzo, Sherwin, and Kraemer (1987) demonstrated a significant reduction in hyperinsulinemia associated with obesity, as well as significant gains in aerobic conditioning. Exercise subjects in this study were moderately obese, 31%–74% over ideal body weight; their plasma insulin response was approximately twice as great as the normal weight-control group.

For both those with IDDM and NIDDM, other exercise benefits include a reduction of blood pressure (Schneider et al., 1984), a decreased incidence of macrovascular disease and intermittent claudication, and decreased mortality risk after 25 years of diabetes (LaPorte, Dorman, & Tajima, 1986; Chazan, Balodimos, & Ryan, 1970).

Cancer

With the notable exception of MacVicar, Winningham, and Nickel (1989), who found that interval training was effective in improving the functional capacity of Stage-II breast cancer patients on chemotherapy, there is little reported work on the effects of exercise therapy for persons with cancer. Oncologists have speculated that there should be beneficial psychological effects that may influence recovery. However, some may be concerned that exercise will be harmful for people with an illness such as cancer. Historically, people with acute illnesses such as infections have been put on bed rest to help promote recovery. However, there is extensive literature on the deleterious effects of inactivity, even for a short time, and an emerging body of literature suggests that even for patients with chronic infections traditionally treated with rest, such as hepatitis B and chronic infectious mononucleosis, engaging in "normal" activity results in faster recovery than restricted activity.

Chronic Obstructive Pulmonary Disease

We are aware of very few controlled studies of exercise for persons with chronic airflow obstruction, and virtually no randomized controlled studies. Gift and Austin (1992) compared characteristics of persons with COPD who participated in a pulmonary exercise program (PEP) with patients who did not, but the study design did not permit conclusions to be drawn. Breslin and her colleagues (Breslin, 1992; Breslin, Celli, & Roy, 1992) have studied unsupported arm exercise for persons with COPD and conclude that unsupported arm exercise training increases unsupported arm endurance, important for many functional activities.

More research is needed in this area. In the meantime, individualization is important. If respiratory weakness is identified, respiratory muscle training should be helpful. If whole body training is conducted, high-intensity exercise for short periods may be useful if dyspnea limits usual aerobic training.

Mental Health and Illness

There is considerable anecdotal and epidemiologic evidence linking exercise and physical activity to positive mental health. As is often the case, however, there is a relative paucity of controlled experiments on the effects of exercise on psychological variables, and those studies that have been done often provide results that are less impressive than those obtained in correlational studies.

A variety of different mechanisms by which physical activity and exercise may influence mental health have been proposed. These mechanisms can be divided into the following categories:

1. psychological and physiological explanations of stress reduction,
2 effects of exercise on psychiatric symptoms, and
3. effects of exercise on cognitive function.

Psychological and Physiological Explanations of Stress Reduction. One way in which exercise or physical activity may affect mental health is by increases in cardiovascular endurance (an indicator of physical fitness), which result in an increase in the individual's ability to respond to psychosocial stressors, both in terms of physiological reactivity (as indicated by heart rate) and in terms of psychological variables, through increased feelings of self-efficacy. However, although correlational studies suggesting these links are numerous, the experimental data to support them are quite weak. Sinyor, Golden, Steinert, and Seraganian (1986) reported an experiment in which 38 untrained men were randomly assigned to aerobic exercise, nonaerobic exercise, or a waiting list control condition for 10 weeks. Measures of heart-rate response and subjective arousal to three different types of psychological tests were obtained before, during, and after the exercise. None of the three groups differed in autonomic or subjective reactivity to the tasks. However, within the aerobic group, increases in estimated VO_2 max were associated with enhanced heart-rate recovery following stress. The authors speculated that the stressors may have been too great to be influenced by such a small training intervention (10 weeks).

Goldwater and Collis (1985) also conducted a controlled experiment to compare the psychological effects of a 6-week aerobic exercise program with the effects of a sham intervention. Fifty-one subjects between the ages of 19 and 30 participated in the study. Aerobic exercise subjects improved more than controls on the Taylor Manifest Anxiety Scale, and on the measure of subjective well-being, but the differences were not statistically significant.

Brown (1991) concludes that there are not well-designed studies to support the hypothesis that physical activity and exercise exert their effect through reducing reactivity to stressors, although a review by Crews and Landers (1987) presents the opposite conclusion. Emery and Blumenthal's 1991 review of studies on the effects of exercise on autonomic reactivity underscores the fact that the data on the responses to psychological tasks are conflicting.

Reductions in Psychiatric Symptoms: Anxiety and Depression. A considerable amount of work on the relationship between exercise and anxiety reduction has been conducted. Findings from studies looking at the effects of acute exercise (single, experimental bouts) point consistently to the following conclusions:

1. Self-reports of anxiety decrease in response to acute exercise across many populations, including people with both high and low levels of aerobic fitness and different psychiatric patient populations.
2. There is a dose–response effect; that is, intensity of exercise influences the magnitude and duration of reduction in anxiety. Exercise must be vigorous enough to produce a cardiovascular response to be effective. The optimal dosage, however, is not known.
3. Exercise is as effective as other relaxation strategies, such as resting, meditation, hypnosis and biofeedback, but no more so.
4. Some data suggest that exercise-induced reduction of anxiety may last longer than reduction of anxiety through other methods.

The results of studies on the effects of chronic exercise (long-term or continuous) on anxiety reduction are less consistent, but they do suggest that participation in fitness-enhancing exercise programs reduces anxiety and improves mood.

The following findings have been supported in a variety of studies:

1. Chronic exercise is associated with decreased depression.
2. Improved fitness is associated with reduction in depression in experimental studies.
3. Exercise compares to other interpersonal therapies in treating some forms of depression.

Klein et al. (1985) compared the effects of group psychotherapy, meditation, and running on 74 volunteer subjects (mean age 30) who met research diagnostic criteria for unipolar, nonpsychotic depression (Spitzer, Endicott, & Robins, 1978). Response to treatment was assessed by previously developed symptom checklists and standardized questionnaires. In addition, each subject was assessed at the end of treatment by a psychiatrist blind to treatment assignment. The psychiatrist used clinical judgment as well as standardized ratings of symptomatology such as the Research Diagnostic Criteria for Depression and the Hamilton Depression Scale. The somatic therapy groups, running and meditation, did as well or better than the psychotherapy group on many of the outcome measures. The groups were equivalent on the psychiatrist ratings.

Effects on Cognitive Function. Studies of the effects of exercise on neuropsychological test performance have generally been performed on healthy older volunteers. Not surprisingly, improvements in cognitive test performance have been modest, perhaps because of a ceiling effect; that is, healthy community-dwelling older persons who volunteer for such studies are unlikely to have much cognitive impairment. Studies of the effects of exercise on cognitive status in impaired older patients are less numerous and in general, less well designed. However, it is logical to think that older adults with multiple chronic illnesses may experience suboptimal cognitive function and have cognitive improvements with exercise. A recent highly suggestive example is found in the work of Friedman and Tappen (1991), who studied the effect of a structured walking program on the communication abilities of people with Alzheimer's disease, using a pretest– posttest design with random assignment to treatment (n=15) or control group (n=15). The program was administered for 30 minutes, three times per week for 10 weeks; the control subjects received an interpersonal intervention for the same amount of time and at the same frequency. The planned walking group significantly improved on one communication measure, and there was some improvement on the second measure but it was not statistically significant.

Unfortunately, no other controlled experiments reported in the literature have addressed the question of whether patients with cognitive impairment experience improved cognitive function as the result of exercise. There is, however, an emerging body of literature that suggests that even people with dementia benefit from exercise programs. Recently, Fisher and colleagues (1991) reported the results of a trial of exercise therapy for chronically institutionalized nursing home patients, some of whom had chronic cognitive impairments. Anecdotally, these patients reported higher levels of well-being and experienced increased functional independence following the exercise program.

CONCLUSIONS

Persons with chronic illness have often not been encouraged or even allowed to incorporate exercise into their illness management. Health care providers and patients have sometimes held attitudes reminiscent of the notions of the 1920s and 1930s, valuing rest as the prevailing therapy for illness. Concerns about risk–benefit ratio in the use of vigorous exercise for persons with chronic illness continued even after the benefits of exercise became well known in recent years. However, there is a growing body of research on the safety and efficacy of exercise testing and training for adults with several chronic illnesses, including coronary artery disease, essential hypertension, chronic obstructive pulmonary disease, diabetes, arthritis, cancer, and chronic mental health and illness problems. In some areas the number of strong studies is small, but in no reported research is there evidence of harmful results of exercise testing or training for persons with chronic illness. The health benefits of exercise available to persons without chronic illness are also possible for persons of all ages with chronic illness. Although exercise regimens for persons with chronic illness need to be carefully developed, a general, open-ended recommendation for rest is not a benign prescription. Finally, Bland and Cooper (1984, p. 125), in their paper on the pathophysiology of osteoarthritis, wrote, "The weakest ... among us can become some kind of athlete but only the strongest can survive as spectators, only the hardiest can withstand the perils of inertia, inactivity, and immobility."

REFERENCES

Amery, A., Brixko, P., Clement, D., De Schaepdryver, A., Fagard, R., Forte, J., Henry, J. F., Leonetti, G., O'Malley, K., Strasser, T., Birkenhager, W., Bulpitt, C., Deruyttere, M., Dollery, C., Forette, F., Hamdy, R., Joossens, J. V., Lund-Johansen, P., Petrie, J., & Tuomilehto, J. (1985). Mortality and morbidity results from the European Working Party on High Blood Pressure in the Elderly Trial. *The Lancet*, i, 1350–1354.

American College of Sports Medicine. (1986). *Guidelines for exercise testing and prescription* (3rd ed.). Philadelphia: Lea and Febiger.

American College of Sports Medicine. (1990). Position stand. The recommended quantity and quality of exercise for developing and maintaining cardiorespiratory fitness in healthy adults. *Medicine and Science in Sports and Exercise, 22*, 265–274.

American Heart Association Writing Group, Fletcher, G. F., Froelicher, V. F., Hartley, H., Haskell, W. L., & Pollock, M. L. (1991). Exercise standards. A statement for health professionals from the American Heart Association. Dallas: American Heart Association.

Andrew, G. M., Oldridge, M. B., Parker, J. O., Cunningham, D. A., Rechnitzer, P. A., Jones, N. L., Buck, C., Kavanagh, T., Shephard, R. J., & Sutton, J. R. (1981). Reasons for dropout from exercise programs in post-coronary patients. *Medicine and Science in Sports and Exercise, 13*, 164–168.

Beals, C. A., Lampman, R. M., Banwell, B. F., Braunstein, E. M., Albers, J. W., & Castor, C. W. (1985). Measurement of exercise tolerance in patients with rheumatoid arthritis and osteoarthritis. *Journal of Rheumatology, 12*, 458–461.

Berger, M., Hagg, S. A., & Rudderman, N. B. (1975). Glucose metabolism in perfused skeletal muscle. Interaction of insulin and exercise on glucose uptake. *Biochemistry Journal, 146*, 23?–238.

Bjorntorp, P., De Joung, K., & Sjostrom, G. (1973). Physical training in human obesity. II. Effects of plasma insulin in glucose-intolerant subjects without marked hyperinsulinemia. *Scandinavian Journal of Clinical Laboratory Investigation, 32*, 42–45.

Bland, J. H. (1988). Joint, muscle and cartilage physiology as related to exercise. *Arthritis Care and Research, 1*, 99–108.

Bland, J. H., & Cooper, S. M. (1984). Osteoarthritis: A review of the cell biology involved and evidence for reversibility, management rationally related to known genesis and pathophysiology. *Seminars in Arthritis and Rheumatism, 14*, 106–133.

Blumenthal, J. A., Rejeski, W. J., Walsh-Riddle, M., Emery, C. F., Miller, H., Roark, S., Ribisl, P. M., Morris, P. B., Brubaker, P., & Williams, S. (1988). Comparison of high- and low-intensity exercise training after acute myocardial infarction. *American Journal of Cardiology, 61*, 26–30.

Blumenthal, J. A., Siegel, W. C., & Appelbaum, M. (1991). Failure of exercise to reduce blood pressure in patients with mild hypertension. Results of a randomized controlled trial. *Journal of the American Medical Association, 266*, 2098–2104.

Bouchard, C., Shepard, R. J., Stephens, T., Sutton, J. R., & McPherson, B. D. (1990). Excercise, fitness and health. A consensus of current knowledge. Champaigne, IL: Human Kinetics Books.

Brandt, K. D. (1988). Management of osteoarthritis. In W. N. Kelley, E. D. Harris, S. Ruddy, & C. B. Sledge (Eds.), *Textbook of rheumatology* (3rd ed.) (pp. 1501–1512). Philadelphia: W. B. Saunders.

Breslin, E. H. (1992). Dyspnea-limited response in chronic obstructive pulmonary disease: Reduced unsupported arm activities. *Rehabilitation Nursing, 17*, 12–20.

Breslin, E. H., Celli, B. R., & Roy, C. (1992, April). *The effects of unsupported arm exercise training and resistance breathing training on arm exercise endurance, respiratory muscle function, and dyspnea in chronic obstructive pulmonary disease.* Paper presented at Key Aspects of Caring for the Chronically Ill: Hospital and Home, Chapel Hill, NC.

Brown, R. D. (1990). Exercise fitness and mental health. In C. Bouchard, R. J. Shepard, T. Tephins, J. R. Sutton, & B. D. McPherson (Eds.), *Exercise, fitness and health: A consensus of current knowledge.* Champaign, IL: Human Kinetics Books.

Brown, J. D. (1991). Staying fit and staying well: Physical fitness as a moderator of life stress. *Journal of Personality & Social Psychology, 60*, 555–561.

Buchner, D. M., Beresford, S. A. A., Larson, E. B., LaCroix, A. Z., & Wagner, E. H. (1992). Effects of exercise on functional status in older adults II: Intervention studies. *Annual Review of Public Health, 13*, 469–488.

Cade, R., Mars, D., Wagemaker, H., Zauner, C., Privette, D., Cade, M., Peterson, J.,

& Hood-Lewis, D. (1984). Effect of aerobic exercise training on patients with systemic arterial hypertension. *American Journal of Medicine, 77*, 785–90.

Carón, D., Poussier, P., & Marliss, E. B. (1982). The effect of postprandial exercise on meal-related glucose intolerance in insulin-dependent diabetic individuals. *Diabetes Care, 5*, 364–369.

Carson, P., Phillips, R., Lloyd, M., Tucker, H., Neophytou, M., Buch, N. J., Gelson, A., Lawton, A., & Simpson, T. (1982). Exercise after myocardial infarction: A controlled trial. *Journal of the Royal College of Physicians of London, 16*, 147–151.

Caspersen, C. J. (1987). Physical inactivity and coronary heart disease. *Physician and Sportsmedicine, 15*, 43–44.

Caspersen, C. J., Powell, K. E., & Christenson, G. M. (1985). Physical activity, exercise, and physical fitness: Definitions and distinctions for health-related research. *Public Health Reports, 101*, 126–131.

Chalmers, T. C., Eckhardt, R. D., Reynolds, W. E., Cigarroa, J. G., Deane, N., Reinfenstein, R. W., Smith, C. W., & Davison, C. S. (1955). The treatment of acute infectious hepatitis: Controlled studies of the effects of diet, rest, and physical reconditioning on the acute course of the disease and the incidence of relapses and residual abnormalities. *The Journal of Clinical Investigation, 34*, 11–63.

Chazan, B. I., Balodimos, M.C., & Ryan, J. R. (1970). Twenty-five to forty-five years of diabetes with and without vascular complications. *Diabetologia, 6*, 656–659.

Crews, D. J., & Landers, D. M. (1987). A metanalytic review of aerobic fitness and reactivity to psychosocial stressors. *J. Medicine and Science in Sports and Exercise, 19*(Suppl), S114–S120.

Danneskiold-Samsoe, B., & Grimby, G. (1986). Isokinetic and isometric muscle strength in patients with rheumatoid arthritis. The relationship to clinical parameters and the influence of corticosteroid. *Clinical Rheumatology, 5*, 459–467.

Danneskiold-Samsoe, B., Lyngberg, K., Risum, T, & Telling, M. (1987). The effect of water exercise therapy given to patients with rheumatoid arthritis. *Scandinavian Journal of Rehabilitation Medicine, 19*, 31–35.

De Fronzo, R. A., Sherwin, R. S., & Kraemer, N. (1987). Effect of physical training on insulin action in obesity. *Diabetes, 36*, 1379–1385.

de Lateur, B. J., & Lehmann, J. F. (1986). Strengthening exercise. In J. C. Leek & J. F. Lehman (Eds.), *Principles of physical medicine and rehabilitation in the musculoskeletal diseases* (pp. 25–61). Orlando: Grune & Stratton.

Ditchey, R. V., Watkins, J., McKirnan, M. D., & Froelicher, V. (1981). Effects of exercise training on left ventricular mass in patients with ischemic heart disease. *American Heart Journal, 101*, 701–706.

Duncan, J. J., Farr, J. E., Upton, J., Hagen, R. E., Oglesby, M. E., & Blair, S. N. (1985). The effects of exercise on catecholamines and blood pressure in patients with mild essential hypertension. *Journal of the American Medical Association, 254*, 2609–2613.

Emery, C. F., & Blumenthal, J. A. (1991). Effects of physical exercise on psychological and cognitive functioning of older adults. *Annals of Behavioral Medicine, 13*, 99–107.

Fisher, N. M., Pendergast, D. R., Gresham, G. E., & Calkins, E. (1991). Muscle rehabilitation: Its effect on muscular and functional performance of patients with knee osteoarthritis. *Archives of Physical Medicine and Rehabilitation, 72*, 367–374.

Friedman, R., & Tappen, R. M. (1991). The effect of planned walking on communication in Alzheimer's Disease. *Journal of the American Geriatrics Society, 39*, 650–654.

Froelicher, V. F. (1990). Exercise, fitness, and coronary heart disease. In C. Bouchard, R. J. Shephard, T. Stephens, J. R. Sutton, & B. D. McPherson (Eds.). *Exercise, fitness and health. A consensus of current knowledge* (pp. 429–450). Champaign, IL: Human Kinetics Books.

Gerberich, S. G., Erickson, D., Serfass, R., Beard, B., Poulson, E., Ross, S., Wasser-Scott, P., Dauwalter, T., Olson, C., & Lewis, S. (1989). Quadriceps strength training using two forms of bilateral exercise. *Archives of Physical Medicine and Rehabilitation, 70,* 775–779.

Gift, A. G. & Austin, D. J. (1992). The effects of a program of systematic movement on COPD patients. *Rehabilitation Nursing, 17,* 6–10.

Glasgow, M. S., Gardner, K. R., & Engel, B. T. (1982). Behavioral treatment of high blood pressure II. Acute and sustained effects of relaxation and systolic blood pressure biofeedback. *Psychosomatic Medicine, 44,* 155–170.

Goldwater, B. C., & Collis, M. L. (1985). Psychologic effects of cardiovascular conditioning: A controlled experiment. *Psychosomatic Medicine, 47,* 174–181.

Gulanik, M. (1991). Is phase 2 cardiac rehabilitation necessary for early recovery of patients with cardiac disease? A randomized, controlled study. *Heart & Lung, 20,* 9–15.

Hagberg, J. M. (1990). Exercise, fitness, & hypertension, In C. Bouchard, R. J. Shephard, T. Stephens, J. R. Sutton, & B. D. McPherson (Eds.). *Exercise, fitness, and health* (pp.455–466). Champaign, IL: Human Kinetics Books.

Hagberg, J. M., Goldring, D., Heath, G. W., Ehsani, A. A., Hernandez, A., & Holloszy, J. O. (1984). Effect of exercise training on plasma catecholamines and hemodynamics of adolescent hypertensives during rest, submaximal exercise, and orthostatic stress. *Clinical Physiology, 4,* 117–124.

Harkcom, T. M., Lampman, R. M., Banwell, B. F., & Castor, C. W. (1985). Therapeutic value of graded aerobic exercise training in rheumatoid arthritis and osteoarthritis. *Arthritis and Rheumatism, 28,* 32–39.

Harris, K. A., & Holly, R. G. (1987). Physiologic response to circuit weight training in borderline hypertensive subjects. *Medicine and Science in Sports and Exercise, 19,* 246–252.

Horton, E. (1988). Exercise and diabetes mellitus. *Medical Clinics of North America, 72,* 1301–1321.

Hypertension Detection and Followup Program Cooperative Group. (1979). Five year findings of the Hypertension Detection and Followup Program: I. Reduction in mortality of persons with high blood pressure, including mild hypertension. *Journal of the American Medical Association, 242,* 2562–2571.

Ike, R. W., Lampman, R. M., & Castor, C. W. (1989). Arthritis and aerobic exercise: A review. *Physician and Sportsmedicine, 17,* 128–138.

Kaplan, N. (1986). *Clinical hypertension.* Baltimore: Williams & Wilkins.

Kemmer, F. W., Berchtold, P., Berger, M., Starke, A., Cuppers, H. J., Gries, F. A., & Zimmerman, H. (1979). Exercise-induced fall of blood glucose in insulin-treated diabetics unrelated to alteration of insulin mobilization. *Diabetes, 28,* 1131–1137.

Kiveloff, B., & Huber, O. (1971). Brief maximal isometric exercise in hypertension. *Journal of the American Geriatrics Society, 19,* 1006–1009.

Klein, M. H., Greist, J. H., Gurman, A. S., Neimeyer, R. A., Lesser, D. P., Bushnessl, N. J., & Smith, R. (1985). A comparative outcome study of group psychotherapy v. exercise treatments for depression. *International Journal of Mental Health, 13,* 148–177.

Kovar, P. A., Allegrante, J. P., MacKenzie, R., Peterson, M. G. E., Gutin, B., & Charlson, M. E. (1992). Supervised fitness walking in patients with osteoarthritis of the knee. A randomized, controlled trial. *Annals of Internal Medicine, 116*, 529–534.

Kramsch, D. M., Aspen, A. J., Abramowitz, B. M., Kreimendahl, T., & Hood, W. B. (1981). Reduction of coronary atherosclerosis by moderate conditioning exercise in monkeys on an atherogenic diet. *New England Journal of Medicine, 305*, 1483–1489.

LaPorte, R. E., Dorman, J. S., & Tajima, N. (1986). Pittsburgh Insulin-Dependent Diabetes Mellitus Morbidity and Mortality Study: Physical activity and diabetic complications. *Pediatrics, 78*, 1027–1033.

Lilloja, S., Young, A. A., Cutler, C. L., Ivy, J. L., Abbott, W. G. G., Zawadzki, J., Yki-Jarvinen, H., Christin, L., Secomb, T. W., & Bogardus, C. (1987). Skeletal muscle capillary density and fiber type are possible determinants of in vivo insulin resistance in man. *Journal of Clinical Investigation, 80*, 415–424.

Luborsky, L., Crits-Christoph, P., Brady, J. P., Kron, R. E., Weiss, T., Cohen, M., & Levy, L. (1982). Behavioral versus pharmacological treatments for essential hypertension-A needed comparison. *Psychosomatic Medicine, 44*, 203–213.

MacDonald, M. J. (1987). Post-exercise late-onset hpyoglycemia in insulin-dependent diabetic patients. *Diabetes Care, 10*, 584–588.

MacVicar, M. G., Winningham, M. L., & Nickel, J. L. (1989). Effects of aerobic interval training on cancer patients' functional capacity. *Nursing Research, 38*, 348–351.

McCarger, L. J., Tauton, J., & Pare, S. (1991). Benefits of exercise training for men with insulin-dependent diabetes mellitus. *The Diabetes Educator, 17*, 179–184.

McCorkle, R., & Given, B. (1991). Meeting the challenge of caring for chronically ill adults. In P. Chinn (Ed.), *Health policy. Who cares?* (pp. 59–69). Kansas City, MO: American Academy of Nursing.

Martin, J. E., Dubbert, P. E., & Cushman, W. C. (1990). Controlled trial of aerobic exercise in hypertension. *Circulation, 81*, 1560–1567.

Minor, M. A. (1991). Physical activity and management of arthritis. *Annals of Behavioral Medicine, 13*, 117–123.

Minor, M. A., Hewitt, J. E., Webel, R. R., Anderson, S. K., & Kay, D. R. (1989). Efficacy of physical conditioning exercise in patients with rheumatoid arthritis and osteoarthritis. *Arthritis and Rheumatism, 32*, 1396–1405.

Oldridge, N. B., Guyatt, G. H., Fischer, M. E., & Rimm, A. A. (1988). Cardiac rehabilitation after myocardial infarction. Combined experience of randomized clinical trials. *Journal of the American Medical Association, 260*, 945–950.

Paffenbarger, R. S., Hyde, R. T., Hsieh, C. C., & Wing, A. L. (1986). Physical activity, other lifestyle patterns, cardiovascular disease and longevity. *Acta Medica Scandinavica, 711*, (Supplement), 85–91.

Paffenbarger, R. S., Hyde, R. T., Wing, A. L., & Steinmetz, C. H. (1984). A natural history of athleticism and cardiovascular health. *Journal of the American Medical Association, 252*, 491–495.

Parker, J. C., Frank, R. G., Beck, Smarr, K. L., Buescher, K. L., Phillips, L. R., Smith, E. I., Anderson, S. K., & Walker, S. E. (1988). Pain management in rheumatoid arthritis patients: A cognitive behavioral perspective. *Arthritis and Rheumatism, 31*, 593–601.

Perlman, S. G., Connell, K. J., Clark, A., Robinson, M. S., Conion, P., Gecht, M., Caldron, P., & Sinacore, J. M. (1990). Dance-based aerobic exercise for rheumatoid arthritis. *Arthritis Care and Research, 3*, 29–35.

Peters, R. K., Cady, L. D. Jr., Bischoff, D. P., Bernstein, L., & Pike, M. C. (1983). Physical fitness and subsequent myocardial infarction in healthy workers. *Journal of the American Medical Association, 249,* 3052–3056.

Pollock, M. L., & Wilmore, J. H. (1990). *Exercise in health and disease.* Philadelphia: W. B. Saunders.

Rechnitzer, P. A. (1990). Exercise, fitness, and coronary heart disease. In C. Bouchard, R. J. Shephard, T. Stephens, J. R. Sutton, & B. D. McPherson (Eds.). *Exercise, fitness and health. A consensus of current knowledge* (pp. 451–453). Champaign, IL: Human Kinetics Books.

Rechnitzer, P. A., Cunningham, D. A., Andrew, G. M., Buck, C. W., Jones, N. L., Kavanagh, T., Oldredge, N. B., Parker, J. O., Shephard, R. J., Sutton, J. R., & Donner, A. P. (1983). Relation of exercise to the recurrence rate of myocardial infarction in men. *American Journal of Cardiology, 51,* 65–69.

Roman, O., Camuzzi, A. L., Villalon, E., & Klenner, C. (1981). Physical training program in arterial hypertension: A long-term prospective follow-up. *Cardiology, 67,* 230–243.

Schneider, S. H., Amoroso, L.F., Khachsdurian, A. K., & Rudderman, N. B. (1984). Studies on the mechanism of improved glucose control during regular exercise in Type II (non-insulin dependent) diabetes. *Diabetologia, 25,* 355–360.

Seals, D. R., & Hagberg, J. M. (1984). The effect of exercise training on human hypertension: A review. *Medicine and Science in Sports and Exercise, 16,* 207–215.

Shapiro, A. P., Schwartz, G. E., Ferguson, D. C. E., Redmond, D. P., & Weiss, S. (1977). Behavioral methods in the treatment of hypertension. A review of their clinical status. *Annals of Internal Medicine, 86,* 626–636.

Shaw, L. W. (1981). Effects of a prescribed supervised exercise program on mortality and cardiovascular morbidity in patients after a myocardial infarction. *American Journal of Cardiology, 48,* 39–46.

Sinyor, D., Golden, M., Steinert, Y., & Seraganian, P. (1986). Experimental manipulation of aerobic fitness & the response to psychosocial stress: Heart rate & self report measures. *Psychosomatic Medicine., 48,* 324–337.

Skinner, J. S. (1987). *Exercise testing and exercise prescription for special cases. Theoretical basis and clinical application.* Philadelphia: Lea & Febiger.

Spitzer, R., Endicott, J., & Robins, E. (1978). Research diagnostic criteria: Rationale and reliability. *Archives of General Psychiatry, 35,* 773.

Tran, Z. V., Weltman, A., Glass, G. V., & Mood, D. P. (1983). The effects of exercise on blood lipids and lipoproteins: A meta-analysis of studies. *Medicine and Science in Sports and Exercise, 15,* 392–402.

U. S. Senate Special Committee on Aging. (1986). *Aging America: Trends and projections* (1985-86 ed.). Washington, D.C.: U.S. Government Printing Office.

Wallberg-Henriksson, H. R., Gunnarson, R., Henricksson, J., DeFronzzo, R., Felig, P., Ostman, J., & Wahren, J. (1982). Increased peripheral insulin sensitivity and muscle mitochondrial enzymes but unchanged blood glucose control in Type I diabetics after physical training. *Diabetes, 31,* 1044–1050.

Wing, R. R., Epstein, L. H., Paternostro-Bayles, M., Kriska, A., & Norwalk, M. B. (1988). Exercise in a behavioral weight control programme for obese patients with Type II (non-insulin dependent) diabetes. *Diabetologia, 31,* 902–909.

World Health Organization. (1978). *Habitual physical activity and health* (WHO Regional Publications European Series No. 6). Copenhagen: World Health Organization.

Veterans Administration Cooperative Study Group on Antihypertensive Agents. (1967). Effects of treatment on morbidity in hypertension: Results in patients with diastolic blood pressures averaging 115 through 129 mmHg. *Journal of the American Medical Association, 202,* 116–122.

Veterans Administration Cooperative Study Group on Antihypertensive Agents. (1972). Effects of treatment on mortality in hypertension: III. Influence of age, diastolic pressure, and prior cardiovascular disease: Further analysis of side effects. *Circulation, 45,* 991–1004.

Yelin, E., Meenan, R., Nevit, M., & Epstein, W. (1980). Work disability in rheumatoid arthritis: Effects of disease, social and work factors. *Annals of Internal Medicine, 93,* 551–556.

Zinman, B., Murray, F. T., Vranic, M., Albisser, A.M., Leibel, P.A., & Marliss, E. B. (1977). Glucoregulation during moderate exercise in insulin treated diabetecs. *Journal of Clinical Endocrinology and Metabolism, 45,* 641–652.

Zinman, B., Zunuga-Guajardo, S., & Kelly, D. (1984). Comparison of acute and long-term effects of exercise on blood glucose contol in Type I diabetes. *Diabetes Care, 7,* 515–519.

[8]

Evaluating Research Findings for Practice

Linda R. Cronenwett

The ultimate purpose of nursing research is to improve nursing practice. You have the opportunity, in reading the research reports presented here, to consider whether or not the research is relevant and substantial enough to warrant changes in *your* practice. In this chapter I will review the definitions of research use and suggest strategies that you might use to decide whether the findings are ready to move into practice.

DEFINITIONS OF RESEARCH USE

Experts in research utilization have delineated two forms of research use: decision-driven and knowledge-driven (Caplan, 1979; Weiss, 1980). Decision-driven research utilization is the form of research use we commonly think of when we talk about integrating research and practice. The basic assumption is that research is used to formulate a policy, procedure, or program. The crucial point here is that the review and integration of the scientific base lead to some decision, course of action, or outcome.

Many nurses have been exposed to decision-driven models of research use such as the Conduct and Utilization of Research in Nursing (CURN) Project (1983) and the videotapes from Horn Video Productions (1987, 1989). With this approach, a clinical problem is identified, the relevant literature is found and critiqued, and new protocols for practice are developed, implemented, and evaluated. This form of research use is crucial to our profession. It is also complex, involving political, organizational, and attitudinal components in addition to requiring research that is relevant to practice.

The knowledge-driven or conceptual model of research use is characterized by the influence of research findings on *thinking*, as opposed to decisions or immediate actions. From this point of view you use research when you attend a research conference or read a research journal. In the process you expose yourself to new knowledge, not necessarily with a specific practice problem in mind, but to stay abreast of what questions are being asked in your field, what hypotheses are being generated by initial findings, and what innovations have been developed and tested. You might be stimulated by an assessment instrument or a new theory instead of feeling a need to apply the findings of a particular study. Weiss and her colleagues (1980) have referred to this type of research use as "knowledge creep." They propose that research is, in fact, "used," even when there is no immediate application to practice. This form of research use keeps you open to new information and ready to formulate new policies or to question the assumptions of old programs when the need arises.

As you read this book, you will certainly *use* research, looking at it from the knowledge-driven model point of view. You will become aware of the questions being asked about several areas of nursing practice. You may learn about some theory or approach that makes you think about other nursing problems in a new light. If you are not satisfied with the state of the science, you may decide to conduct a study yourself. On the other hand, maybe your current care plans, critical paths, or practice guidelines are soundly based on current knowledge, according to the studies presented. The effect of the book, then, may be for you to redouble your efforts to see that all patients receive the best standard of care. Any of these outcomes will be valuable.

Because this book includes a summary of the science on important areas in caring for the chronically ill—managing the hospitalized chronically ill, assisting with transitions from hospital to home, managing home care, and living with chronic illness—and these summaries are presented along with the newest research, you have an excellent basis for determining whether you want to take some action to change practice in your setting. So let's proceed with a discussion about how to assess new knowledge for its applicability to your practice.

NEED FOR CHANGE IN YOUR SETTING

First of all, does anyone perceive a need for change in practice in your setting? To perceive such a need, someone must be open to the possibility of change. What is the culture among the nurses and managers with whom you work? Is there an openness to the idea of change based on scientific information?

When change is considered, who plans the change? Are the staff who will implement the change involved in the planning? Is anyone in your work group familiar with theoretical models of research utilization (such as those reviewed by Crane, 1985)? Have you talked about what models seem to work best among your colleagues: problem-solving models, linkage models, social interaction models, or research and development models? Have you experimented with research-use activities using guidelines from the CURN Project (1983), Stetler and Marram (1976), Stetler and DiMaggio (1991), or Goode, Lovett, Hayes, and Butcher (1987)? If not, you may decide that the biggest need for change in your setting is the need to change the culture. You may want to pick one innovation and use it to create a model for research-based change in your setting. If so, consider choosing an innovation with these characteristics: a clear advantage over past practice, compatibility with current staff values and norms, low complexity, ease of experimentation on a limited basis, and highly visible outcomes (Rogers, 1983). Pick one important and salable idea and begin the process of changing your culture.

If your colleagues are used to the idea of change, it will still enhance your ability to use research-based findings if there is some pre-existing evidence of a need for change. Have you had a set of patient complaints that struck a common theme? Have your quality assessment activities uncovered a problem? Have you been achieving less than ideal outcomes from certain interventions or critical paths? Have some newly hired staff members mentioned that your approaches to certain practice problems differ from what they did in another setting? Have you been seeing an increase in problems, and thus may have an increased readiness among staff to try something new? Proposed practice changes are likely to be welcomed if a perceived need for change exists. You may want to focus initial planning efforts on activities that will heighten your colleagues' perceptions of the need for change.

READINESS OF THE RESEARCH FOR PRACTICE

The other critical component for change in practice is readiness of the science. Even if everyone agrees that current practice could be improved, you want to be sure there is sufficient scientific evidence for any change you propose. How do you know when the scientific evidence provides a clear rationale for a change in practice? You start formulating your opinion by reading what the investigators say in the opening and concluding sections of their reports. Do they summarize a group of studies from which findings converge to support a change in practice? Or do the investigators indicate that this was the first and only study with the reported findings? How similar are the characteristics of the people studied to the patients with whom you work? How similar is the study's environment to the setting in which you work? If several investigative teams have concluded that the evidence for a change in practice is fairly clear and if studies have been conducted with patients who resemble your own, in settings similar to your own, you have strong support for a change in your practice.

The extent of the evidence required for change may vary depending on the needs of your practice setting. Let's consider, for example, how the evaluation of the research base might differ depending on whether you are trying to affect nurses' sensitivity to patient experiences, methods of assessment, or interventions.

Sensitivity to Patient Experiences

Healthy nurses may have no idea what it feels like to experience a particular illness or surgery, or to care for someone who has that experience. Even when the nurse is knowledgeable about the medical and nursing facts of the situation, he or she may know little about human responses to the illness experience, the symptoms or reactions with which the patient and family have to cope, or the resources available to assist recovery or adaptation. In the last 10 years nurse researchers have studied the experiences of patients and their families using qualitative research methods. When you read these research reports, your practice changes in terms of sensitivity to patient cues, styles of assessment or teaching, and even intervention. In this book, for example, you will see a report by Eakes and colleagues that introduces the concept of chronic sorrow as a normal response to the abnormal situation of chronic illness.

There is rarely a large body of replicated work about patient experiences. But you *will* use what you read because the impact comes from reading the report. You see the actual words of patients and families, and these words lead you to do a better job of eliciting your own patients' experiences and perceptions. As a result, you will understand your patients and families better than you have in the past, and you will plan your nursing care differently—and thus change your practice. There are few risks to such use of research; and your increased sensitivity should benefit your practice.

Methods of Assessment

The primary aim of some studies is to establish the reliability and validity of various methods of assessment. Some instruments are developed solely for research purposes, but most are designed to serve clinical purposes. To assess the readiness of these instruments for use in practice, you need to know how to evaluate the reliability and validity of the instruments. The researchers give you that information in their reports. If you do not understand, write to the authors and ask whether, and under what conditions, the instrument is ready for clinical assessment purposes.

If you are interested in trying an instrument in practice, you can write and ask the researcher if further data are being collected or desired. Usually you can obtain a copy of the instrument and directions for its use in exchange for forwarding your data to the investigator. If your patients differ from the sample used by the investigator, there would be benefits to collaboration for both of you. Perhaps the investigator would analyze your data using the same techniques as were used in the original study. Both you and the investigator would then know whether the instrument works as well with your patients and in your environment as it did with other patient samples.

A final issue regarding instruments is how much will be gained at what cost; that is, what are the relative benefits of making the assessment compared to the costs in patient and staff time that will be necessary to perform and document the assessment? One also has to ask if the assessment will affect some outcome. Data collected for data collection's sake alone will be unlikely to be worth the labor costs; however, if the assessment will lead to new interventions, and these interventions improve patient outcomes, the instrument can be considered ready for use in terms of its cost/benefit ratio.

Interventions

Generally, scientific findings that appear to provide a rationale for changing nursing interventions require the most careful critique and evaluation of the research base. Again, particular attention must be paid to the issues of fit between the settings and samples studied and the populations and settings in which the findings will be applied. In addition you should consider the following questions (Stetler & Marram, 1976) as you decide the extent of further effort that you can or must devote to evaluating the research base:

1. Do you have a theoretical or scientific basis for your current practice?
2. How effective is your current method of practice?
3. What degree of potential risk could be associated with the implementation of the new findings?

For example, let's consider the early findings of Holtzclaw (1990) about the effect on the shivering associated with a patient's chemotherapy of terry cloth wraps to the extremities. Certainly her early report was unreplicated and pertained only to a small sample of patients. Should the results of such a study be used?

First you could ask if there is a theoretical or scientific rationale for current methods of helping patients with the discomforts of shivering. Are nurses experimenting with comfort measures or providing only medications as ordered? If no interventions are currently being tried or if the current interventions are ineffective (that is, not diminishing the shivering), you can move to consideration of risk. What level of risk would be associated with wrapping a patient's arms and legs with terry cloth? If the risk is minimal, then it is reasonable to consider applying these research findings yourself and evaluating the results of your trial in the same way you would evaluate an idea that came from any other source or way of knowing, such as intuition, logic, or problem-solving.

Your ideas for research-based changes in practice will require significantly more evidence and evaluation if the current basis for practice is effective and risk-free and is believed to be based on scientific evidence. Recently, for example, multiple investigators have studied the relative effectiveness of heparinized saline versus saline as a flushing solution for intermittent infusion devices (Goode et al., 1991). Because providers believed that there was scientific evidence demonstrating the benefit of using heparinized saline, and because there is always risk involved in a clogged line, nurses needed evidence to demonstrate the effectiveness of saline, even though the change would decrease both supply and labor costs. At this point we even have the editor of a nursing research journal calling for this well justified change in practice (Downs, 1991).

Depending on the characteristics of the change in practice you are considering, your need for evaluation of the research base may be accomplished by the work presented in this book. However, if your innovation is perceived as risky, if it involves withholding care that is currently considered standard practice, if implementation would require changes in policies or procedures, if new equipment or supplies would be required, or if implementation would be impossible without the support of other health care providers, then you are likely to have to expend greater effort to collect, evaluate, and make a case for the quality of the research base that supports your innovation.

Integrating a body of research literature into a coherent argument for a practice innovation is no small task. If you have had training to critique a research base as a part of your education and you have some flexibility regarding how you spend your work time, follow up on the ideas you gain from this book by conducting your own review and critique of the literature. In our society in particular, nothing establishes expertise on a topic as well as an intimate familiarity with the research base. By reviewing the literature yourself, you also have the advantage of being exposed to other ideas, other nuances of the same idea, or other strategies or suggestions for practice that perhaps have not yet occurred to you.

If you feel uncomfortable with your ability to find or critique a research base, does that mean you can not use your ideas for changing practice? No. Just choose different strategies for this phase of the process. Here are some ideas:

1. Find a colleague in your setting who *is* responsible for reviewing research and proposing research-based innovations—a clinical nurse specialist, a director of research, the chair of your practice or standards committee, a staff development instructor, or a nurse with advanced education who works on your unit. Share your ideas with this person and request help in evaluating the research base. Offer to call the investigators whose studies set you thinking about change and ask them to assist in finding the studies that deserve consideration. Ask your colleague to lead a discussion of the articles with you and other nurses on your unit.
2. Contact a faculty member in your specialty at your local School of Nursing. See if you can set up a process whereby a student is assigned to assist in evaluating a specified research base as a part of fulfilling the requirements for a research course. If that is not possible, maybe the faculty member would do the evaluation for you in return for your giving one or two lectures to his or her students.
3. If you have no access to nursing colleagues who are able and willing to assist you in the review process, do the best job you can to collect all the pertinent articles related to the innovation. Then ask a colleague from another discipline to validate your understanding of the implications for practice to be derived from this research base.

Although this chapter includes a number of ideas about when and how to evaluate the research base for a change in practice, and although you are encouraged to try innovations that are low risk and do not compete with current practices that are effective and well supported by scientific findings, there is one caveat that must be considered. Practices once adopted are difficult to change (Dixon, 1990). You should be cautious about implementing an expensive intervention without a full evaluation of its effectiveness. Just as we are today reluctant to take the heparin out of flushing solutions, we might be reluctant someday to remove your innovation from practice.

CONCLUSION

The challenge to you as you read the chapters of this book is to think broadly about your practice. As you read, make notes about all the ideas that come to mind. Without a doubt, you will use research in at least one of the ways described here. We hope that you will evaluate the science base for one or more practice changes you are willing to consider. When you complete your reading and evaluation of the science, you may be ready to make a specific practice change. A list of references on the "how-tos" of research utilization is appended to this chapter. Remember to keep notes on your experiences so that you can share the results with others. In the next decade, how we *use* research will be as important as the knowledge generation activities themselves.

REFERENCES

Caplan, N. (1979). The two-communities theory and knowledge utilization. *American Behavioral Scientist, 22*, 259–470.

Crane, J. (1985). Research utilization: Theoretical perspectives. *Western Journal of Nursing Research, 7*, 261–268.

CURN Project (Horsley, J. A., Crane, J., Crabtree, M. K., & Wood, D. J.) (1983). *Using research to improve nursing practice: A guide*. New York: Grune & Stratton.

Dixon, A. S. (1990). The evolution of clinical policies. *Medical Care, 28*, 201–220.

Downs, F. S. (1991). How to make a difference. *Nursing Research, 40*, 323.

Goode, C. J., Lovett, M. K., Hayes, J. E., & Butcher, L. A. (1987). Use of research-based knowledge in clinical practice. *Journal of Nursing Administration, 17*(12), 11–18.

Goode, C. J., Titler, M., Rakel, B., Ones, D. S., Kleiber, C., Small, S., & Triolo, P. K. (1991). A meta-analysis of effects of heparin flush and saline flush: Quality and cost implications. *Nursing Research, 40*, 324–330.

Holtzclaw, B. J. (1990). Effects of extremity wraps to control drug-induced shivering: A pilot study. *Nursing Research, 39*, 280–283.

Horn Video Productions. (1987). *Using research in clinical nursing practice* [film]. Ida Grove, IA: Horn Video Productions.

Horn Video Productions. (1989). *Research utilization: A process of organizational change* [film]. Ida Grove, IA: Horn Video Productions.

Rogers, E. M. (1983). *Diffusion of innovations*. New York: Free Press.

Stetler, C. B., & DiMaggio, G. (1991). Research utilization among clinical nurse specialists. *Clinical Nurse Specialist, 5*, 151–155.

Stetler, C., & Marram, G. (1976). Evaluating research findings for applicability in practice. *Nursing Outlook, 24*, 559–563.

Weiss, C. H. (1980). Knowledge creep and decision accretion. *Knowledge: Creation, Diffusion, Utilization, 1*, 381–404.

ADDITIONAL REFERENCES

ANA Commission on Nursing Research. (1981). *Guidelines for the investigative function of nurses*. Kansas City, MO: ANA.

Barnard, K. E. (1980). Knowledge for practice: Directions for the future. *Nursing Research, 29*, 208–212.

Beal, J. A., & Love, C. F. (Eds.). *Nursing Scan in Research*. Hagerstown, MD: J.B. Lippincott (1988-present, bimonthly).

Bock, L. R. (1990). From research to utilization: Bridging the gap. *Nursing Management, 21*(3), 50–51.

Brett, J. L. (1987). Use of nursing practice research findings. *Nursing Research, 36*, 344–349.

Brett, J. L. (1989). Organizational integrative mechanisms and adoption of innovations by nurses. *Nursing Research, 38*, 105–110.

Breu, C., & Dracup, K. (1976). Implementing nursing research in a critical care setting. *Journal of Nursing Administration, 6*(12), 14–17.

Briones, T., & Bruya, M. A. (1990). The professional imperative: Research utilization in the search for scientifically based nursing practice. *Focus on Critical Care, 17*(1), 78–81.

Buckwalter, K. C. (1985). Is nursing research used in practice? In J. C. McCloskey & H. K. Grace (Eds.), *Current issues in nursing* (2nd ed., pp. 110-123). London: Blackwell Scientific Publishers.

Burns, N., & Grove, S. K. (1987). *The practice of nursing research: Conduct, critique and utilization*. Philadelphia, PA: W.B. Saunders.

Champion, V. L., & Leach, A. (1989). Variables related to research utilization for nursing: An empirical investigation. *Journal of Advanced Nursing, 14*, 705–710.

Connelly, C. E. (1986). Replication research in nursing. *International Journal of Nursing Studies, 23*, 71–77.

Coyle, L. A., & Sokop, A. G. (1990). Innovation adoption behavior among nurses. *Nursing Research, 39*, 176–180.

Crane, J. (1985). Research utilization–nursing models. *Western Journal of Nursing Research, 7*, 494–497.

Cronenwett, L. R. (1986). Research contributions of clinical nurse specialists. *Journal of Nursing Administration, 16* (6), 6–7.

Cronenwett, L. R. (1987). Research utilization in practice settings. *Journal of Nursing Administration, 17* (7–8), 9–10.

Cronenwett, L. R. (1988). Disseminating research to clinicians. *CNR* (Newsletter of the ANA Council of Nurse Researchers), *15* (1), 1, 3.

Cronenwett, L. R. (1990). Improving practice through research utilization. In S. Funk, E. Tornquist, M. Champagne, L. Copp, & R. Wiese (Eds.), *Key aspects of recovery: Improving nutrition, rest, and mobility* (pp. 7–22). New York: Springer Publishing Co.

Cruise, M. J., Alderman, M. C., & Gorenberg, B. D. (1989). Facilitating research utilization: A model for nurse managers. *Nursing Connections, 2*, 53–61.

Curlette, W. L., & Cannella, K. S. (1985). Going beyond the narrative summarization of research findings: The meta-analysis approach. *Research in Nursing & Health, 8*, 293–301.

Edwards-Beckett, J. (1990). Nursing research utilization techniques. *Journal of Nursing Administration, 20* (11), 25–30.

Fetter, M. S., Feetham, S. L., D'Apolito, K., Chaze, B. A., Fink, A., Frink, B. B., Hougart, M. K., & Rushton, C. H. (1989). Randomized clinical trials: Issues for researchers. *Nursing Research, 38*, 117–120.

Firlit, S. L., Kemp, M. G., & Walsh, M. (1986). Preparing master's students to develop clinical trials. *Western Journal of Nursing Research, 8*, 106–109.

Firlit, S. L., Kemp, M. G., & Walsh, M. (1987). Nursing research in practice: A survey of research utilization content in master's degree programs. *Western Journal of Nursing Research, 9*, 612–617.

Funk, S. G., Champagne, M. T., Wiese, R. A., & Tornquist, E. M. (1991). Barriers to using research findings in practice: The clinician's perspective. *Applied Nursing Research, 4*, 90–95.

Funk, S. G., & Tornquist, E. M. (1992). The listener's guide to research presentations. *Journal of Pediatric Nursing, 7*, 141–144.

Funk, S. G., Tornquist, E. M., & Champagne, M. T. (1989). A model for improving the dissemination of nursing research. *Western Journal of Nursing Research, 11*, 361–367.

Haller, K. B., Reynolds, M. A., & Horsley, J. A. (1979). Developing research-based innovation protocols: Process, criteria, and issues. *Research in Nursing and Health, 2*, 45–51.

Havelock, R. G. (1969). *Planning for innovation through dissemination and utilization of knowledge*. Ann Arbor: Center for Research on Utilization of Scientific Knowledge, ISR, University of Michigan.

Havelock, R. G. (1972). *Research-user linkage and social problem solving*. Ann Arbor: Center for Research on Utilization on Scientific Knowledge, ISR, University of Michigan.

Havelock, R. G. (1973). *The change agent's guide to innovation in education*. Englewood Cliffs, NJ: Education Technology Publications.

Hickey, M. (1990). The role of the clinical nurse specialist in the research utilization process. *Clinical Nurse Specialist, 4*(2), 93–96.

Horsley, J. A. (1985). Using research in practice: The current context. *Western Journal of Nursing Research, 7*, 135–139.

Horsely, J. A., & Crane, J. (1986). Factors associated with innovation in nursing practice. *Family and Community Health, 9*, 1–11.

Janken, J. K., Dufanlt, M. A., & Yeaw, E. M. S. (1988). Research roundtables: Increasing student/staff nurse awareness of the relevance of research to practice. *Journal of Professional Nursing, 4*, 186–191.

Ketefian, S. (1975). Application of selected nursing research findings into nursing practice: A pilot study. *Nursing Research, 24*, 89–92.

King, D., Barnard, K. E., & Hoehn, R. (1981). Disseminating the results of nursing research. *Nursing Outlook, 19*, 164–169.

Kirchhoff, K. T. (1982). A diffusion survey of coronary precautions. *Nursing Research, 31*, 196–201.

Kirchhoff, K. T. (1983). Should staff nurses be expected to use research? *Western Journal of Nursing Research, 5*, 245–247.

Kirchhoff, K. T. (1991). Who is responsible for research utilization? *Heart & Lung, 20*(3), 308–9.

Krueger, J. C. (1978). Utilization of nursing research: The planning process. *Journal of Nursing Administration, 8*(1), 6–9.

Krueger, J. C., Nelson, A. H., & Wolanin, M. O. (1978). *Nursing research: Development, collaboration and utilization*. Germantown, MD: Aspen Publishers, Inc.

Larson, E. (1989). Using the CURN project to teach research utilization in a baccalaureate program. *Western Journal of Nursing Research, 11*, 593–599.

Lindeman, C. A. (1988). Research in practice: The role of the staff nurse. *Applied Nursing Research, 1*, 5–7.

Lindquist, R., Brauer, D. J., Lekander, B. J., Foster, K. (1990). Research utilization: Practical considerations for applying research to nursing practice. *Focus on Critical Care, 17*(4), 342–347.

Lobiondo-Wood, G., & Haber, J. (1986). *Nursing research: Critical appraisal and utilization*. St. Louis: C.V. Mosby.

Loomis, M. E. (1985). Knowledge utilization and research utilization in nursing. *Image: Journal of Nursing Scholarship, 17*, 35–39.

MacGuire, J. M. (1990). Putting nursing research findings into practice: Research utilization as an aspect of the management of change. *Journal of Advanced Nursing, 15*, 614–620.

Mallick, M. (1983). A constant comparative method for teaching research critiquing to baccalaureate nursing students. *Image: Journal of Nursing Scholarship, 15*, 120–123.

Massey, J., & Loomis, M. (1988). When should nurses use research findings? *Applied Nursing Research, 1*, 32–40.

Maurin, J. T. (1990). Research utilization in the social-political arena. *Applied Nursing Research, 3*, 48–51.

Miller, J. R., & Messenger, S. R. (1978). Obstacles to applying nursing research findings. *American Journal of Nursing, 78*, 632–634.

Phillips, L. R. F. (1986). *A clinician's guide to the critique and utilization of nursing research*. Norwalk, CT: Appleton-Century-Croft.

Roberts-Gray, C., & Gray, T. (1983). Implementing innovations: A model to bridge the gap between diffusion and utilization. *Knowledge: Creation, Diffusion, Utilization, 5*, 213–232.

Rothman, J. (1980). *Social R & D: Research and development in the human services*. Englewood Cliffs, NJ: Prentice Hall.

Stark, J. L. (1989). A multiple-strategy based research program for staff nurse involvement. *Journal of Nursing Administration, 19*, 7–8.

Stetler, C. B. (1985). Research utilization: Defining the concept. *Image: Journal of Nursing Scholarship, 17*, 40–44.

Stokes, J. E. (1981). Utilization of research findings by staff nurses. In S.D. Krampitz & N. Pavlovich (Eds.), *Readings for nursing research*. St. Louis: C.V. Mosby.

Tanner, C. A. (1987). Evaluating research for use in practice: Guidelines for the clinician. *Heart & Lung, 16*, 424–431.

Topham, D. L., & DeSilva, P. (1988). Evaluating congruency between steps in the research process: A critique guide for use in clinical nursing practice. *Clinical Nurse Specialist, 2*, 97–102.

Part II

CARING FOR CHRONICALLY ILL ADULTS

[9]

A Special Care Unit for the Chronically Critically Ill

Barbara J. Daly and Ellen B. Rudy

The restricting of federal reimbursement for escalating health care costs to a prospective payment system has made hospitals acutely aware of the need to cut costs. In fact, the survival of tertiary care facilities will rest on the ability of administrators to ferret out disproportionately expensive services and alter or eliminate them altogether. One of the most costly services provided by hospitals is the care that requires the specialized skill and technology of intensive care units (ICUs). The increased availability of life-saving and life-prolonging treatment modalities has stimulated rapid expansion of critical care services in U.S. hospitals through the last two decades. In 1984 the Office of Technology Assessment estimated that total national hospital expenditures were $136 billion; of this, $13 to $15 billion were spent in adult ICUs (Berenson, 1984). These high-cost environments are now under increased scrutiny to decrease their costs, and of particular concern are those patients who stay beyond their reimbursement limit and become financial burdens to the hospital.

Although the typical ICU patient is assumed to have a short length of stay (3 to 4 days), stays of more than a month are not uncommon (Berenson, 1984). At one end of the spectrum are patients who receive concentrated intensive medical and nursing care and various forms of life support. They enter the ICU during a particularly vulnerable period of their illness, are monitored closely, and generally recover within a relatively short period of time and are transferred out of the intensive care environment. At the other end of the spectrum are patients whose stay in the ICU is prolonged because of complications or underlying chronic health conditions that are exacerbated by a critical illness (General Accounting Office, 1986). These long-term patients have recovered from the most acute phase of critical illness but still require intensive nursing care for several weeks or even months, and may be described as "chronically critically ill." This particular group of patients is usually well beyond the diagnosis-related group (DRG) cost allocation, and each day of care is an additional financial burden to the hospital. They are costly to hospitals both in terms of actual dollars and in terms of costs to ICU personnel. These long-term patients take up needed ICU beds and become a burden to both nurses and physicians because their recovery is slow and difficult to see day-to-day.

More and more chronically critically ill patients are creating a financial and caseload crisis in hospitals, and a group of patients have developed who are unpopular with both physicians and nurses and strain the already diminishing supply of nurses. This chapter describes the development of a special care unit (SCU) to address this situation.

THE CHRONICALLY CRITICALLY ILL PATIENT POPULATION

To obtain a measure of the demands of the chronically critically ill population at our hospital, we made a retrospective analysis of patients who were in the ICU longer than 3 weeks in 1987. Although this cutoff was somewhat arbitrary, we reasoned that the majority of patients who stayed in the ICU for this length of time would probably have reached the stage of their illness at which their condition was no longer medically unstable and their needs would not be served by the intensive, technologically focused environment of the traditional ICU. Of the 46 patients with length of stay (LOS) of 21 days or longer, 57% of the patients were in the surgical intensive care unit (SICU) and 43% were in the medical intensive care unit (MICU). The majority were female (52%), and the average age was 66. They had spent an average of 64 days in the hospital and 52 days in the ICU. Thirty-two percent were discharged home and 20% were discharged to other institutions; 48% died.

The International Classification of Diseases (ICD 9) codes on the patient charts were used for documentation of diagnoses and procedures. Thirty-six (78.3%) of the patients had documentation of infection. Of the 28 patients who had an ICU LOS of 22 to 53 days, 20 (71%) had documentation of infection. Of the 18 patients who had an ICU LOS of more than 53 days, 16 (88%) had documentation of infection. Ninety-one percent of the patients had a respiratory diagnosis, and 61% of these required a tracheostomy.

Although the 46 patients with LOS 21 days or longer represented only 3% of the total number of patients admitted to the MICU and SICU in 1987, they used 28% of the total patient days of care in these two units. A similar analysis of 1988 patients showed that, again, patients with a length of stay greater than 21 days represented only 3% of all admissions. However, in 1988, they used 38% of all available patient days.

Although respiratory problems were common, the principal diagnoses of these chronically critically ill patients varied widely. Included were such entities as chronic obstructive pulmonary disease, Guillain-Barre syndrome, cardiac surgery, vascular graft procedures, meningitis, and pneumonia. Clinical characteristics that were similar among the patients included the existence of chronic diseases in addition to the problem necessitating critical care; complications of their primary disease, such as postoperative respiratory failure and sepsis, malnutrition, and muscle wasting resulting from prolonged hospitalization; and patient and family psychosocial disturbance caused by the stress of the lengthy illness. It was these characteristics, rather than the primary critical event, that created the care needs so difficult to meet in traditional ICU settings. Consistent weaning plans, nutritional support, muscle retraining, and restoration of normal sleep-wake cycles all were difficult to manage in the ICU.

In addition, when these patients reached the point in their illness when the medical therapy for their primary condition was completed and their condition stabilized, they became "low priority" in the ICU. Interns and residents did not view them as good "teaching cases" and the ICU nurses did not feel challenged by their slow progress or equipped to meet their rehabilitative needs. Yet these patients remained in the ICU because of continued need for some limited technologic support, such as arterial line monitoring or mechanical ventilation, or because the intensity of their nursing needs could not be met on a general division.

THE SPECIAL CARE UNIT CONCEPT

Because the data from the retrospective chart reviews clearly established that this population of patients was using a significant proportion of critical care beds in an environment that was not designed to meet their needs, a plan was initiated to create a Special Care Unit (SCU). The primary purpose of opening a new unit was to provide an environment designed to meet the specific needs of these patients. At the same time, this seemed the ideal opportunity to create an environment designed to address the factors that create dissatisfaction among professional nurses, such as lack of autonomy and dissatisfaction with traditional management structures, which ultimately contribute to increased turnover rates.

To obtain approval for the plan to open the SCU, a proposal was developed setting forth the potential benefits. Most important to gaining approval was the projection of significant cost savings because of the ability to staff the SCU at a lower nurse/patient ratio than that used in the ICU. Because the unit would accept only medically stable patients transferred from other ICUs, we did not have to plan for routinely providing a one-to-one ratio for some patients or for the unexpected emergency department admission, as occurs in most ICUs. Most important, we proposed that this unit not have any involvement of physician house staff, thus reducing the demand for intern and resident coverage. These advantages, in conjunction with releasing ICU beds for use for the more typical short-term ICU patients, were sufficient to convince the hospital administrators to approve the creation of the SCU.

Although we would have preferred to have at least a full year to plan for opening the unit, it was decided that the SCU had to be opened earlier, to coincide with other cost-reduction initiatives of the hospital. Consequently we concentrated over the next few months on recruiting staff, choosing a unit on which to house the SCU, purchasing monitoring equipment, writing the initial treatment protocols, and establishing a multidisciplinary advisory group to oversee the design and functioning of the unit.

THE SCU ENVIRONMENT

The SCU environment is composed of a physical design that accommodates limited technology, with care aimed at family involvement and rehabilitation, a case management practice model, and a shared governance management model. These features are considered to be in dynamic interaction with one another and as a whole influence nurse and patient outcomes.

Key features of the SCU include the exclusive use of private rooms, which open from a central hallway and have an exterior view. All rooms are large enough to accommodate family members overnight in patient rooms if desired, and a spacious family lounge is located on the unit. The entire unit has been painted and furnished to produce a homelike atmosphere. Physiologic monitoring of patients is limited to electrocardiographic monitors and occasional arterial pressure monitoring. Ventilators are the most common technologic support system used. Family involvement in the recovery process is encouraged by the staff and facilitated by the physical setting. In addition to a physical setting that promotes rest, privacy, and limited technology, the case management patient care delivery system and the shared governance management model promote a social system for the nursing staff that is intended to foster autonomy and self-regulation.

The case management practice model is defined as expanded and extended management of an episode of care by nurses who are accountable clinically and financially for each patient's outcomes. Care is built on case-type specific protocols that result in the development of critical pathways for specific types of patients or patient conditions. The patient and family are actively involved in the planning and decision making about the patient's care (Zander, 1988). The shared governance management model vests authority and responsibility for managing the work environment in the staff and uses collaboration and consensus for decision making.

In contrast, features of the typical ICU includes a majority (80%) of bed spaces that are open or curtained off from a central circular nursing station. Lighting and noise from the overall unit cannot be excluded from patient bed spaces, and family members are not accommodated for overnight stays. Visitor lounges are outside the physical space of the unit and family visiting is controlled. Many types of technology for physiologic monitoring and life support are in evidence. The goal of the ICU is to monitor patients closely to intervene when life-threatening events occur.

A primary nursing delivery system and a bureaucratic management model are in place in ICUs, and they represent the traditional systems for both care delivery and management in most ICUs. The primary nursing practice model defines the nursing delivery system as the distribution of nursing care such that total care of an individual is the responsibility of one nurse, who plans the individual's care with that individual (Loveridge, Cummings, & O'Malley, 1988). The bureaucratic management model is defined as a centralized decision-making model at the unit level, with organizational responsibility and authority descending within the unit through a distinct chain of command. In our institution the traditional ICUs include an 18-bed SICU and a 12-bed MICU.

SCU OPERATIONS

The SCU is an eight-bed unit, budgeted for 15 registered nurses, 3 patient care assistants, and 1 secretary. One of the registered nurses is an MSN-prepared nurse with experience as a clinical nurse specialist (CNS) in critical care. She has the title of Project Leader and fulfills some traditional head nurse and some CNS responsibilities. She acts as the liaison for the unit with the rest of the hospital bureaucracy, coordinates many of the operational details, such as preparing reports and providing a contact person for other units and departments, and serves as a clinical teacher.

The staff members are all experienced critical care nurses with an average experience of 8 years. All either attended a formal program about the goals and organizational structure of the SCU or actually spent a day observing the unit after it was opened and before accepting a position. Therefore, all the staff members are committed to the care of these long-term patients, to the case management model of care delivery, and to participating in the responsibilities of shared governance. The characteristics of professional maturity and interest in this patient population have been crucial to the staff's ability to accept the responsibilities of their roles.

All full-time registered nurses act as case managers. Their responsibilities begin when the patient is accepted for admission to the SCU. Once the patient has met the admission criteria (described in the next section), the case manager goes to the unit where the patient is at that time, meets with the patient, family, and care givers; explains the purpose and operations of the SCU to the patient and family; gives the family a tour of the SCU if possible; takes a thorough history; and initiates a beginning case management plan. Of special importance in the plan, given the severity of these patients' illnesses, is the resuscitation status and the goals of the patient and family related to discharge placement.

Once the patient is in the SCU, the case manager directs the nursing care and coordinates the involvement of all other disciplines. He or she presents the patient at the weekly interdisciplinary meetings, arranges family conferences as often as necessary, and obtains consultation from other disciplines, such as the gastrointestinal service if a gastrostomy tube is necessary or ophthalmology if an eye examination is needed. Nursing interventions in the SCU are guided by management plans developed by the case manager, by patient care protocols, and by critical pathways developed by the SCU staff in consultation with the medical director. Examples of patient care protocols include ventilator weaning, nutrition, and emergency situations. These protocols could be equated with physician standing orders. Protocols allow each specialist, such as the nutritionist or speech therapist, as well as consulting physicians, to write orders that are clarified, integrated in the plan, and implemented by the case manager. Disagreements or conflicts are resolved by the case manager, with assistance from the project leader if needed.

Critical pathways identify patient progress (outcomes) as standards or goals to be met in specified periods of time. For example, the critical pathway for "failure to wean" (see Table 9.1) indicates the day the weaning is to begin, the method to be used, and the outcomes to be achieved at various times during hospitalization (e.g., without the ventilator all day). The medical director reviews patient progress each day, collaborates with the case manager in planning, and is called for critical changes in patient condition and for necessary medication orders.

Because the SCU represents a new approach to care, a great deal of communication and education of others has been necessary to explain the purpose and operation of the unit. In addition, the education and adjustments required have not been just on the part of those outside the SCU. The staff members themselves have had to undergo a process of learning, trial and error, and growth as the role of case manager and the responsibilities of shared governance have been experienced. As with any learning situation, efficiency has suffered as we have tried different communication methods and made changes in the operational routines. Most important, however, the changes have stemmed from the experiences and ideas of the staff

TABLE 9.1 Failure to Wean: Critical Pathway

	SCU day						
	1	2	3	7	14	21	28 (Discharge)
Teaching/ discussion	Purpose of SCU, case management, SCU routines		DNR[a] status, patient goals, including weaning plan	Placement/ discharge goal	Confirmation of discharge goal		
Tests	Chem 23 CBC[b] Prealbumin Cardiac monitor I&O/weight	Cardiac monitor I&O/weight	Cardiac monitor I&O/weight	Chem 23 CBC Prealbumin UUN[c] Cardiac monitor I&O/weight Pulse oximetry for weaning	Chem 23 CBC Prealbumin UUN Cardiac monitor I&O/weight Pulse oximetry for weaning	Chem 23 CBC Prealbumin UUN I&O[d]/weight	
Treatments	Assist/control ventilator Postural drainage and clapping	Assist/control ventilator Postural drainage and clapping	Assist/control ventilator Postural drainage and clapping	Wean on T-piece, 30 min, x 2 Postural drainage and clapping	Wean 4 hr x 2 Postural drainage and clapping	Without ventilator 24 hr Postural drainage and clapping	
Activity	Bed rest	Bed rest	Lift to chair (1 hr)	Lift to chair (2hr)	Dangle, two-person assist to chair	Up to chair with one person assist	
Nutrition	Per SCU nutritionist or as in ICU	Per SCU nutritionist	Half strength TF[e], 50 ml/hr	Full strength TF, 90 ml/hr	Beginning PO/maintained with TF	PO[f], supplement with TF, if necessary	
Consultations	OT[g] PT[j]	Nutrition Social work		Neurology, if disorientation persists	GI[h] if PEG[i] necessary		

[a]Do not resuscitate.
[b]Complete blood cell count.
[c]Urinary urea nitrogen.
[d]Intake and output.
[e]Tube feeding.
[f]By mouth.
[g]Occupational therapy.
[h]Gastroenterology.
[i]Percutaneous endoscopic gastrostomy.
[j]Physical Therapy.

themselves. Although this approach has sometimes slowed the process of change, it has been an essential element in the development of the unit.

RESULTS

We believe it is important that the success or failure of this newly created environment for the care of the chronically critically ill be carefully evaluated. The potential for changing the way in which care is delivered to this vulnerable and increasing population is great and it requires rigorous testing with a well-designed prospective procedure for capturing both patient and nurse outcomes.

A research project was initiated with the opening of the SCU. The purpose of the study is to compare the effects of the SCU with the effects of traditional ICUs on nurse and patient outcomes. The nurse outcomes to be compared are satisfaction, absenteeism, and retention; the patient outcomes are length of stay, complications (respiratory and infections), mortality, readmission rate, cost, and patient and family satisfaction with care. Figure 9.1 reflects the study design.

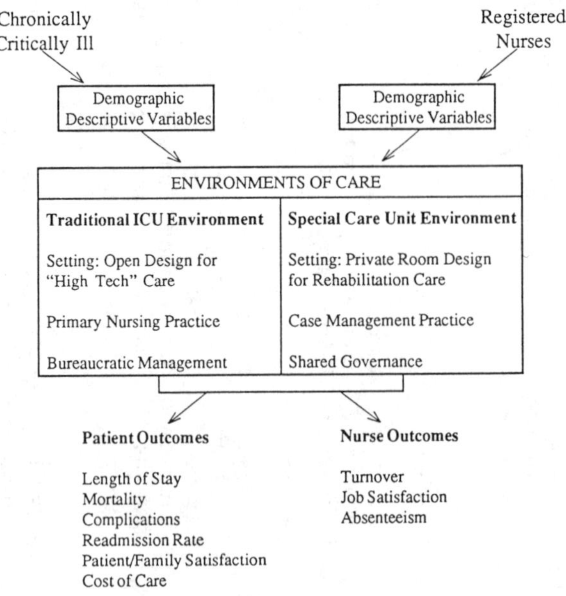

FIGURE 9.1 SCU study design.

Note: Reprinted from B. Daly, E. Rudy, K. Thompson, & M. Happ, 1991, "Development of a special care unit for chronically critically ill patients," *Heart & Lung*, *20*, 45-51. Copyright 1991 by Mosby. Reprinted by permission.

Twice a week every patient in the MICU and SICU is assessed for eligibility for transfer to the SCU by use of the admission algorithm (see Figure 9.2). Subject criteria include:

Length of stay in ICU > 7 days,
Not currently receiving IV vasopressors (low-level maintenance drip is an exception),
No pulmonary artery monitor required,
No arterial monitor required,
No acute event (arrest, unstable event) in past 3 days,
APACHE (Acute Physiology and Chronic Health Evaluation) II 15 or less,
TISS (Therapeutic Intervention Scoring System) Class II or III (10–39 points), and
Unable to be cared for on general nursing unit.

Once it has been established that the patient meets the criteria for eligibility, he or she is randomly assigned by the flip of a coin either to remain in his or her present unit (control group) or to be transferred to the SCU (experimental group). The usual requirements for informed consent apply.

The study results to date are summarized in the tables. At the 2-year point we had had 144 patients. The patients were evenly divided in terms of gender. They were predominantly white, matching the demographics of our hospital, and older, much like the initial pilot group we examined (see Table 9.2).

Patient outcomes are shown in Table 9.3. We are getting SCU patients out of the hospital 6 days earlier than patients in the ICU. The difference between SCU and ICU patients is not statistically significant yet, because there is a very wide range in patient stays. Some of our patients stay 190 days. Note the mortality rates on this table. That was a surprise to us. We monitored mortality rates because we were taking people out of a traditional ICU, away from all the usual monitoring, and we wanted to be sure we were not putting them at increased risk. We did not expect, however, that we were going to make this dramatic a difference in mortality rates.

Complications are another category of outcome. We monitor three kinds: infections, respiratory complications, and what we call "other life threatening complications" (see Table 9.4). There is no significant difference in the total frequency of any of these. Each group is a little higher in one category or other, but not significantly. The figures remind us, again, that these are very sick people.

We have seen a significant difference show up in the incidence of sepsis. There have been significantly fewer episodes of sepsis in the SCU than in the ICU, and we are convinced that is because the first thing we do for these patients is get out all invasive lines. We take out their CVP and take out

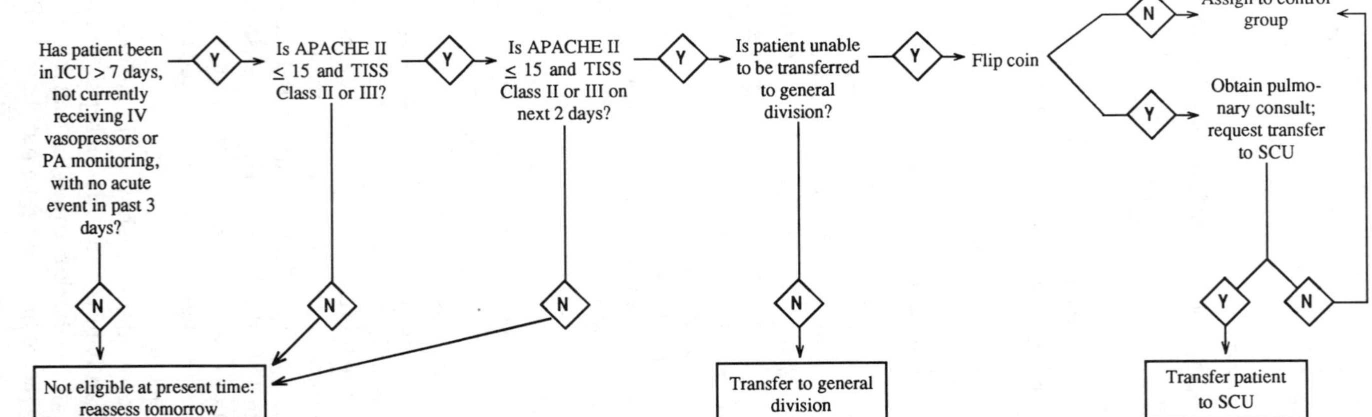

FIGURE 9.2 Algorithm for patient selection. APACHE, Acute Physiology and Chronic Health Evaluation; IV, intravenous; PA, pulmonary artery; TISS, Therapeutic Intervention Scoring System.

Note: Reprinted from B. Daly, E. Rudy, K. Thompson, & M. Happ, 1991, "Development of a special care unit for chronically critically ill patients," *Heart & Lung*, *20*, 45-51. Copyright 1991 by Mosby. Reprinted by permission.

TABLE 9.2 Subject Characteristics

Variables		Special Care Unit (n = 96t)		Intensive Care Units (n = 48)		Total (n = 144)	
		N	Percentage	*N*	Percentage	*N*	Percentage
Sex:	female	47	49	24	50	71	49
	male	49	51	24	50	73	51
Race	black	27	28	15	31	42	29
	white	69	72	33	69	102	71
Age:	mean	65.0		62.6		64.2	
	S.D.	16.4		15.8		16.2	
	range	16–90		17–85		16–90	
Previous ICU (patients come from):							
	CICU	10	10.4	3	6.3	13	9.0
	MICU	27	28.1	17	35.4	44	30.6
	SICU	53	55.2	22	45.8	75	52.1
	NSU	6	6.3	6	12.5	12	8.3
Prestudy ICU LOS (days)							
	mean	18.4		16.6		17.8	
	S.D.	16.3		13.5		15.4	
	range	3–99		6–60		3–99	
Medical diagnosis							
	cardiovascular	47	49.0	16	33.3	63	43.8
	respiratory	35	36.5	20	41.7	55	38.2
	neurologic	9	9.4	8	16.7	17	11.8
	GI & other	5	5.1	4	8.4	9	6.3

TABLE 9.3 Clinical Outcomes

Variables	Special Care Unit (n = 96)		Intensive Care Units (n = 48)		Total (n = 144)	
	N	Percentage	*N*	Percentage	*N*	Percentage
Discharge disposition from hospital						
died	32	33.3	24	50.0	56	38.9
other hospital	4	4.2	1	2.1	5	3.5
long–term care	15	15.6	8	16.7	23	16.0
rehabilitation	12	12.5	2	4.2	14	9.7
home	31	32.3	13	27.1	44	30.6
home ventilator	2	2.1	0		2	1.4
Discharge disposition from hospital						
died	32	33.3	24	50.0	56	38.9
institutions	31	32.3	11	22.9	42	29.2
home	33	34.4	13	27.1	46	31.9
Discharge disposition of ICU[a]						
died	30	31.3	15	31.3	45	31.3
in hospital	26	27.1	31	64.6	57	39.6
institutions	20	20.8	1	2.1	21	14.6
home	20	20.8	1	2.1	21	14.6

Length of hospital stay (days)						
mean	51.6		57.3		53.5	
S. D.	30.3		38.5		33.3	
range	9–160		8–176		9–176	
Days in study						
mean	25.9		25.0		25.6	
S.D.	19.0		26.0		21.6	
range	1–76		1–140		1–140	
Survival status on discharge from hospital (% mortality)[b]						
died	32	33.3	24	50.0	56	39.0
lived	64	66.7	24	50.0	88	61.0
Survival status on discharge from ICU/SCU (% mortality)						
died	30	31.0	15	31.0	45	31.0
lived	66	69.0	33	69.0	99	69.0

[a]$X^2(3) = 26.8, p < .001$.
[b]$X^2(1) = 3.74, p = .053$.

TABLE 9.4 Complication Outcomes

Variables	Special Care Unit (n = 96)		Intensive Care (Units n = 48)		Total (n = 144)	
	N	Percentage	*N*	Percentage	*N*	Percentage
Infectious Complications						
Total number of infections						
mean	1.84		1.94		1.88	
S.D.	2.46		2.53		2.47	
range	0–10		0–10		0–10	
No	46	48	22	46	68	47
Yes	50	52	26	54	76	53
Number of respiratory infections						
mean	0.65		0.85		0.72	
S.D.	1.1		1.22		1.14	
range	0–4		0–4		0–4	
No	64	67	28	58	92	64
Yes	32	33	20	42	52	36
Number of urinary infections						
mean	0.64		0.48		0.58	
S.D.	1.05		0.77		0.96	
range	0–4		0–2		0–4	
No	63	66	33	69	96	67
Yes	33	34	15	31	48	33
Number of blood infections[a,b]						
mean	0.13		0.35		0.20	
S.D.	0.46		0.86		0.63	
range	0–3		0–4		0–4	
No	88	92	38	79	126	87.5
Yes	8	8	10	21	18	12.5

Number of wound infections									
mean		0.11			0.08			0.10	
S.D.		0.41			0.35			0.39	
range		0–2			0–2			0–2	
No	88		92	45		94	133		92
Yes	8		8	3		6	11		8
Number of other infections									
mean		0.32			0.17			0.27	
S.D.		0.69			0.63			0.67	
range		0–3			0–4			0–4	
No	75		78	43		90	118		82
Yes	21		33	5		10	26		18
Total Number of respiratory complications									
mean		1.99			2.27			2.08	
S.D.		1.69			2.00			1.80	
range		0–7			0–7			0–7	
Atlectasis									
No	80		83	38		79	118		82
Yes	16		17	10		21	26		18
Hypoxia									
No	39		41	27		56	66		46
Yes	57		59	21		44	78		54
Respiratory infection[b]									
No	75		78	30		62	105		73
Yes	21		22	18		38	39		27
Pulmonary emboli									
No	94		98	48		100	142		99
Yes	2		2	0		0	2		1
Failure to Wean[c]									
No	86		90	37		77	123		85
Yes	10		10	11		23	21		15

[a]ANOVA for mean differences: $F(1,142) = 4.3, p = .040$
Chi Square for group differences: $X^2(1) = 4.571, p = .033$

[b]$X^2(1) = 3.96, p = .047$
[c]$X^2(1) = 4.01, p = .045$

their arterial line; we do not use these unless we absolutely have to. So, with less invasive technology, of course, we expose the patient to less risk. And since that is the most important kind of infection, we think this is a very important finding.

Respiratory outcomes vary a bit. The SCU patients are lower in atelectasis, a little higher in hypoxia. We think that is because we very aggressively wean these patients. We approach weaning from a ventilator as something that will happen with every patient. We assume that living on a ventilator is not an acceptable outcome for most patients, and we just assume that all patients are weanable. Thus the idea that a patient is "unweanable" is something we do not consider. The incidence of pulmonary edema reflects the fact that most patients have coexisting heart disease. Their heart disease is clearly the most important factor in getting them off the ventilator. We think we have fewer episodes of failure to wean because we pay attention to patient readiness. Ours is not a "cowboy" approach such as you might see in surgical ICUs. We very carefully monitor and adjust fluid balance and we are very conservative with interventions. We correct anemia and malnutrition and have very good success with weaning.

The financial or cost outcomes are shown in Table 9.5. We do a detailed analysis of costs, looking at charges (hospital bill), payment (reimbursement), and actual costs. These are expensive patients, with an average bill of $154,335. The average actual cost to the hospital per patient is $6,000 less for the SCU group. The margin is, literally, the bottom line. It is the difference between what we were paid to take care of the patient, and what it cost us. You can see that for the average patient in the ICU, we show a positive margin or a profit of $1,313 and for each control patient who stays in the ICU, the hospital loses an average of $11,066.

If we take that margin and multiply it by the number of patients in the study thus far, the Special Care Unit has been associated with a profit of $106,353 and the ICU patients have produced a loss of $453,706 for the hospital. This tends to be very convincing data. Now, as you know, almost all patients in this age group are paid for through a DRG system. One significance of this is that we have to think about the fact that some DRGs are, in a sense, more costly or more profitable than others. To control for that, we use a derived figure called "standard." We take the patient's payment and cost and divide it by the DRG weight, to make sure that these good results have not happened just because we happened to get the more "profitable" patients. In fact, we found that the difference was even more marked when we used standard figures and factored out the influence of the DRG. This just confirms our results.

The question now is, why is the SCU less costly? Remember, this is cost, not charge, so it is not just that we bill the patient for less; it actually costs less. To analyze this we took the hospital bill and looked only at the period

TABLE 9.5 Patient Cost Data[a]

Parameter	Special Care Unit $n = 81$	Intensive Care Units $n = 41$
Average charges/patient		
mean	154,335	176,487
S.D.	84,275	123,572
range	30,404–413,460	40,109–548,829
Average payments/patient		
mean	70,642	65,291
S.D.	46,722	47,933
range	3,698–212,452	4,699–199,771
Average cost/patient		
mean	68,458	74,765
S.D.	39,556	44,928
range	1,420–228,885	13,880–207,151
Margin (payment–cost)		
mean	1,313	–11,066
S.D.	35,197	36,101
range	–68,215–103,184	–131,911–53,668
DRG weight		
mean	8.24	6.73
S.D.	5.133	5.34
range	.454–14.1506	.5123–14.1506
Standard payment (payment/DRG weight)		
mean	11,608	15,686
S.D.	11,617	20,380
range	1,901–60,368	3,847–117,837
Standard cost/patient (cost/DRG weight)[b]		
mean	13,114	23,731
S.D.	13,111	39,496
range	536–82,566	2,764–245,292
Margin x # of patients		
estimated net profit	106,353	0
estimated net loss	0	453,706

[a]Due to varying *N*s the mean differences do not equal the difference of the means.
[b]$F(1,120) = 4.79$, $p = .031$

when the patient was in the study, separating out charges for the different services. There was a significant difference in X-ray charges and laboratory charges, which says that we are actually changing the pattern of care. We are doing different things—and mostly fewer things—for these people. For example, when our patients have a headache, we do not do a CAT scan, we give them an aspirin. That illustrates our approach nicely. Our view is that these are very fragile patients, they have multiple system problems, and probably the less we do to them, the better. Pharmacy charges are also quite different because we use the same approach with medications. One of the things we do in addition to getting lines out is to stop prescribing many drugs. These patients are on multiple medications when they come to us and we stop many of them. Respiratory therapy is significantly different because we rarely do blood gases. Blood product charges are less, not because we give fewer red cells, but because we do not use albumin, which is heavily used by surgeons in our institution.

We also take another approach to cost. We look at each patient in the 7 days before he entered the study and the 7 days after he entered, and we simply count the number of CBCs, electrolytes, blood gases, and chest X-rays. The week before the patients come to us they are getting more than one CBC a day, more than one set of electrolytes, three blood gases a day, and one chest X-ray. Those of you who work in ICUs know how this happens; it's just the routine. It doesn't have to be ordered, everybody does it because it is expected. When patients come to us, we cut down on all of that, especially the blood gases. In the week after the patients transfer to the SCU, diagnostic testing rates decrease to about 3 CBC's, one electrolyte panel, one blood gas, and two chest X-rays a week. In contrast, when they stay in the ICU, there is almost no change. This is not because the patients need the tests, it is because that is the unwritten protocol in ICUs.

DISCUSSION

The preliminary conclusions on our SCU are clear. First, although we have another year of data collection, we are convinced that we have enough data now to say that the special care unit model is associated with care that is less costly and equally, if not more, effective than care in traditional ICUs for this population. Second, job satisfaction has increased in some respects for the nurses in the special care unit, as reflected in reduced absenteeism and reduced turnover.

There are many additional questions raised by this study. For example, we do not know if this model can be utilized in community hospitals. We have submitted a request for supplemental funding to test it in two community hospitals to see if the patterns that we have found hold in different settings. We also do not know if this model has implications for the organization of care for other kinds of patients. It fits these people, but we do not know about other kinds of patients. Also, we do not know what happens to these people when they go home. Overall they have about a 30% to 40% hospital mortality rate, and they are still quite sick when we send them out.

Finally, the most important question is, how can we stop producing patients who are this sick? Although we are able to send some patients home, a third of them go to nursing homes, and a third die in the hospital. Of the two-thirds who survive at hospital discharge, an additional third die in the first year post-discharge. This clearly raises questions both about better treatment approaches that can prevent "chronic critical illness" and about the tremendous costs, both personal and financial, of treating these patients.

ACKNOWLEDGMENT

The opening section of this chapter is reprinted from "Development of a special care unit for chronically critically ill patients," by B. Daly, E. Rudy, K. Thompson, & M. Happ, 1991, *Heart & Lung, 20,* pp. 45–51. Copyright 1991 by Mosby. Reprinted by permission. This research was funded by the National Center for Nursing Research, NIH, Grant # ROI NR 02248–02.

REFERENCES

Berenson, R. A. (1984). Health technology case study 28: Intensive care units—clinical outcomes, costs and decision making. Congress, OTA-HCS-28. Washington, DC: Office of Technology Assessment.

General Accounting Office. (1986). Past overuse of intensive care services inflate hospital payments. (GAO/HRD-86-25). Washington, DC: Government Printing Office.

Loveridge, C., Cummings, S. H., & O'Malley, J. (1988). Developing case management in a primary nursing system. *Journal of Nursing Administration, 18*(10), 36–39.

Secretary's Commission on Nursing: Final report. (1988). Washington, DC: Office of the Secretary, U.S. Department of Health and Human Services publication, Vol 3v:iII.

Zander, K. (1988). Nursing case management: Strategic management of cost and quality outcomes. *Journal of Nursing Administration, 18*(9), 23–30.

[10]

Special Care Units for Persons with Alzheimer's Disease: A Successful Intervention?

Kathleen Coen Buckwalter, Meridean L. Maas, Elizabeth A. Swanson, and Geri Richards Hall

Recent studies indicate that currently over 4 million persons may be afflicted with Alzheimer's disease (AD), the leading cause of dementia (Evans et al., 1989); about 70% of new admissions to nursing homes are demented (Rovner et al., 1990). Despite recent efforts to improve the quality of long-term care, there continue to be problems with the care of residents with dementing illness (U. S. Congress, Office of Technology Assessment [OTA], 1987).

The concept of special care units (SCUs) designed especially for persons with dementia is not a new one; in fact, the first such unit was opened at the Philadelphia Geriatric Center almost 20 years ago. In the past decade, however, SCUs have become the most rapidly growing segment of the health care industry (Coons, 1991). A 1987 survey found that approximately 1700 nursing homes in this country had special care units or programs for persons with dementia (Leon, Potter, & Cunningham, 1990). Nearly a third of those nursing homes were planning to expand their programs, whereas another 1400 facilities were planning to open new special care units within the next year. The research reported here represents an initial effort to address the question, "Is segregating persons with Alzheimer's disease a successful intervention strategy?" (Maas & Buckwalter, 1990).

Alzheimer's disease is characterized by progressive, inexorable deterioration of cognitive skills and functional status. The average length of time from diagnosis to death is around 10 years. Throughout the course of the illness, persons with AD present increasingly difficult care problems because of behavioral dysfunction, and usually nursing home placement is eventually required. Although persons with dementia constitute 65% of nursing home residents (Hing, 1987), many facilities are not equipped to deal with the heavy care demands of the demented resident. Most still integrate confused and nonconfused residents, which may not be in the best interest of lucid residents (Hall, Kirschling, & Todd, 1986; Johnson, 1989; Kane, 1987; Wiltzius, Gambert, & Duthie, 1981). Many have staff who are unprepared to deal with the complex and ever-changing emotional, behavioral, and physical needs of demented patients (Chambers, 1990; Sbordone & Sterman, 1988).

Prior to implementation of the regulations of the Omnibus Budget Reconciliation Act in October of 1990, chemical and physical restraints were the prevailing treatment for behavioral dysfunctions in AD patients. Although structured environmental strategies, such as special care units, have been proposed as a key to providing better care both for persons with Alzheimer's disease and related disorders (ADRD) and for nondemented residents of long-term care facilities (Benson, Cameron, Humback, Servino, & Gambert, 1987), there remains much controversy about the critical and most beneficial characteristics of SCUs (Berg et al., 1991). The question, "What makes a special care unit special?" is essential to understanding the nature of the research reported here and is a compelling reason for conducting this type of evaluative research as special care units proliferate in this country.

Quite simply, the best answer to the question of what makes a special care unit special is now, regrettably, "It depends," or, "We don't know." At present there is no standard definition of a special care unit, there is no uniform terminology used nationally, and there are no standard criteria by which to evaluate or regulate SCUs (Maas & Buckwalter, 1988; Schultz, 1987). Literally, a facility could put a Lazy-Boy recliner and an afghan in a room and hang out a shingle marketing this as a "Special Care Unit." There would be very little that concerned health care providers, state agencies, or family members could do, because the facility would not be violating any national statutes, and licensure of SCUs and related regulatory mechanisms are only available now in six states (Alzheimer's Association, 1992). This is of particular concern because the AD population is extremely vulnerable to promises of "special care," in that caregivers are often in crisis, feel very guilty about "abandoning" their loved one, and are looking for the best possible type of institutional placement. Thus, without uniform standards for SCUs, the potential for abuse of this vulnerable population is great, and there is no way to avoid or correct inappropriate use of the concept of special care, or to prevent marketing of SCUs which may have no beneficial effects or may even be harmful.

DEFINITIONS AND CRITERIA OF AN SCU

A specialized environment and program(s) of care distinguish SCUs from merely "segregated" units (Buckwalter, 1991). Iowa was the first state to develop licensure for special care units, and we used the state's definition for our study, although, as noted earlier, definitions vary from state to state. In our research a special care unit was defined as a "distinct part of the health care facility, clearly identifiable, containing contiguous rooms in a separate wing or building, or on a separate floor of the facility, and for which a special program of care has been approved" (ADRDA Unit Rules Committee, 1988).

The literature suggests that at least five characteristics are "special" about special care units. These are: 1) special staff selection and training; 2) unique physical environment and decor, including separation of the cognitively impaired from lucid residents; 3) specialized admission criteria (Buckwalter, 1991); 4) family programming; and 5) activity programming. Each of these will be briefly reviewed in this chapter; interested readers are referred to the article "Special Care Units for Persons with Dementia" (Berg et al., 1991) for a more detailed account.

Staff Selection and Training

With regard to staff selection and training, the literature suggests that requirements and content vary dramatically from unit to unit, with, on average, 10 hours of specialized training per staff member (Greene, Asp, & Crane, 1985). The unit on which we conducted our research is somewhat unique in that SCU staff were required to complete 40 hours of didactic training and another 40 hours of experiential training (for a total of 80 hours), whereas some units require no specialized training whatsoever. Staff members (level of preparation/professional discipline) and staffing patterns also vary considerably, although SCUs tend to be staffed like skilled units or skilled nursing facilities, with staff/patient ratios ranging from about 1:4 to 1:6 (Ackerman, 1985). Hours of care per patient per day range anywhere from 2 to 5 (Schultz, 1987). A consistent theme in the literature on SCUs is that staff morale is an extremely important variable for the success of the unit, and the most critical characteristics to look for in hiring somebody to work on an SCU are common sense, flexibility, and knowledge (Peppard, 1989).

Physical Environment and Decor

Although there is no set formula for constructing an SCU, most provide comfort, security and safety for the cognitively impaired resident while allowing freedom of movement (Beitler, 1988). Many special care units also have some sort of lower or managed stimuli. This concept is not to be interpreted as the *absence* of stimuli, in that the environment is not sterile; rather it is an environment of controlled stimuli. Environmental modifications are designed to reduce noxious and confusing stimuli and extraneous noise, such as "busy" patterned fabrics, blaring public address systems, mirrors, and congregate dining. The rationale for this approach is that people who are cognitively impaired have increasing difficulty in interpreting and processing normal levels of stimuli (Maas, 1988) as a result of progressive cerebral pathology and associated cognitive and functional decline (Hall & Buckwalter, 1987). Both environmental and internal stressors constitute demands that make the person with dementia anxious and agitated, and if the stressful stimuli are allowed to continue or increase, behavior becomes more dysfunctional and often catastrophic.

For safety and security, secured doorways, alarmed exits, and other special precautions are used to prevent elopement or injury. The philosophy of care often is that remaining functional abilities should be enhanced while supporting those domains in which there is loss, such as conative or planning abilities, functional abilities, cognitive abilities, and the affective domain (Hall & Buckwalter, 1987). Many units seek to optimize freedom and flexibility through adequate lighting, design of innovative wandering patterns or outdoor courtyards, for example, and provision of interesting but safe objects for exploration. Indoor decor varies greatly among units, although many employ moderate color schemes with bright colors for emphasis/contrast, and encourage the use of possessions from home to personalize the environment and make common areas more homelike (Beitler, 1988).

The literature suggests that rooms in most SCUs are single or double occupancy (Greene, Asp, & Crane, 1985), and optimum unit size for both staff and patients is around 20 beds (Johnson, 1989). However, there is great variability in this as well: Some SCUs are very small, consisting of only four or five beds, others are "cluster units" at the end of a hallway, and some of the larger units range all the way up to 40–60 beds (Hepburn, Severance, Gates, & Christensen, 1989; Schultz, 1987).

Admission Criteria

Although there are no standard admission criteria for SCUs, most units admit residents with dementia who are ambulatory or wheelchair bound. Many SCUs make an effort to rule out reversible dementias such as acute confusional states (delirium) and dementias that may mimic a chronic dementia but are caused by infections, acute metabolic disorders, hypoxia, vitamin/mineral deficiencies, or other etiologies. Some units report using more standardized criteria, such as Reisberg, Ferris, deLeon, & Crook's (1982) Global Deterioration Scale (GDS), to "stage" residents. Using this scale, the majority of admissions rate around a 5 or 6, meaning they are in the middle to late confusional stage, at which time families commonly seek placement. Higher functioning residents are not recommended for special care units (Buckwalter, 1991).

A pre-admission assessment is highly recommended to determine the appropriateness of placement on the SCU, as is a comprehensive neurological work-up to diagnose dementia by ruling out other reversible or confounding conditions. Some nursing homes have specialized units designed to be most therapeutic for particular stages of dementia, and individuals are moved to another unit once their functional and cognitive status deteriorates beyond a certain point. For example, residents are relocated to a "bed-fast" unit in the later stages of the disease when they become immobile (Buckwalter, 1991). However, strict criteria for relocating residents to another unit are still not used in most settings.

Family Programming

The role of family vis-à-vis the special care unit and its staff remains quite unclear and confusing (Buckwalter & Hall, 1987). Recently the National Institute on Aging funded two projects to address this important but neglected issue, and the authors have recently completed pilot work to test an intervention creating a new role for family members as partners with staff caregivers. Clearly some family-specific programming exists in many units, but it varies a great deal in intensity, frequency, and quality. Many units are developing visitor training programs because they have found that when the family is trained to visit appropriately, staff do not have to deal with negative sequelae after the family leaves—that is, disruptive behaviors such as "Oh, I want to go home" and similar agitated verbalizations, as well as nighttime wakefulness. Support groups and education/information groups for family members are also increasing in special care units. These are potentially important in enhancing family involvement and level of satisfaction, which vary greatly from unit to unit (Maas, Buckwalter, Kelley, & Stolley, 1991).

Activity Programming

Most special care units have some sort of specialized activity programming that is geared to the cognitive and functional level of persons with dementia. Many SCUs, in fact, employ a part-time activities coordinator. However, the amount and nature of the activities differ depending on the unit's philosophy of care. For example, some units are very rehabilitation oriented, whereas others have more of a custodial/maintenance orientation. Some facilities stress continuity and routinization in their programming, although most successful activity programs allow for greater creativity and flexibility (Hall et al., 1986; Schultz, 1987). Flexibility appears to be an essential characteristic—not everyone is going to want to play bingo or make leather coin purses just because they are old and demented. Certainly there is need for attention to issues of cultural sensitivity in planning activities. For example, the special care unit where we conducted our study is located in rural Iowa and serves primarily a retired farmer population. Thus cooking and various housekeeping-type activities (e.g., folding linen, setting the table), which are often very successful activities in other settings, are simply not of interest to these residents, whereas woodworking, gardening, and other kinds of large muscle group activities are extremely well received. The benefits of reality orientation for the demented population remain controversial and without empirical support for any long-lasting effects.

The philosophy of care advanced by the American Association of Homes for the Aged (Beitler, 1988) supports the highest level of resident functioning while accommodating individual differences, responding to changing abilities over time, and compensating for losses while supporting remaining abilities. As with all the key characteristics of special care units, much more systematic research on programming is needed.

SCUS: PROS AND CONS

The major argument against special care units presented in the literature is that no dramatic difference in outcomes has been observed between segregated and integrated units (Holmes et al., 1990; Mathew, Sloan, Kilby, & Flood, 1988). This may be because many units lack diagnostic precision, they use inconsistent admission and discharge criteria, and the staff have inadequate training. Further, costs of care in SCUs are reported to be generally higher, on balance about $10 more per patient per day (U. S. Congress OTA, 1987), although Maas and Buckwalter (1990) found no difference in nursing care costs.

The argument for special care units includes the fact that there is at least anecdotal evidence that nondemented (lucid) residents suffer from close proximity to persons with cognitive impairment, that is, other residents rummaging in their closets, sleeping in their beds, and urinating in their philodendrons. Staff consistently report that they believe they provide better care on a specialized unit (Grossman, Weiner, Salamon, & Burrows, 1986). Family satisfaction is reported to be higher on SCUs, and there has been a documented decrease in the use of chemical and physical restraints, as well as less weight loss among residents with dementia housed on a special care unit (Cleary, Clamon, Price, & Shullaw, 1988; Hall et al., 1986).

To expand a bit more on the point that housing lucid and demented residents together is harmful to the former, the problems reported most frequently for lucid residents include invasion of privacy, lost or damaged personal property, decreased socialization, interrupted sleep patterns, and fear of physical harm from agitated residents. Also, there may be problems for demented residents. For example, they tend to get more than their fair share of tranquilizing medication, which has negative sequelae associated with it, and they are often excluded from traditional planned activities and subsequently experience decreased socialization (Hall et al., 1986; Johnson, 1989; Kane, 1987; Wiltzius, Gambert, & Duthie, 1981). It has been suggested that persons with dementia may not really understand why they cannot go on a particular outing or event that all the other residents are attending, but they know at some affective level that they have been excluded, which has implications for their self-esteem and feelings of self-worth. Of course, this is a very difficult dimension to operationalize and measure, and therefore very few studies have systematically investigated the problems posed by having demented and lucid elders live together.

Problems Associated with Research on SCUs

As noted earlier, there has been little empirical support reported for special care units. There is a paucity of systematic evaluation, and most of the research has been conducted on single units without adequate controls (Ohta & Ohta, 1988). The research conducted in single-unit settings may suffer from bias and lack of generalizability because staffing patterns, training, and other unit characteristics vary so dramatically. Also, a difficult problem with research of this nature is getting an adequate sample size with sufficient power to detect differences in outcomes, because of the high level of attrition in this frail population.

THE STUDY

The purpose of this study was to assess the effects of special care units on patient, family, staff, and cost variables. The aims of the study were: 1) to document differences between experimental and control groups on a variety of dependent variables; 2) to document clinical and cost effectiveness differences between experimental and control groups; and 3) to describe differences over time within the experimental and control groups. Patients in the special care unit served as the experimental group and those on traditional integrated nursing home units in the same facility served as the control group.

The fit and interactions between person and environment served as the general framework for the study (Kahana, 1975; Lawton, 1975). Silverstone and Burach-Weiss (1983) contend that dysfunctional and socially inappropriate behaviors of AD patients can be explained by person-environment interactions. The impairment of ego-sensory, perceptual, and cognitive processes affects AD patients' overall ability to interact successfully with their environment. Because of these disease-related impairments, AD patients exhibit behaviors that indicate disordered person-environment interactions, including repetitive, dysfunctional, and catastrophic behaviors (Roberts & Algase, 1988).

Based on the premise that disordered AD patient-environment interactions occur when environmental demands exceed the AD patient's abilities to adjust, Hall and Buckwalter (1987) formulated the Progressively Lowered Stimulus Threshold (PLST) Model. They proposed that persons with AD need environmental conditions to be modified because of their declining cognitive and functional abilities and their increasing difficulty in dealing with stress. If the stress level continues or increases as a result of environmental and internal demands, the patient's behavior becomes more dysfunctional and often catastrophic. Most importantly, the PLST model suggests that stress can be reduced with modification of the patient's environmental demands, and functional adaptive behavior can be promoted. Patients on special care units can thus be expected to exhibit less inappropriate behavior and to maintain cognitive and functional skills (Hall & Buckwalter, 1987).

Specifically, an environment with reduced stimuli is postulated to create less demand on the cognitive processing abilities of AD patients, so they can use their remaining cognitive abilities more effectively. In turn, the more effective use of cognitive abilities should result in greater retention of the functional abilities of dressing, grooming, toileting, and eating and in less agitation and fewer socially unacceptable behaviors. Thus in the study reported here, a slower rate of cognitive and functional decline with fewer adverse behaviors and less use of chemical and physical restraints was expected for patients with AD on the SCU than for patients on traditional integrated units.

Specific research questions posed were these:

1. Are there slower rates of deterioration (both functional and cognitive) for patients in the special care unit?
2. Do they have fewer falls?
3. Do they have less injurious falls?
4. Do they consume more or less health care resources?
5. Are fewer medications and lower drug costs required for patients with AD on the special care unit?
6. Is there a difference in the level of restraint use?
7. What are the family members' perceptions of care, and are families of patients on an SCU more satisfied?

8. What are the differences in staff on the experimental and control units, in terms of knowledge, job satisfaction, absenteeism, and stress levels? (One important argument against special care units is that they are too stressful for the staff and attrition rates are therefore increased in an industry with too much staff turnover to begin with.)

METHOD

Design, Sample, and Setting

A field quasi-experiment with repeated measures was used to compare the effects of an SCU on AD patients, staff, and families with the effects of care provided on traditional integrated units at a large state veterans' home in the Midwest. The design for the study and data collection points are illustrated in Table 10.1.

The Iowa Veterans' Home (IVH) is a state-owned long-term care facility serving veterans and their spouses. It provides residential, intermediate, skilled, and comprehensive rehabilitative care to 764 residents, 120 of whom are women and 100 of whom are nonveterans. Services available at the IVH include nursing; dentistry; physical, occupational, and speech therapy; pharmacy; radiology; clinical psychology; medicine; optometry; social services; recreation therapy; dietician care; and audiology.

The SCU is a 20-bed self-contained unit designed to segregate AD residents from nondemented residents and to allow unrestricted safe wandering on the unit and in a fenced-in courtyard contiguous with the SCU. Staff are selected to work on the SCU based on seniority and demonstrated ability to work with the cognitively impaired. All staff who care for residents with AD receive 80 hours of formal training (40 didactic and 40 supervised clinical practicum). The content areas addressed in the training program

TABLE 10.1 Study Design and Data Collection Points

Study Design (Patient, Staff, and Family Members)													
E	O1	O2	O3	O4	O5	O6	X	O7	O8	O9	O10	O11	O12
C	O1	O2	O3	O4	O5	O6		O7	O8	O9	O10	O11	O12

Phase 1	(Pretreatment measures January–December, 1986)	Phase II	(Posttreatment measures May 1987–June 1988)

Where: O = bimonthly measurements before and after the Special Unit was created
X = Special Care Unit
E = Experimental Group
C = Comparison Group

include the AD disease process; cognitive and functional sequelae; rationale for a controlled, therapeutic environment and programming interventions; actions and recommended use of psychotropic medications; and behavioral approaches that employ concepts of unconditional positive regard, managed stimuli, flexibility, diversion, avoidance of physical and chemical restraints, and use of psychosocial rehabilitative modalities such as reminiscence, art, music, and recreational therapies. Staff assigned on the SCU remain on the unit and are not rotated to other units. Similarly, staff from other units are not rotated to the SCU.

A full-time activities specialist assigned to the SCU coordinates therapeutic and diversional activities. Activities are designed around the individual needs of the residents to maximize cognitive and functional abilities and to prevent agitated and dysfunctional behaviors. Rest is an important therapy and is combined with activity.

Family programming includes an active family support group coordinated by the social worker and primary nurses. SCU policies outline an orientation for family members to the SCU philosophy, program objectives, the roles of staff, and education regarding visitation.

The SCU is designed according to Hall and Buckwalter's (1987) Progressively Lowered Stress Threshold Model, and emphasizes the management of environmental stress based on the individual abilities of the residents (Maas, 1988). The SCU is not devoid of sensory stimuli, but stimuli are managed and tailored to the progressively lowered cognitive and functional abilities of individual residents. Noise, shadow, traffic from other areas in the setting, and sensory overload are avoided while providing an environment that is pleasing to the senses, with cues to foster orientation and optimum functioning. Soothing music is played, and the decor is interesting in design, texture, and color. Furnishings and appointments are selected for safety and to withstand repetitive handling. Closets and drawers are kept locked except for one bedside drawer for each resident's use.

The SCU has specific admission criteria that include 1) diagnosis of irreversible dementia, confirmed by comprehensive psychoneurological examination; 2) middle stages of dementia as assessed by a score of 4–6 on the Global Deterioration Scale (GDS) (this scale is scored from 1 to 7 based on seven distinct clinically identifiable stages of the disease process) (Reisberg et al., 1982); and 3) ability to walk. Residents with psychoses, mental retardation, or reversible dementias are not admitted. Thus, all subjects in our study had scores on the GDS between 4 and 6 (mid-stage dementia) and none had reversible dementia or major psychiatric or developmental disorders.

All staff on both the SCU and the traditional units who cared for patients with AD were included in the study. Staff subjects in both groups received 80 hours of training (40 hours of didactic and 40 hours of experiential), prior to the collection of baseline measures. There were 42 staff assigned to the special care unit, 4 RNs, 6 LPNs, 25 nursing assistants, 1 unit clerk, 1 physician, 1 social worker, 1 dietician, and 1 recreation activities therapist, as well as 2 housekeeping staff. Comparison subjects with AD were housed on 14 other intermediate and skilled units where they were integrated with nondemented residents. Staffing on these units varied depending upon whether they were skilled or intermediate. SCU staffing was comparable to the staffing on skilled units. One important difference on traditional units was that staff (nursing and other disciplines) could not focus their programming on the special needs of the demented. One family member per patient was invited to participate in the study. The family member had to be 18 years of age or older and have at least monthly contact with the relative with AD.

Data Collection

Data on a broad range of dependent measures were collected bimonthly for 1 year prior to and 1 year following the opening of the SCU. Data to describe falls, restraints, medications, activities, behaviors, and morbidity were collected from patient records or staff observations. Staff observations were collected for one-half of the days in each 2 month period and were randomly selected. We measured a variety of patient, family and staff variables using standardized instruments as well as investigator-developed and psychometrically tested instruments. Table 10.2 lists the instruments used in the study and their purposes.

Patient Measures

Alzheimer's Disease Assessment Scale (ADAS) The ADAS was used to collect data on cognitive and noncognitive functioning of AD patients. The ADAS is designed specifically to evaluate the severity of cognitive and noncognitive behavioral dysfunctions characteristic of persons with AD (Rosen, Mohs, & Davis, 1984).

Geriatric Rating Scale (GRS) Activities of daily living (ADL) were assessed by the GRS, a 31-item rating scale of resident behavior. It is an observational scale that can be completed by members of the nursing staff (Plutchick et al., 1970).

Functional Abilities Checklist (FAC) The FAC was used to measure the functional abilities of AD patients in relation to ADLs including grooming, hygiene, toileting, bathing, eating, sleeping, exercising, and interacting with others in the environment. The five areas of functional abilities included in the scale are self-care activities, inappropriate behaviors, cognitive status, agitation, and sexual behaviors. The FAC was developed by

Maas and Buckwalter (1990) because other instruments in the literature did not include all of the areas relevant to the functional abilities of residents with AD.

Individual Incident Record (IIR) The IIR was developed to record daily occurrences of incidents that might be indicative of impaired AD patient safety and/or that were cost intensive for the institution and staff. AD patient behaviors indicating interaction with other patients and staff and participation in activities were also documented on the IIR. The incidents on the IIR include AD patient falls; psychotropic, hypnotic, and sedative medication use and response; use of physical restraints; 1:1 staff surveillance; wandering; participation in activities; and catastrophic reactions.

Family Measures

Demographic data were collected at the first observation point in the posttest only.

Family Perceptions Tool (FPT) A 36-item self-report FPT was developed by Maas and Buckwalter (1990) to measure four areas of family member perceptions: (1) satisfaction with overall care of the AD patient; (2) appropriateness of the patient unit environment; (3) quality of staff relation-

TABLE 10.2 Phases I and II Instruments

Purpose	Instrument	Rater	Time
Patients:			
Eligibility criteria	Global Deterioration Scale (GDS)	RN RA	15 min
Demography	Patient Demographic Tool	RN RA	5 min
Cognitive status	GDS	RN RA	
	Alzheimer's Disease Assessment Scale (ADAS)	RN RA	30 min
Functional status	Functional Abilities Checklist (FAC)	Primary RN	10 min
	Geriatric Rating Sale (GRS)	Primary RN	10 min
Falls, medications, restraints, behaviors, activities, morbidity	Individual Incident Report (IIR)	RN RA Nurse Staff	15 min
Family Members:			
Demography	Family Demographic Tool	Self	5 min
Satisfaction	Family Perceptions Tool (FPT)	Self	10 min
Staff:			
Demography	Staff Demographic Tool	Self/RA	5 min
Job satisfaction	Nursing Satisfaction Questionnaire (NSQ)	Self	15 min
Knowledge	Knowledge of Alzheimer's Test (KAT)	Self	10 min
Stress	Caregiver Stress Inventory (CSI)	Self	10 min
Burnout	Maslach Burnout Inventory (MBI)	Self	10 min
Absenteeism	Agency Records	RA	5 min

ships with patients and family members; and (4) the family member's satisfaction with physical care of the AD patient.

Staff Measures

Each staff member was assigned a code number known only to the investigators. Several of the staff measures were paper and pen instruments. In order to follow each subject, each staff person's code number was placed on the cover sheet of the questionnaires. All other information collected about the staff member was identified by this number. Demographic information about each staff member was collected at the initial contact. The other variables describing staff that were measured were knowledge about AD, job satisfaction, job stress, burnout, and absenteeism.

Maslach Burnout Inventory (MBI) The Maslach Burnout Inventory (Maslach & Jackson, 1981) was developed to measure the frequency and intensity of perceived burnout among people in helping professions. It assesses three aspects of burnout: emotional exhaustion, depersonalization, and (lack of) personal accomplishment. The Emotional Exhaustion subscale contains nine items addressing feelings of being emotionally over-extended and worn out by one's work. The five-item Depersonalization subscale measures the degree of impersonal responses toward the recipients of care. The Personal Accomplishment subscale uses eight items to assess feelings of competence and achievement in one's work with people. A high degree of burnout is reflected by high scores on Emotional Exhaustion and Depersonalization and low scores on Personal Accomplishment.

Caregiver Stress Inventory (CSI) There is evidence that stress is related to burnout, and much speculation that handling residents who have Alzheimer's disease is particularly stressful work. The purposes of the stressor questionnaire were two-fold: to determine whether staff on the SCU experienced less stress than those on integrated units in handling people with AD; and to determine which resident behaviors were reported as occurring less often and/or being less stress-inducing on each type of unit (Maas & Buckwalter, 1990). Given that the SCU housed only demented residents, certain stressors were expected to increase in spite of some behavior improvements. The questionnaire was used to document differences in types of stress experienced by staff for the treatment and control group.

Nursing Satisfaction Questionnaire (NSQ) The NSQ is a standardized tool with established reliability and validity reported by McCulloch (1974). The NSQ was revised by deleting inappropriate items for this study, such as those related to compensation. The original 120-item instrument was reduced to 83 items measuring six domains: 1) working conditions; 2) professional considerations; 3) professional preparation; 4) emotional climate; 5) supervision; and 6) social significance.

Knowledge of Alzheimer's Test (KAT) The original 20-item tool was pretested using parallel forms with 20 nursing home staff, yielding a reliability coefficient of .80. Content validity was assessed from a review of the literature and by a panel of gerontological nurses expert in the care of AD patients. Because high scores were consistently obtained, it appeared that the tool did not discriminate levels of knowledge; therefore, the instrument was expanded to include 33 items (Maas & Buckwalter, 1990).

Staff Absenteeism Absenteeism was assessed from the Iowa Veterans' Home's daily records of the number of hours each staff person was absent from work without sick pay and absent with sick pay.

The two pretests and two posttests reported here represent the 2 bimonthly periods immediately prior to the opening of the SCU (05 & 06 in Table 10.1) and the 2 bimonthly periods beginning with the fifth month after the opening of the SCU (07 & 08 in Table 10.1). The 12 months of posttest data collection began in the fifth month after the SCU was opened to allow effects of relocation to dissipate.

Repeated measures analysis of variance was used to examine differences between experimental and control groups over time, as well as changes within each group over time.

RESULTS

Results for Residents with AD

A total of 100 residents with AD met the inclusion criteria for the study during the 28-month study period. Because of a high attrition rate, mostly due to death, repeated measures analysis could only be conducted for 22 subjects for whom we had complete data from 2 pretests and 2 posttests. The mean age of these 22 subjects (13 experimental and 9 control) was 72.5 years. The majority were male (91%) reflecting the mostly male population of veterans. More than 70% of the AD patients had been institutionalized less than 12 months before their admission to the SCU. For about two-thirds of the patients, the most frequent family member contact was the spouse.

Behavioral Dysfunction While there were no significant differences in cognitive or noncognitive behavioral abilities between the groups or over time, a consistent pattern of change from pretest to posttest was noted in both groups. The experimental group's cognitive (ADAS) mean score increased from 56.67 to 59.69, while the control group's mean score increased from 45.38 to 53.88, indicating a decrease in cognitive functioning of the AD patients in both groups. However, the non-cognitive ADAS scores decreased for both groups over the study period. For the experimental group, non-cognitive scores dropped by 2 points from 18.83 (pre) to 16.83 (post) and for the control group, the non-cognitive scores dropped from 13.75 (pre) to 7.88 (post) indicating that both groups increased in social accessibility. One possible explanation for the greater improvement in non-cognitive function among control subjects is that perhaps the groups were not comparable, with more highly agitated patients placed on the special care unit.

Functional Abilities No significant differences were found between groups on either the FAC or GRS total scores. Further, the scores did not change significantly over time. Additionally, there were no significant differences between groups or time periods for any of the FAC or GRS subscales. Both experimental and control groups exhibited an increase in GRS mean scores from pretest to posttest, indicating a slight decrease in functional ability from the baseline assessment period to the last data collection period. In addition, when cognitive status was held constant, there was no significant difference between groups on the FAC total scores.

Using the IIR, catastrophic reactions were observed and recorded. A catastrophic reaction was defined as a reaction (mood change) of the resident in response to what might appear to staff to be minimal stimuli. A sign test ($p = .035$) showed that AD patients on the SCU had significantly fewer catastrophic reactions post intervention than at baseline and significantly fewer than AD patients on traditional units. AD patients on the SCU also interacted more with staff and other residents, had fewer disruptive and catastrophic behaviors, and participated more in pet therapy and other therapeutic activities. During the first 4 months following the opening of the SCU, AD patients on this unit were restrained less often but fell more often than AD patients on the traditional units (see Table 10.3 & 10.4). Despite no injurious falls, AD patients on the SCU were restrained more during months 5 and 6 following the opening of the SCU. The SCU patients were also restrained more and fell more during these 2 months than AD patients on the traditional units (see Table 10.4). SCU patients were given significantly fewer laxatives than AD patients on traditional units. The slight difference in the number of antipsychotic medications used for patients on the SCU and those on traditional units was not statistically significant. Residents on the SCU had fewer acute illnesses than residents on the traditional units during the baseline period but had more illnesses than residents on traditional units during the posttreatment phase. The average number of illnesses was less than one per month for both groups. Cost of nursing care ranged from $34 to $57 per day for average SCU patients

TABLES 10.3 Falls Per Patient Week

	Pretest				*Posttest*[a]					
	Time 5		Time 6		Time 7		Time 8		Time 9	
Group	*M*	*SD*	*M*	*SD*	*M*	*SD*	*M*	*SD*	*M*	*SD*
Experimental (N = 13)	0.15	0.38	0.23	0.44	1.31	2.02	1.54	1.46	1.39	1.39
Control (N = 9)	0.44	1.33	0.11	0.33	0.56	0.88	0.33	0.77	0.33	0.71

[a] Experimental and control groups differed significantly on posttest falls: [$F(1,20) = 4.54, p < .05$].

throughout the study and from $47 to $58 for residents on traditional units. These costs did not differ significantly between groups or over time.

Results for Staff Caregivers

Of the 186 staff in the original sample, only 76 (21 experimental, 55 control) were included in the analysis because of attrition or missing data. Staff were assigned to the SCU and traditional units according to study site policies and procedures and were therefore not randomized to groups. The majority of staff were female, between 20 and 39 years of age, and worked full-time. Staff on the SCU and traditional units tended to be comparable in age but staff on traditional units had a shorter tenure at the facility. There were fewer registered nurses (RNs) in the SCU group than on traditional units because of the need to distribute professional nursing staff among all of the units in this long-term care facility.

TABLE 10.4 Use of Restraints Per Resident: Average Number of Times Restrained per Day

	Pretest				*Posttest*[a]					
	Time 5		Time 6		Time 7		Time 8		Time 9	
Group	*M*	*SD*	*M*	*SD*	*M*	*SD*	*M*	*SD*	*M*	*SD*
Experimental (N = 13)	2.92	2.78	2.69	2.21	3.53	2.96	3.30	2.40	4.15	2.76
Control (N = 9)	3.56	2.69	2.44	2.29	3.88	2.93	4.33	2.74	3.77	2.99

[a]Experimental and control groups differed significantly in the pattern of restraint use across posttest times 7–9 [$F(2,40) = 3.72, p < .05$].

Not surprisingly, RN knowledge about AD was consistently higher throughout the study than non-RN staff knowledge [Mean knowledge scores = 29.4 and 27.1 out of 33, respectively; $t(60) = 3.24$, $p < .001$]. However, all staff on the SCU consistently had slightly higher knowledge scores (mean [*M*] = 28.26) than staff on traditional units (*M* = 27.42), even though the proportion of RNs was greater among staff on the traditional units and all staff who cared for patients with AD had the same specialized training. It is likely that the SCU environment provided staff with more opportunities to use and thus reinforce the special knowledge they were given. RNs working on the SCU were significantly more satisfied with their preparation than were other nursing staff [$F(1,62) = 4.09$, $p = .047$], whether on the SCU or traditional units. Overall, throughout the study period, all staff were moderately to highly satisfied with their work. SCU nursing staff experienced significantly less stress because of their knowledge, abilities, and resources, while stress for staff on traditional units increased over time [$F(2,62) = 2.28$, $p = 0.12$]. SCU nursing staff also had significantly less depersonalization and burnout than staff on traditional units [$F(1,62) = 4.81$, $p = .032$]. People who were working in this unit felt that they were a therapeutic instrument. There was also a significant reduction in sick time and absenteeism on the SCU. So, to all who say it is not cost effective to train people or to have an SCU, our data suggest that staff are less stressed, more satisfied, and absent less from work.

Results for Family Members

Of the 52 family members who participated in the study, the majority were female (81%), married (79%), the patient's spouse (52%) and 60 years of age or older (64%). Patients with AD on the SCU generally had been institutionalized longer than patients on other units and their family members had been aware of their relative's mental deficits for a longer period than family members of patients on the traditional units. Although family members were moderately to highly satisfied with the care of their AD relatives [*M* = 5.5 to 5.8], they were most satisfied with overall care (*M* = 6.1 to 6.4) and with the AD patient's environment (*M* = 5.5 to 5.8) and least satisfied with the physical care provided by nursing staff (*M* = 4.3 to 5.1). Results of repeated measures MANOVA showed that there were no statistically significant differences in perception of care by family members of the SCU group and the group on traditional units, nor did these perceptions change significantly over time. Examination of individual items showed that family members with relatives on both the SCU and traditional units were most dissatisfied with their lack of involvement in the care of their AD relatives (*M* = 2.9 to 3.5), with activities provided for the AD patients (*M* = 3.0 to 5.1), and with the amount of staff resources available for the care of AD patients

(M = 3.3 to 4.2). Family members' dissatisfaction in these areas tended to increase over the study period. We have piloted a new family/staff partnership protocol to try and address these very troubling findings about family member dissatisfaction with nursing care and have submitted a proposal to NIH to test the intervention in multiple SCUs.

DISCUSSION

Although several recent studies suggest that segregation of persons with AD from non-cognitively impaired residents is desirable and leads to better behavioral and quality of life outcomes, much more research is needed in the planning and design of SCUs. One important area to target is the effect of specific programming on patient outcomes. We also need to be able to operationalize the optimum role of family members; as noted earlier, our research team is currently working on that. We must be able to isolate, define, and evaluate those elements of the physical environment that make a special care unit "special." We must also strive to define clearly what are optimal levels of staff training and what is the best staff mix and staffing pattern. Certainly more research on the cost-effectiveness of SCUs is important, and we clearly need more multi-site studies with larger and more diverse samples.

Our policy-related recommendations include funding a national registry for special care units (not unlike a cancer registry) where the typologies of special care units would be developed, defined, and refined, because they vary so greatly. More research related to constructing taxonomies is needed in order to be able to define outcomes according to types of special care units. For example, if one SCU has a 1:4 staff ratio and another has a ratio of 1:10, how can investigators conclude that the outcomes are due to the unit itself rather than staffing variables? We need to develop and evaluate standardized training programs. When we have this body of research—and then and only then—we can develop standards that will provide the basis for effective regulatory mechanisms.

ACKNOWLEDGMENT

This research was funded by the National Center for Nursing Research, NIH, Grant # R01 NR01689.

REFERENCES

Ackerman, J. O. (1985). Separated, not isolated—as basic as administrative backing and commitment. *The Journal of Long Term Care Administration, 13,* 90–94.

Alzheimer's and Related Disorders Unit Rules Committee Meeting, State of Iowa, minutes of the February 18, 1988, meeting.

Alzheimer's Association. (1992). Request for proposal. Evaluation of Special Care Units. Chicago, IL.

Beitler, D. (1988, November). *Observable criteria for judging quality of care for dementia patients in nursing homes.* Symposium presented at Gerontological Society of America, 41st Annual Scientific Meeting, San Francisco, CA.

Benson, D. M., Cameron, D., Humback, E., Servino, L., & Gambert, S. (1987). Establishment and impact of a dementia unit within the nursing home. *Journal of the American Geriatrics Society, 35*, 319–323.

Berg, L., Buckwalter, K. C., Chafetz, P. K., Gwyther, L. P., Holmes, D., Koepke, K. M., Lawton, M. P., Lindeman, D. A., Magaziner, J., Maslow, K., Morley, J. E., Ory, M. G., Rabins, P. V., Sloane, P. D., & Teresi, J. (1991). Special care units for persons with dementia. *Journal of the American Geriatrics Society, 39*, 1229–1235.

Buckwalter, K. C. (1991). Segregating the cognitively impaired: Are dementia units successful? In P. Katz, R. Kane, & M. Mezey (Eds.), *Advances in long-term care, Vol 1*, New York: Springer Publishing Co.

Buckwalter, K. C., & Hall, G. R. (1987). Families of the institutionalized older adult: A neglected resource. In T. H. Brubaker (Ed.), *Aging, health and family: Long-term care*, (pp. 176–196). Beverly Hills, CA: Sage.

Chambers, J. D. (1990). Predicting licensed nurse turn-over in skilled long-term care. *Nursing and Health Care, 11*, 474–477.

Cleary, T., Clamon, C., Price, M., & Shullaw, G. (1988). A reduced stimulus unit: Effects on patients with Alzheimer's disease and related disorders. *The Gerontologist, 28*, 511–514.

Coons, D. H. (1991). *Specialized dementia care units.* Baltimore: The Johns Hopkins University Press.

Evans, L., Funkenstein, H. H., Albert, M. S., Scherr, P. A., Cook, N. R., Chown, M. J., Herbert, L. E., Hennekens, C. H., & Taylor, J. O. (1989). Prevalence of Alzheimer's disease in a community population of older persons: Higher than previously reported. *Journal of the American Medical Association, 262*, 2551–2556.

Greene, J. A., Asp, J., & Crane, N. (1985). Specialized management of the Alzheimer's disease patient: Does it make a difference? A preliminary progress report. *Journal of the Tennessee Medical Association, 78*, 559–563.

Grossman, H., Weiner, A. S., Salamon, M. J., & Burrows, L. (1986). The milieu standard for care of dementia in a nursing home. *Journal of Gerontological Social Work, 9*, 73–98.

Hall, G. R., & Buckwalter, K. C. (1987). Progressively lowered stress threshold: A conceptual model for care of adults with Alzheimer's disease. *Archives of Psychiatric Nursing, 1*, 399–406.

Hall, G. R., Kirschling, M. V., & Todd, S. (1986). Sheltered freedom: An Alzheimer's unit in an ICF. *Geriatric Nursing, 7*, 132–137.

Hepburn, K., Severance, J., Gates, B., & Christensen, M. (1989). Institutional care of dementia patients: A state-wide survey of long-term care facilities and special care units. *The American Journal of Alzheimer's Care and Related Disorders Research, 4*(2), 19–23.

Hing, E. (1987). Use of nursing homes by the elderly: Preliminary data from the 1985 National Nursing Home Survey. *National Gerontological Nursing Association Newsletter* (pp. 4–6).

Holmes, D., Teresi, J., Weiner, A., Monaco, C., Ranch, J., & Vickers, R. (1990). Impacts associated with special care units in long term care facilities. *The Gerontologist, 30*, 178–183.

Johnson, C. J. (1989). Sociological intervention through developing low stimulus Alzheimer's wings in nursing homes. *The American Journal of Alzheimer's Care Related Disorders and Research*, 4(2), 33–41.

Kahana, E. (1975). A congruence model of person-environment interaction. In P. Windley, T. Byerts, & F. Ernst (Eds.), *Theory development in environment and aging*. (pp. 181–214) Washington, DC: Gerontological Society.

Kane, R. (1987, May). *Considerations before developing a special care unit for Alzheimer's patients. Beyond folklore III: Standard of care in managing Alzheimer's patients.* Paper presented at symposium conducted by the University of Minnesota and the Veterans' Administration. Minneapolis, MN.

Lawton, M. P. (1975). Competence, environmental press and the adaptation of older people. In P. Windley, T. Byerts, & F. Ernst (Eds.), *Theory development in environment and aging* (pp. 13–83). Washington DC: Gerontological Society.

Leon, J., Potter, D., & Cunningham, P. (1990). Current and projected availability of special nursing home programs for Alzheimer's disease patients. Rockville, MD: Public Health Service, (DHHS Publication No. [PHS] 90–3463). National Medical Expenditure Survey Data Summary 1, Agency for Health Care Policy and Research.

Maas, M. (1988). Management of patients with Alzheimer's disease in long-term care facilities. *Nursing Clinics of North America, 23*(1), 57–68.

Maas, M., & Buckwalter, K. (1988, November). *Methodologic issues in the study of specialized units (special care units) in nursing homes.* Panel presentation, Gerontological Society of America, 41st Annual Scientific Meeting, San Francisco.

Maas, M., & Buckwalter, K. C. (1990). *Final report, nursing evaluation research: A special Alzheimer's unit.* National Institutes of Health, National Center for Nursing Research (#NR0689).

Maas, M., Buckwalter, K. C., Kelley, L. S., & Stolley, J. M. (1991). Family members' perceptions: How they view care of Alzheimer's patients in a nursing home. *The Journal of Long Term Care Administration, 19*, 21–26.

Maslach, C., & Jackson, S. (1981). *Maslach burnout inventory.* Palo Alto, CA: Consulting Psychologists Press, Inc.

Mathew, L., Sloan, P., Kilby, M., & Flood, R. (1988, March/April). What's different about a special care unit for dementia patients: A comparative study and research. *The American Journal of Alzheimer's Care and Related Disorders Reasearch, 3*, 16–23.

McCulloch, E. S. (1974). Nurse satisfaction questionnaire. In M. J. Ward & M. Fetler (Eds.), *Instruments for use in nursing education resaearch.* (pp. 297–304) Boulder, CO: WICHE.

Ohta, R. J., & Ohta, B. (1988). Special units for Alzheimer's disease patients: A critical look. *The Gerontologist, 28*, 803–808.

Peppard, N. R. (1989, April). *Point-counterpoint. Session on special needs units.* American Society on Aging. Washington, DC.

Plutchick, R., Conte, H., Leiberman, M., Baker, M., Grossman, J., & Lehrman, N. (1970). Reliability and validity of a scale for assessing the functioning of geriatric patients. *Journal of the American Geriatrics Society, 18*, 491–500.

Reisberg, B., Ferris, M. J., deLeon, M., & Crook, T. (1982). The global deterioration scale (GDS): An instrument for the assessment of primary degenerative dementia. *American Journal of Psychiatry, 139*, 1136–1139.

Roberts, B. L., & Algase, D. L. (1988). Victims of Alzheimer's disease and the environment. *Nursing Clinics of North America, 35*(2), 113–118.
Rosen, W. G., Mohs, R. C., & Davis, K. L. (1984). A new rating scale for Alzheimer's disease. *American Journal of Psychiatry, 141*, 1356–1364.
Rovner, B. W., German, P. S., Broadhead, J., Morriss, R., Brant, L., Blaustein, J., & Folstein, M. (1990). The prevalence and management of dementia and other psychiatric disorders in nursing homes. *International Psychogeriatrics, 2*, 13–24.
Sbordone, R. J., & Sterman, L. T. (1988). The psychologist as a consultant in a nursing home: Effect on staff morale and turnover. *Professional Psychology: Research and Practice, 14*, 240–250.
Schultz, D. J. (1987). Special design considerations for Alzheimer's facilities. *Contemporary Health Care, 10* (11), 49–56.
Silverstone, B., & Burach-Weiss, A. (1983). *Social work practice with the frail elderly and their families: The auxiliary function model.* Springfield, IL: Thomas.
U. S. Congress, Office of Technology Assessment. (1987). Losing a million minds: Confronting the tragedy of Alzheimer's disease and other dementias. OTA–BA–323. Washington, DC: U.S. Government Printing Office.
Wiltzius, F., Gambert, S., & Duthie, E. (1981). Importance of resident placement within a skilled nursing facility. *Journal of the American Geriatrics Society, 29*, 418–421.

[11]

Managing Acute Exacerbations of Chronic Illness in the Elderly

Denise M. Kresevic, C. Seth Landefeld, Robert Palmer, and Jerome Kowal

Over half of the acute care admissions in hospitals are for people over age 65. Most patients come to the hospital with strength and resiliency, though with acute medical problems. Many leave less able to function (Applegate, 1990; Gillick, Serrell, & Gillick, 1982; McVey, Becker, Saltz, Feussner, & Cohen, 1989). Dysfunction has been in the literature since around 1963 (Katz, Ford, Muskowitz, Jackson, & Jaffee, 1963); it points to functional decline or decline in the ability to carry out activities of daily living, and it may lead to loss of independence and to institutionalization. For many years it has been known that 20% to 40% of all patients who enter a hospital decline in this way, despite what we think is appropriate medical and nursing care. The pulmonary embolus resolves, the congestive heart failure gets better, the myocardial infarction gets better, the pneumonia gets better, the urinary tract infection gets better, but the patient is now confused, eating poorly, and may even be unable to walk, though the patient was clear-headed, eating, and walking prior to the hospitalization (Boyer, Lane, Chaung, & Gipner, 1986; Fretwell et al., 1990; Gillick et al., 1982; McVey et al., 1989).

A host of factors may interact to cause the dysfunctional syndrome. Not least of these is what we have come to call the hostile hospital environment—the cold, shiny, uninviting floors; the gowns that were designed for physicians and medical students to do a head to toe exam, but provide no dignity; the nursing routines of vital signs every 4 hours, sometimes at midnight and 4:00 a.m.; NPO—hospitals are the only institutions that can get away with starving patients in the name of cure; and an environment that is perhaps without any cues such as clocks, calendars, or newspapers. There are probably multiple factors that cause dysfunction.

Geriatric units in acute care hospitals have been widely advocated but little studied. Meissner, Andolsek, Mears, and Fletcher (1989) and Boyer et al. (1986) reported improved functioning at discharge from a geriatric unit. Teasdale, Shuman, Snow, and Luchi (1983), Meissner et al. (1989), and Boyer et al. (1986) also noted markedly prolonged lengths of stay. Fretwell et al. (1990), however, found no significant effects on physical function, mental function, death rate, length of stay, or hospital charges. While these results are consistent with the hypothesis that functional decline cannot be lessened in acutely ill older patients, there are alternative explanations. The intervention may have been inadequate. Perhaps, for example, the physical environment was not extensively modified to meet the needs of older patients, or patients' primary physicians were rarely involved in team meetings, and consultative recommendations were not followed. Moreover, the outcome measures used in the study may have been insensitive to important changes. For example, functioning was reported 6 weeks after inclusion in the study, but not at discharge.

Based on our conceptual model of dysfunctional syndrome, our preliminary studies, and the work of others, we developed the "Prehab Program of Patient-Centered Care" to prevent functional decline in acutely ill medical patients and to rehabilitate patients whose functioning has already begun to decline (Figure 11.1). Maintaining function is key because the amount of energy to maintain someone's walking is a third less than what it takes to help the person regain the ability to walk. So our interventions are both preventive and restorative. The Prehab Program has been developed, implemented, and pilot tested on a 15-bed unit for the Acute Care of the Elderly (the ACE Unit) at University Hospitals of Cleveland (Landerfeld, Palmer, Kresevic, & Kowel, 1991). The ACE Unit was implemented to prevent functional decline through attention to three major areas: physical environment, collaborative team building, and development of nurse-initiated clinical protocols for prevention and restoration of cognitive function, continence, mobility, and nutrition. Our primary goal for the study reported here was to ascertain whether the dysfunctional syndrome can be ameliorated or prevented by a special unit.

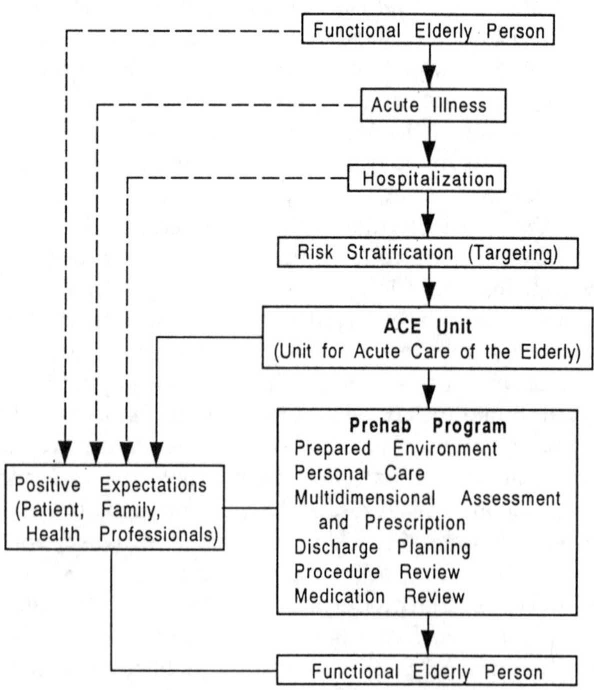

FIGURE 11.1. Unit for Acute Care of the Elderly (ACE) Model.

METHOD

A 29-bed medical surgical nursing unit was renovated in preparation for the study. Clinicians worked with designers to plan adaptations that would enhance function; for example, soft and calming colors were chosen for patient rooms while hallway carpeting was geometrically designed to help patients pace activity. The activity room for congregate meals, visiting, and art and music therapy was decorated in vivid colors. Doorknobs were replaced with levers for easy access. Low beds with automatic night lights and recliners were purchased.

Collaborative team building began with interdisciplinary inservices and workshops. All team members—nurses, physicians, social workers, nutritionists, and therapists—reviewed core gerontological content including aging demographics, attitude exploration, physiological aging changes, environmental adaptations for aging, communication skills, and ethical decision making. A major goal of the sessions was the creation of interdisciplinary guidelines for preventive and restorative care for nutrition, mobility, mood, skin, and toileting. Unlike previous models using gerontological experts as consultants, this model used the geriatric medical director and clinical nurse specialists in dual roles. These experts provided direct clinical care, managing a caseload of patients as well as facilitating daily interdisciplinary rounds. Rounds included the primary nurse, CNS, medical director, resident, physician, social worker, home care nurse, nutritionist, and rehabilitative specialist. Nurses described the medical functional status of the patients, progress in the protocols, and discharge planning efforts. The physician reviewed the medical work-up and treatment goals. Thus the team functioned both as consultants and providers of care.

Four hundred medical patients age 70 years or older were randomly assigned at the time of admission to an intervention group receiving Prehab and ACE Unit (n = 198) or to a control group receiving usual care on a conventional ward (n = 202). The study sample of 400 patients was 18% of all medical patients ≥ 70 years admitted to University Hospitals during the study period; 36% of medical patients ≥ 70 years were eligible but not randomly assigned because beds were not available for random assignment, and the remaining 46% of patients ≥ 70 years were not eligible (most often because they were admitted to an intensive care or oncology unit). Thus, the study sample was representative of 54% of all acutely ill patients ≥ 70 years admitted to the medical service of University Hospitals. Patients, family, and nurses were interviewed on admission, discharge, and 90 days after discharge. The main outcome measure was the number of independent ADLs reported at discharge; 360 patients were discharged alive.

INTERVENTIONS

Restoring Cognition

The environment of the ACE Unit contains basic cues such as clocks and calendars that are not standard in an acute care unit. Patients also bring familiar objects from home, including pets. We've all known that pet therapy makes a difference. What our staff said in the beginning was, "Can we do that?" What we've taught them is to ask first, "What does the patient need?" and then, "How do we do that?" We have a videotape of a woman who had an acute stroke, and who was aphasic for 3 days. We brought her dog up to our activity room and she said, "My Gigi, my Gigi." There wasn't a dry eye in that room. We're not sure that all of the speech therapy in the world could have made such fast progress.

Socialization is perhaps the most important intervention for maintaining and restoring cognitive function. The congregate room on the nursing unit is the center of many activities such as meals, art, music, pet therapy, and physical therapy as well as the room for family conferences. Large recliners, books, and tapes are available. Seeing elders interacting with each other and even trying out new activities like listening to tapes with headphones has given nurses a new perspective. Initially patients are reluctant to get out of bed and even out of their rooms. However, once they get to the activity room, the majority continue to request to come back. It is important to have someone coordinate activities and to have a support person like a nurse's aide to assist with ambulation and toileting; this has been a constant challenge for us on a busy medical unit where nurses may be overwhelmed with intravenous medications, blood administration, or documentation.

Medications are reviewed daily in team rounds. However, ongoing analysis of medications needs to be done as patients often go off the floor for procedures and may get premedications. After 2 years of the ACE Unit, it is wonderful to watch primary nurses taking the lead in questioning medications when agitation and confusion initially develop and then persuading, sometimes not so gently, the medical caregivers not to add more medications that could complicate care without really addressing the problems of anxiety, hypoxia, or malnutrition.

Maintaining Cognition

Maintaining patients' individualized *routines* is important—not everybody takes a bath at 7:00 a.m. Also, not everybody takes a bath every day, nor should they, perhaps, with dry aging skin. Being flexible is the key to good nursing care.

Assessing cognition is also important. There is one question a nurse can ask on a very busy day that will give her a true picture: "How did you come to be in the hospital?" It will provide a wealth of information. Some patients will say, "Oh, am I in a hospital?" Other patients will give you a vivid story. Cognitive status may be the most sensitive and critical indicator of a myocardial infarction, or the most sensitive indicator of fluid imbalance. But acute care nurses are not used to asking questions to assess cognitive status.

Mood should be monitored daily. Although we need the support of psychiatrists and mental health workers to assess mood and depression, we also need the bedside nurse. At 3:00 a.m. on a Friday morning it is the nurse who is there. What questions should she ask? The questions about mood are: "How are you feeling?" "Are you sad?" "Are you depressed?" These questions should be part of the daily assessment, important indicators to share with the team.

Attention to sensory needs is critical because hearing-impaired patients are a high percentage of our population. We have experimented with hearing aids ranging from very expensive amplifiers purchased from our local Hearing and Speech Center to an economical device purchased for under $10 at local drug stores called the Whisper 2000, which is also advertised on TV. Interestingly enough, both seem to work equally well. It is incredible what health histories you can get when the patients can hear the questions. We've had patients who were acting out and delirious, screaming out. When we put the Whisper 2000 on them, they could not stand to hear themselves yelling and they got much quieter.

Maintaining Mobility

Of all our protocols, probably the two most important ones are for mobility and nutrition. Bed rest is an appropriate order only for people who are dead, or during the first 24 hours of a stroke. There is little literature providing compelling evidence that bed rest is a therapy in and of itself. Everyone on our unit is encouraged to be up and moving. What we have done is make people put shoes on, and that is one of the most important things for safe mobility. If you can't change anything else in your hospital environment, have the patients bring in their tennis shoes.

Patient and family teaching are also a part of our intervention. Our nurses are very, very busy and we're using a self-care model. From Day 1 patients are told in a little handout, not to take it easy, but rather, that exercise is a part of their entire hospitalized care and they will be asked to exercise twice a day. They choose the times and we teach them and their families range of motion exercises, balance, and gait training.

Physical therapy has worked very closely with primary nurses and patients and their families to pilot several balance and gait training exercises with elders. Patients are instructed by the nurse on basic range of motion exercises to maintain function. In high risk patients with poor balance and gait, a physical therapy consult and usually an occupational therapy consult are sought. Exercises are developed for individual patients and implemented by the therapist and nurse, who then instruct the family. Having nurses and therapists work in such a close collaborative relationship has greatly increased consistency for patients and enhanced nurses' assessment skills and knowledge about exercise.

Physicians have commented on several striking differences evident to them when they care for patients on the ACE Unit. First, nurses are aggressive about getting patients out of bed. Second, patients are often out of their rooms, with many walking in the hallway. Finally, consults for therapy are ordered very early.

Some of our protocols allow us to empower primary nurses to get assistive devices for patients. We know that the patient's first 24 hours are critical, so our interventions should be maximized in that period. Under the old system the nurse had to talk to the physician in order to get a physical therapy consult to get an assistive device for a patient. That's a ludicrous system and it certainly isn't good for the patient. The nurse should be expected to have the knowledge and skill to make an assessment; we ascertained that our nurses could do this and then created within the structure the ability to obtain walkers and begin gait training. When we call in physical therapy and occupational therapy, it is because our protocols aren't working or the patient isn't progressing.

Carpeting is another intervention. We went back and forth on this; the housekeeping department said, "It's too hard to clean, it's too expensive, it's not safe." What the hospital wasn't used to was clinicians designing a therapeutic environment. In our view the first question is not cleaning, and it is not cost, it is: What is good for patients? What will promote mobility? If carpeting will do it, then we need to find the right carpeting, and we need to figure out how to clean it. We've had carpeting on our unit for 18 months now, and we do not regret that decision at all.

Continence

Continence has been one of the hardest areas to deal with. Avoiding catheters and restraints is critical. We moved to prompted toileting on a schedule. The schedule was based not on the nurse and the nurse's aide, but on the elderly patient. We believe that their bladders should never catch them by surprise. It is important to have information on medications, fluid balance, and post-void residual; nurses routinely collect this information when they assess for continence. If the information is available, the physician, when called, can make educated interventions. If we have older people walk and we give them enough fluid, we will probably keep them more continent. Also, we do not need a pretty bathroom, but a functional bathroom, with side rails and elevated toilet seats. After we saw an old lady actually wet her pants while trying to turn a door knob, we put levers on bathroom doors.

Nutrition

Nutrition is probably the single most important intervention in acute care—but it is not paid a lot of attention. Congregate dining is a critical factor. We persuaded the staff to split their lounge in half and share it with patients as a dining/activity room. Incredible things have happened here—trading of food, helping one another open packages, all the social skills that keep cognition intact. Every hospital should have a dining room. Also, how much should people eat or drink? We settled on a minimum of 1200 calories, 1200 ccs. The majority of our patients were drinking only about 800 ccs of fluid, even with prompting. Also, it is important to teach patients oral hygiene, even if they have dentures.

Restoring nutrition is crucial. Nobody wants to have a box of Ensure left at the bedside and to be told that this will improve nutrition. It's ludicrous, but we do this all the time. We talked our dietary department into making what we call the ACE cookie. It's made with jevity (high fiber soy based supplement), it has 200 calories, and it is high in protein. We put it on people's pillows, similar to the way candy is left on your pillow in a hotel. It's a nice thing to do and the patients love it. We don't take feeding tubes and hyperalimentation lightly. Education and consent are important prerequisites.

Appropriate clinical protocols are initiated on admission by the primary nurse and a daily flow sheet is used to target assessment and track function.

Results

Our preliminary data indicte that ACE Unit patients had a shorter mean length of stay (7.5 days vs 8.7 days) and lower mean hospital charges ($10,450 vs $12,580) than did usual care patients; these differences were not statistically significant ($p > .1$), however, because of the widely skewed distributions of length of stay and charges. We also found promising trends toward ameliorating functional decline.

Further, prior to our intervention, the nursing group on the ACE Unit had the lowest perceived professional status. After 18 months the study nurses' mean scores on all components of Stamp and Piedmonte's work

TABLE 11.1 Nurses' Outcomes: Satisfaction - Attitudes[a]

Item	*Control* $n = 29$	*ACE* $n = 14$
Work satisfaction	4.67	4.83
Autonomy	5.39	5.62
Professional status	5.91	5.93
Interaction	5.04	5.39
Attitudes	3.15	3.25

[a]Standardized mean scores on Stamps and Piedmonte (1986) scale.

satisfaction scale (work satisfaction, autonomy, professional status interaction, and attitudes) (1986) were higher than those of the nurses on the control units (see Table 11.1).

These encouraging preliminary results have important limitations. Few differences at discharge between usual care and ACE Unit care groups achieved levels of statistical significance. Efficacy of the ACE Unit has been examined for only a 2-year period of time and analyses are incomplete. The unit clearly will need ongoing evaluation.

DISCUSSION

The implementation of a specialty unit with nurse-initiated guidelines is clearly feasible. Trends toward ameliorating functional decline and shortening length of stay are promising. Early experience suggests that nurses enjoy working in this kind of environment, and adverse consequences such as falls and overuse of medications have declined.

Given our experiences, both intuitively and based on data trends, we would recommend that nurses and physicians begin to evaluate current environments of care for elders. Many of our interventions, like a congregate room and interdisciplinary rounds, could be done anywhere. Whenever environmental renovation is planned, it provides an excellent opportunity to have clinicians critically evaluate the proposed designs and bring to the project clear goals of patient safety and function. It is our hope that as we continue to evaluate our nurse-initiated protocols within our acute care setting and share these with other acute care, home care, and long-term settings, refinement and ongoing research will be able to demonstrate the effectiveness of targeted interventions.

REFERENCES

Applegate, M. B., Miller, S. T., Graney, M. J., Elam, J. T., Burns, R., & Akins, D. E. (1990). A randomized, controlled trial of a geriatric assessment unit in a community rehabilitation hospital. *New England Journal of Medicine, 322,* 1572–1578.

Boyer, N., Lane, J., Chaung, C., & Gipner, D. (1986). An acute care geriatric unit. *Nursing Management, 17,* 22–25.

Fretwell, M. D., Raymond, P. M., McGarvey, S. T., Owens, N., Traines, M., Silliman, R. A., & Mor, V. (1990). The senior care study: A controlled trial of a consultative/unit-based geriatric assessment program in acute care. *Journal of the American Geriatrics Society, 38,* 1073–1081.

Gillick, M. R., Serrell, M. A., & Gillick, L. S. (1982). Adverse consequences of hospitalization in the elderly. *Social Science and Medicine, 16,* 1033–1038.

Katz, S., Ford, A. B., & Muskowitz, R. W., Jackson, B. A., & Jaffee, M. W. (1963). Studies of illness in the aged. The index of ADL, a standardized measure of biological and psychosocial function. *Journal of the American Medical Association, 185,* 914–919.

Landerfeld, C., Palmer, R., Kresevic, D., & Kowal, S. (1991, November). The dysfunctional syndrome. Paper presented at the meeting of the Gerontological Society of America, San Francisco, CA.

McVey, L. J., Becker, P. M., Saltz, C. C., Feussner, J. R., & Cohen, H. J. (1989). Effect of a geriatric consultation team on functional status of elderly hospitalized patients. *Annals of Internal Medicine, 110,* 79–84.

Meissner, P., Andolsek, K., Mears, P. A., & Fletcher, B. (1989). Maximizing the functional status of geriatric patients in an acute community hospital setting. *The Gerontologist, 29,* 524–528.

Stamp, P. L., & Piedmonte, F. B. (1986). *Nurses and work satisfaction: An index for measurement.* Ann Arbor: Michigan Health Administration Press Perspectives.

Teasdale, T. A., Shuman, L., Snow, E., & Luchi, R. J. (1983). A comparison of placement outcomes of geriatric cohorts receiving care in a geriatric assessment unit on general medicine floors. *Journal of the American Geriatrics Society, 31,* 529–534.

[12]

Meeting the Discharge Needs of Hospitalized Elderly and Their Caregivers

Mary D. Naylor, Roberta L. Campbell, and Janice B. Foust

At any given time the elderly occupy more than 40% of hospital beds (National Center for Health Statistics, 1985). They are experiencing earlier discharge as a result of the prospective payment system (PPS) (Prospective Payment Commission, 1989) and are a high risk group for poor post-discharge outcomes (Johnson & Fethke, 1985; Jones, Densen, & Brown, 1989). Thus they represent a population in great need of post-discharge services (Johnson & Fethke, 1985; Jones et al., 1989). The primary need is for cost-effective interventions that facilitate the discharge of hospitalized elderly to their homes and improve their discharge outcomes. Indeed, a panel of experts in the care of the elderly has identified discharge planning as a major priority in delivering quality health care to the elderly (Fink, Siu, Brook, Park, & Solomon, 1987).

While the post-discharge needs of the elderly and their caregivers have changed dramatically since the introduction of the PPS, there is little information on the impact of these changes on the discharge planning done by nurses. There is some indication, however, that preparation of the elderly and their caregivers for discharge is not receiving the attention it requires because of shortened hospital stays, increased complexity of patients' needs, and inadequate preparation of most nurses to meet the special needs of this population (Floyd & Buckle, 1987).

Several studies have demonstrated the efficacy of interventions by master's prepared clinical nurse specialists in enhancing post-hospitalization outcomes for vulnerable populations (Brooten et al., 1986; Burgess et al., 1987; Kane et al., 1989). However, the actual time devoted to discharge planning for the elderly has been reported in only one study. Kennedy, Neidlinger, and Scroggins (1987) examined the effectiveness of a comprehensive discharge planning protocol implemented by geriatric clinical nurse specialists (GCNSs) in meeting the post-discharge needs of elderly patients. For subjects in the treatment group, length of hospital stay was reduced by a mean of 2 days and the mean time between hospital admission and readmission was increased by 11 days. The average difference in total hospital costs was $1,311, with the control group being significantly more costly (Neidlinger, Scroggins, & Kennedy, 1987). The GCNSs devoted an average of 80 minutes per subject to comprehensive discharge planning. The study reported here extended the work of these researchers and examined the nature of the interactions and activities and the time devoted by GCNSs to meet the discharge planning needs of hospitalized elderly and their caregivers.

METHOD

Study Design

This research was conducted as part of a larger study of comprehensive discharge planning for hospitalized elderly. Building on the discharge planning protocol for the elderly developed by Kennedy, Neidlinger, and Scroggins (1987) and the discharge planning portion of the Quality Cost Model of Early Hospital Discharge and Nurse Specialist Transitional Care devised by Brooten and colleagues (1988), the larger study was designed to compare the effectiveness of a comprehensive discharge planning protocol developed specifically for hospitalized elderly and implemented by GCNSs with the effectiveness of the hospital's general discharge planning procedure (Naylor, 1990). Two master's prepared GCNSs provided comprehensive discharge planning services to 123 experimental subjects and their caregivers.

Setting and Sample

The study was conducted on both medical and surgical intensive care and general units of a large tertiary care institution located in a major city on the East Coast. To be eligible for the study, patients had to be age 70 or older, alert and oriented at admission, able to speak English, able to respond to questions, admitted from home, and with a primary DRG classification of coronary artery bypass graft (CABG), cardiac valve replacement, congestive heart failure (CHF), myocardial infarction (MI), or angina/percutaneous transluminal coronary angioplasty (PTCA). The patient's caregiver, that is, the person the subject believed would assume primary responsibility for his/her care after discharge, was also asked to participate in the study.

The Intervention

The GCNSs completed an initial assessment of the post-discharge needs of subjects and their caregivers within 24 hours of each subject's hospital admission. Plans to meet these needs were developed in consultation with subjects, caregivers, and other members of the health team. The discharge plans were documented by the GCNSs on subjects' progress notes. The GCNSs then implemented the discharge plans, evaluated their effectiveness, and followed up for 2 weeks after discharge on the needs and care of the subjects and their caregivers.

The GCNSs were expected to make a minimum of four visits (admission, discharge, and two "other" hospital visits) during each subject's hospital stay (see Figure 12.1). In addition, throughout each subject's hospitalization and for 2 weeks post-discharge, the GCNSs were available by telephone for any questions or concerns of subjects or caregivers. The GCNSs initiated two telephone contacts with subjects and/or caregivers during the 2 weeks immediately following discharge (the first at 48 hours and the other at 7 days post-discharge). Table 12.1 outlines the components of the discharge planning protocol completed by the GCNSs.

Data Collection

The total time the GCNSs devoted to discharge planning through both direct and indirect care of subjects and caregivers was examined. Direct care was defined as the time spent by GCNSs in interactions with subjects and their caregivers that were associated with subjects' discharge plans. Indirect care was defined as the time spent by GCNSs in interactions with other

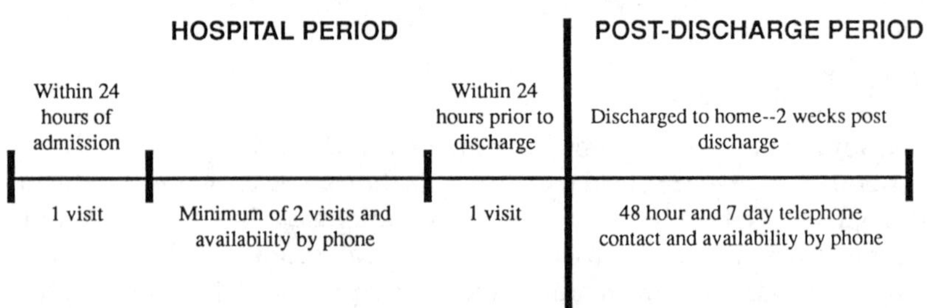

FIGURE 12.1. Comprehensive discharge planning protocol for hospitalized elderly by GCNS.

TABLE 12.1 Components of Discharge Planning Protocol

I. Assessment

A. *Patient*
1. sociodemographics
2. subjective health rating
3. mental status
4. functional status
5. housing
6. supportive devices
7. social supports
8. resource use
9. perceived needs
10. self-esteem
11. stress level

B. *Caregiver*
1. sociodemographics
2. subjective health rating
3. functional status
4. caregiving demands
5. perceived needs
6. stress level
7. family functioning

II. Development of Discharge Plan

A. Project teaching needs
B. Project home care needs
C. Involve patient/family/health care team members
D. Documentation

III. Implementation of Discharge Plan

A. Teaching
B. Validation of learning
C. Collaboration
D. Communication
E. Coordination
F. Documentation

IV. Evaluation

A. Ongoing evaluation
B. Modification as needed

---

members of the health care team or in other activities related to the subjects' discharge plans (e.g., documentation, coordination of services).

All GCNS interactions with subjects and their caregivers during the hospitalization and the 2-week post-discharge period were recorded in standardized logs. The following data on direct care activities were recorded: date; initiator (subject, subject's caregiver, or GCNS); person contacted (subject, subject's caregiver); purpose of interaction or activity; method of contact (personal visit or telephone); and length of interaction (in minutes).

The following data on indirect care activities associated with discharge planning were also recorded: date; initiator (e.g., subject's primary nurse, physician, or GCNS); person(s) contacted (e.g., subject's primary nurse, physician, social worker); purpose of interaction or activity (e.g., coordination of services, referrals, documentation); method of contact; and length of interaction/activity (in minutes). On the daily log, the GCNSs also documented the subject's and caregiver's needs and progress made in addressing those needs. The GCNSs were oriented to the use of this format, and subjects' logs were reviewed by the principal investigator and project director throughout the study to assure quality documentation.

RESULTS

The comprehensive discharge planning protocol designed for the elderly and implemented by GCNSs was received by 123 subjects. The age range of these subjects was 70–92 with a median of 74. Sixty-nine percent were male; 90% were either married or widowed. The majority of subjects were white, with at least a high school education, retired, and with an annual income greater than $10,000. Subjects were equally divided among four DRG categories: CABG, cardiac valve replacements, CHF/MI, and angina/PTCA.

Caregivers for 70 of the subjects (57%) were also enrolled in the study. Their age range was 30 to 83; 44% were over 70. The subjects' caregivers were predominantly female (primarily wives or daughters), white, married, with at least a high school education, and unemployed.

Major Findings

The GCNSs spent a mean of 4-¼ hours (256.5 minutes) per patient and caregiver in interactions and activities associated with discharge planning. The average number of contacts between the GCNS and each subject, caregiver, and other health care professional was seven. This included contacts made through personal visits and telephone calls. A mean of 207 minutes, or approximately 3 hours (81%), was spent while subjects were hospitalized. The remaining 49 minutes (19%) were spent in activities and interactions during the 2 week post-discharge period (see Figure 12.2). Direct care time per subject and caregiver was 139 minutes (54% of the total), while indirect care time was 117 minutes (46%) (see Figure 12.3).

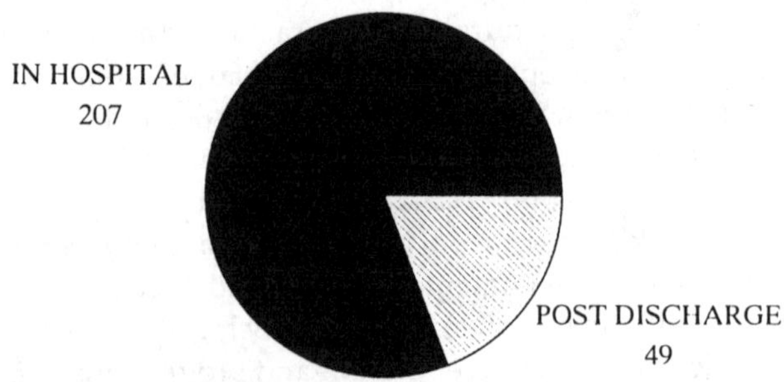

FIGURE 12.2. Mean total time (in minutes) that GCNSs spent in discharge planning activities.

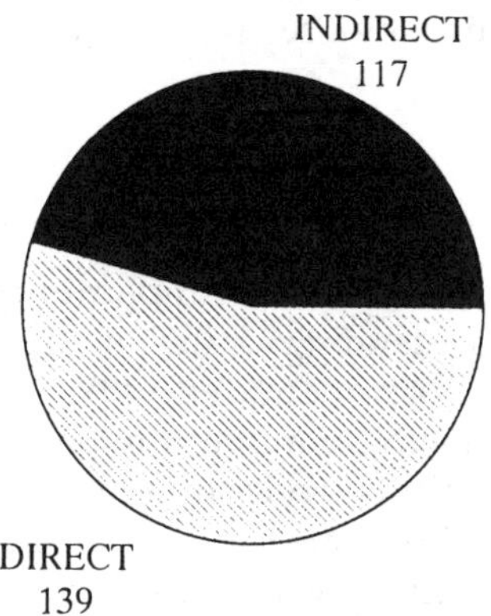

FIGURE 12.3. Mean time (in minutes) that GCNSs spent in direct and indirect discharge planning activities per subject.

Interestingly, there was a large difference in the total time devoted by GCNSs to medical and surgical subjects; surgical subjects received approximately an hour more time than medical patients. For medical patients, 41% of the total hospital time was spent on the admission visit, 34% during "other" visits, and 25% at the discharge visit. In contrast, for surgical patients, 56% of the total hospital time was devoted to "other" hospital visits, while the remaining time was split equally between the admission and discharge visits.

The admission visit focused on the need for and availability of post-discharge health and social services for subjects and their caregivers, the ability of subjects and caregivers to manage the health problem that had resulted in the current admission, the psychosocial adaptation of subjects and caregivers, and the need for information and skills to prevent and/or address health problems.

The "other" hospital visits focused on teaching subjects and caregivers to manage health care problems and needs post-discharge, coordinating the discharge planning teams and services, consulting with staff, referring to other health care providers and/or community services, providing emotional support, and monitoring changes in health status.

The discharge visit and post-discharge follow-up focused on validating that the subject and caregiver understood and could demonstrate the skills necessary to manage the subject's care after discharge, providing reinforcement and reassurance, ensuring that home health and social services were available, and monitoring changes in the health status of the subject and caregiver to determine the effectiveness of the discharge plan and detect complications.

DISCUSSION

The findings of this study have several implications for practice. The most obvious is that discharge planning for hospitalized elderly and their caregivers requires a great deal of time and effort. While it is true that the protocol in this study prescribed a minimum number of contacts, the actual amount of time invested in this service was determined by the GCNSs. The GCNSs devoted most of their time to direct care interactions with patients and their caregivers, including health care teaching, providing emotional support, and validating that patients and caregivers understood and could demonstrate the skills necessary to manage their health care.

Indirect care activities such as collaboration with other health team members, coordination of care, referral for home health care and/or community services, and documentation also required a considerable investment of time. These components are essential for effective discharge planning.

How much do hospital staffing patterns take into account the time that is required, not just to meet the immediate needs of patients and caregivers, but also to think critically about and plan for the transition that patients must make as they move from hospital to home? If discharge planning is factored into staffing patterns, are both the direct and indirect care components considered? Is the investment of time with caregivers included?

In our study, the vast majority of GCNS time was spent on interactions and activities related to discharge planning while patients were hospitalized. Still, post-discharge follow-up required 19% of the total time. The nature of the interactions during this period suggests that elderly patients have major concerns and needs that necessitate breaking down traditional hospital boundaries. Nurses need to be given the opportunity and support for providing post-discharge follow-up to patients and their caregivers.

The difference in the time devoted to discharge planning for medical and surgical patients is very interesting. The shorter time devoted to elderly medical patients may reflect the fact that for many elderly patients, health problems are chronic. These patients have had multiple hospitalizations and, thus, they may be better prepared for the post-discharge experience. The time difference may also reflect patient and caregiver need for additional knowledge and skills after a major surgical procedure such as coronary artery bypass grafting.

The GCNS possesses both advanced knowledge and skills in the care of the elderly and an understanding of the maze of community health and social services that are often needed by the elderly after discharge. The nature of interactions and activities and the time devoted to discharge planning in this study suggest that nurse specialists are the appropriate people who should be providing discharge planning and home follow-up to a vulnerable population with complex health problems.

ACKNOWLEDGMENT

This study was supported by the National Center for Nursing Research (Grant # NR02095-03).

REFERENCES

Brooten, D., Kumar, S., Brown, L., Butts, P., Finkler, S., Bakewell-Sachs, S., Gibbons, A., & Delivoria-Papadopoulos, M. (1986). A randomized clinical trial of early hospital discharge and home follow-up of very low birthweight infants. *New England Journal of Medicine, 315*, 934–939.

Brooten, D., Brown, L. P., Munro, B. H., York, R., Cohen, S., Roncoli, M., & Hollingsworth, A. (1988). Early discharge and specialist transitional care. *Image: Journal of Nursing Scholarship, 20*, 64–68.

Burgess, A. W., Lerner, D. J., D'Agostino, R. B., Vokonas, P. S., Hartman, C. R., & Gaccione, P. (1987). A randomized clinical trial of cardiac rehabilitation. *Social Science and Medicine, 24*, 359–370.

Fink, A., Siu, A., Brook, R., Park, R., & Solomon, D. (1987). Assuring the quality of health care for older persons: An expert panel's priorities. *Journal of the American Medical Association, 258*, 1905–1908.

Floyd, J., & Buckle, J. (1987). Nursing care of the elderly. *Journal of Gerontological Nursing, 13*(2), 20–25.

Johnson, N., & Fethke, C. (1985). Post-discharge outcomes and care planning for the hospitalized elderly. In E. McClelland, K. Kelly, & K. Buckwalter (Eds.), *Continuity of care: Advancing the concept of discharge planning* (pp. 229–240). New York: Grune and Stratton, Inc.

Jones, E. W., Densen, P. M., & Brown, S. D. (1989). Posthospital needs of elderly people at home: Findings from an 8 month follow-up study. *Health Services Research, 24*, 644–664.

Kane, R. L., Garrard, J., Skay, C. L., Radosevich, D. M., Buchanan, J. L., McDermott, S. M., Arnold, S. B., & Kepferle, L. (1989). Effects of a geriatric nurse practitioner on process and outcomes of nursing home care. *American Journal of Public Health, 79*, 1271–1277.

Kennedy, L., Neidlinger, S., & Scroggins, K. (1987). Effective comprehensive discharge planning for hospitalized elderly. *The Gerontologist, 27*, 577–580.

National Center for Health Statistics. (1985). Utilization of short-stay hospitals, United States, 1983. Annual Summary. *Vital and health statistics survey* (Series 13, No. 83, DHHS Publication No. PHS 85-1744). Washington, DC: U. S. Government Printing Office.

Naylor, M. (1990). A special feature: An example of a research grant application: Comprehensive discharge planning for hospitalized elderly. *Research in Nursing and Health, 13*, 327–347.

Neidlinger, S., Scroggins, K., & Kennedy, L. (1987). Cost-evaluation of discharge planning for hospitalized elderly. *Nursing Economics*, *5*, 225–230.
Prospective Payment Commission. (June, 1989). *Medicare prospective payment and the American health care system*. Report to the Congress. Washington, DC: Author.

[13]

Effect of a Self-Help Course on Adaptation in People with Arthritis

Ann Mabe Newman

One of the greatest challenges facing nurses and other health care providers is how to best support the adaptive behaviors of people living with chronic illnesses such as arthritis. Educational programs emphasizing self-management have become an important part of the support for these individuals, and evaluation of the programs suggests that self-management results in improved health status (Lorig, Konkol, & Gonzoles, 1987).

The Arthritis Self-Help Course (ASHC), which is endorsed by the Arthritis Foundation, is designed to help people adapt to their illness. The course is an experiential, cognitive-behavioral, self-management course in which participants learn principles of self-management, receive information on medications and nutrition, and learn about the relationship between pain and depression. The leader engages participants in problem solving, practice of communication skills, relaxation techniques, and physical exercises. Participants are given homework assignments to complete between sessions. The program is prescriptive in nature, but the course leader is encouraged to tailor the material to meet the needs of each group being taught. The content and process of the ASHC are standardized, as outlined in the *ASHC Leader's Manual* (Lorig, 1986) and the supplementary textbook, *The Arthritis Helpbook*, by Lorig and Fries (1986). A summary of the Self-Help Course is given below.

THE ARTHRITIS SELF-HELP COURSE

Program Description

The ASHC is a group education program that provides an opportunity for mutual peer support. Self-help involves willingness to learn about and to assume responsibility for one's arthritis. It includes all the decisions a person must make, and actions he or she takes to control the arthritis and to maintain independence. Consistent with this self-help philosophy, the Arthritis Self-Help Course is designed to give people with arthritis the knowledge and skills needed to take a more active part in their arthritis care.

Program Goals

The Arthritis Self-Help Course is designed to:

1. Inform participants about basic aspects of arthritis and joint anatomy.
2. Teach participants principles of exercise and provide an opportunity to practice stretching and strengthening exercises.
3. Teach principles of joint protection and energy conservation and provide an opportunity to share ideas about improving one's functional ability.
4. Teach participants the appropriate utilization of arthritis medications.
5. Encourage informed decisions about the use of special diets and nontraditional forms of treatment.
6. Encourage participants to take an active role in arthritis management and make appropriate use of arthritis care providers.
7. Encourage sharing of experiences and group problem solving.
8. Provide an opportunity for learning and practicing stress management and other self-help behaviors designed to decrease stress, pain, and depression.

Course Content and Process

The ASHC is taught over 6 consecutive weeks in sessions lasting 2 – 2½ hours per week. The instructional methods include lecture/discussion,

role-playing, brainstorming, and demonstration. Active participation by the course members and experiential learning are emphasized.
The course includes:

- Arthritis/Joint Anatomy
- Self-Help Principles
- Pain Control
- Exercise
- Relaxation
- Dealing with Depression
- Communicating with Your Caregiver
- Nutrition
- Nontraditional Treatment

(Arthritis Foundation, 1987)

ASHC participants have shown improvements in both health status and perceived ability to manage symptoms (Lorig, Mazonson, & Holman, 1989). This perceived ability to manage symptoms and make changes, termed self-efficacy, is associated with adaptation to arthritis and has been identified as one of the mechanisms by which the arthritis education program improves health status (Lorig, Chastain, Ung, Shoor, & Holman, 1989). Three other factors identified as affecting adaptation are the perceived level of and satisfaction with social support received from others, the degree to which persons experience life as meaningful, and disability status (Broadhead et al., 1983; Kobasa, Maddi, & Kahn, 1982; Phillips, 1980; Thompson & Janigan, 1988; Weinert, 1987).

The study reported here investigated the effects of the ASHC on the following factors related to adaptation in arthritis: arthritis self-efficacy, perceived social support, purpose and meaning in life, and arthritis impact, or disability status. *Arthritis self-efficacy* was defined as the belief that one can achieve a behavior or state of mind in relation to a specific task. (It is not an actual measure of accomplishment [Bandura, 1986].) *Perceived social support* was defined as the psychological and tangible aid from the social network perceived by the person. *Purpose and meaning in life* were considered to affirm a common purposefulness of human existence. *Arthritis impact* was a measure of physical functioning, which helps to determine the level of disability.

METHOD

Subjects

The sample consisted of 130 people, over age 18, English-speaking, with a diagnosis of arthritis, and not currently experiencing an episode of an acute or chronic illness other than arthritis. They were recruited from a multipurpose arthritis center, from a national group sponsoring day-long programs for the elderly, and from the community in a large Southeastern city.

Data Collection Tools

The instruments were self-report, paper-and-pencil tests. The Arthritis Self-Efficacy Scale was developed by Lorig and colleagues (Lorig, Chastain, et al., 1989). This is a 20-item scale divided into three subscales. The self-efficacy pain subscale consists of five items reflecting one's perceived ability to control pain. Reliability is reported as .87. The subscale on self-efficacy for other symptoms measures self-efficacy for controlling symptoms of arthritis such as fatigue and frustration. Reliability is reported as .90. The subscale on self-efficacy for function contains nine items and measures one's self-efficacy for performing daily activities. Reliability is reported as .85 (Lorig, Chastain, et al., 1989). Each of the 20 questions is followed by a horizontal line anchored at either end by "very uncertain" and "very certain" with "moderately uncertain" in the center. Responses are marked on the line, which represents a scale calibrated from 10 to 100.

The Personal Resources Questionnaire, PRQ85, measuring social support, was developed by Weinert and Brandt in 1981 (Weinert, 1988) and revised in 1985 (Weinert, 1987). Part 1 addresses various aspects of network structure and provides descriptive data regarding situational support. Part 2 is a scale based on the work of Robert Weiss (1969) which was developed to measure the level of perceived relational support. Since perceived support was the variable of interest in this study, only Part 2 was used. Part 2 contains 25 items scored on a 7-point Likert scale. Scores may range from 25 to 175, with higher scores indicating higher levels of perceived social support. Cronbach's alpha is reported as .91.

The Purpose in Life Test is a 20-item scale which measures how much an individual experiences life as meaningful, how much an individual "feels like somebody who matters," and how strongly an individual has developed a sense of purposeful direction in life (Crumbaugh & Maholick, 1964). Scores may range from 20 to 140. Higher scores suggest a stronger sense of life-meaning, with scores above 112 indicating definite purpose and meaning in life, and scores below 92 indicating a lack of clear meaning and purpose.

The short version of the Arthritis Impact Measurement Scales, or AIMS, is a 10-item functional impairment index which measures mobility, physical activity, dexterity, household role, and activities of daily living. The higher the score, the greater the impairment. The authors (Wallston, Brown, Stein, & Bobbins, 1989) report that the overall internal consistency of the short version is as adequate as the longer, widely used version by Meenan, Gertman, Mason, and Dunaif (1982). Alpha for the short version is reported as .83; for the long version, .88. A demographic data sheet was used to collect information on medication use, length of arthritis affliction, prior arthritis education, and coexistence of other illnesses.

Procedure

Subjects were randomly assigned to an experimental or control group. All subjects took the pretest (consisting of the four instruments) and completed the demographic data sheet. The experimental group received the *Arthritis Helpbook* to introduce and reinforce the material to be presented in class. Then, in groups of 10–20, the experimental group participated in the ASHC once a week for 2½ hours for 3 weeks. (Because of scheduling constraints at one of the study sites, the course was taught in 3 weeks instead of the usual 6 weeks. Consultation with the local Arthritis Foundation director indicated that the ASHC had previously been taught in this shorter time frame without compromising the integrity of the course content [E. Parley, personal communication, February 23, 1990].) The course used experiential, cognitive-behavioral, self-management techniques and covered the information described earlier. After the course, participants were mailed a posttest. The control group received a brochure on self-management (Arthritis Foundation, 1989) and were mailed a posttest at the end of 3 weeks. They were then offered the opportunity to take the course after the study period (42 did so).

RESULTS

Of the 130 subjects, 71 were in the experimental group and 59 in the control group. The majority were Caucasian females with rheumatoid arthritis (RA) or osteoarthritis (OA) (RA = 58.2%, OA = 32.9%; 8.9% did not know the type of arthritis); their age range was 27–87 with a mean of 68.5 years; and the mean duration of arthritis was 12.9 years. Seventy per cent took NSAIDS (non-steroidal anti-inflammatory drugs); 92% had not participated in previous arthritis education.

An analysis of covariance (ANCOVA) of posttest scores with the pretest as the covariate was used to look at the effect of the self-help course on the variables. The ASHC participants' scores on arthritis self-efficacy for pain management were significantly higher at posttest than the scores of those who did not participate [$F(1,128) = 6.89$, $p = .01$]. The self-help course group had a mean score of 68 at pretest and 76 at posttest; the control group's mean score was 67 at pretest and 67 at posttest.

Posttest scores of the treatment and control groups also differed on self-efficacy for managing other symptoms such as fatigue, controlling activity, doing something to help themselves feel better when feeling depressed, doing things they enjoyed, and dealing with frustration. The ASHC increased the perceived ability to deal with these symptoms. The posttest scores of participants in the self-help course were significantly higher than the scores of those who did not take the course [$F(1,128) = 7.84$, $p = .006$]. Self-help course participants had a mean score of 73 at pretest and 81 at posttest; non-participants had a mean of 73 at pretest and 73 at posttest.

The mean score on perceived social support for the self-help course participants was 139 on the pretest and 140 at posttest; the control group had a pretest mean of 138 and a posttest mean of 141. The mean purpose in life score for the ASHC participants was 114 at pretest and 115 at posttest; the mean for the control group was 111 at pretest and 111 at posttest. Like those scores, the Arthritis Impact scores showed little or no change; for participants in ASHC the mean was 20 at pretest and 21 at posttest; the mean for the control group was 20 at both points. Thus, no statistically significant differences were noted between the experimental and control groups in perceived social support, meaning and purpose in life, or functional ability.

In an end-of-course evaluation, 97% of those responding indicated that they intended to make changes in their arthritis care as a result of the course. Specifically, 90% said they would practice relaxation, 93% said they intended to do more stretching exercises, and 86% indicated that they would do more strengthening exercises.

DISCUSSION

The findings provide confirmation that the ASHC, using self-management techniques and experiential activities, can improve aspects of arthritis that are both physiological and psychological, particularly in terms of symptom management. The program failed to produce improvements on some measures of adaptation to arthritis; however, in arthritis, symptoms tend to wax and wane, and it may be that these subjects were adapting well to their disease. (Also, my colleagues who work in arthritis care tell me that a finding of *no change* on the disability score is a positive one, since most people with RA experience an increase in disability over time.) The goal of the Arthritis Self-Help Course is to teach persons with arthritis how to best manage the disease activity themselves and the program seemed to be successful in doing that for the majority of the participants. Assessment of those who would benefit from health education programs such as the ASHC would help the nurse target for special attention those behaviors or tasks with which the assessment indicates the client needs help.

People with arthritis who received the educational intervention had significantly higher self-efficacy scores than people in the control group. Research supports a high correlation between one's confidence in the ability to do a task and actually doing it. Clinicians can adapt the self-efficacy tool for use in their practice. Using the stem "At this time, how certain are you that you can . . . ," the expert clinician in any area can fill in the task or behavior needing assessment.

With its emphasis on self-management, the ASHC can be used as a prototype for nursing interventions to help people with arthritis and other chronic illnesses feel more confident in managing their illnesses. The *Self-Help Course Manual* and *The Arthritis Helpbook* are available from the Arthritis Foundation in all 50 states. These sources provide information on making or ordering relaxation tapes, as well as a variety of clever inexpensive items clients can make (I effectively used exercise bands made from discarded panty hose). Both in a previous study (Dulski & Newman, 1989), and in this one, I have demonstrated that simply teaching relaxation techniques, which all nurses are familiar with, can decrease the client's perception of pain.

Some clients only need nurses' support and encouragement to manage their arthritis. From the anecdotal notes I kept, I would like to share a comment from a participant that summarizes how these brave people face their daily tasks *despite* their pain: "Most people with arthritis don't want pity, just understanding; I've learned that I have to help myself, let other people help me, move a little at a time, and just keep on keepin' on."

ACKNOWLEDGMENT

This research was supported by a Doctoral Dissertation Award from the Arthritis Foundation.

REFERENCES

Arthritis Foundation. (1987). *The arthritis self-help course.* Atlanta, GA: Author.

Arthritis Foundation. (1989). *Self-help tips to help you combat arthritis.* Atlanta, GA: Author.

Bandura, A. (1986). *Social foundation of thought and action: A social cognitive theory.* Englewood Cliffs, NJ: Prentice Hall.

Broadhead, W., Kaplan, B., James, S., Wagner, E., Schoenbach, V., Grimson, R., Heyden, S., Tibbin, G., & Gehlbach, S. (1983). The epidemiologic evidence for a relationship between social support and health. *Journal of Epidemiology, 117,* 521–536.

Crumbaugh, J., & Maholick, L. (1964). An experimental study in existentialism: The psychometric approach to Frankl's ogenic neurosis. *Journal of Clinical Psychology, 20,* 200–207.

Dulski, T., & Newman, A. (1989). The effectiveness of relaxation in relieving pain of women with rheumatoid arthritis. In S. Funk, E. Tornquist, M. Champagne, L. Copp, & R. Wiese (Eds.), *Key aspects of comfort: managing pain, fatigue, and nausea* (pp. 150–154). New York: Springer Publishing Co.

Kobasa, S., Maddi, S., & Kahn, S. (1982). Hardiness and health: A prospective study. *Journal of Personality and Social Psychology, 42*, 168–177.

Lorig, K. (1986). *Arthritis self-help course leader's manual and reference materials.* Atlanta, GA: Arthritis Foundation.

Lorig, K., Chastain, R., Ung, E., Shoor, S., & Holman, H. (1989). Development and evaluation of a scale to measure perceived self-efficacy in people with arthritis. *Arthritis and Rheumatism, 32*, 37–44.

Lorig, K., & Fries, J. (1986). *The arthritis helpbook (revised ed.).* Reading, MA: Addison-Wesley.

Lorig, K., Konkol, L., & Gonzoles, V. (1987). Arthritis patient education: A review of the literature. *Patient Education Counseling, 10*, 207–252.

Lorig, K., Mazonson, P., & Holman, H. (1989). Four-year clinical and service utilization benefits of arthritis patient education. *Arthritis Care and Research, 2*, 58.

Meenan, R., Gertman, P., Mason, J., & Dunaif, R. (1982). The Arthritis Impact Measurement Scales: Further investigations of a health status measure. *Arthritis and Rheumatism, 25*, 1048–1053.

Phillips, W. (1980). Purpose in life, depression, and locus of control. *Journal of Clinical Psychology, 36*, 661–667.

Thompson, S., & Janigan, A. (1988). Life schemes: A framework for understanding the search for meaning. *Journal of Social and Clinical Psychology, 7*, 260–280.

Wallston, K., Brown, G., Stein, M., & Bobbins, C. (1989). Comparing the short and long versions of the Arthritis Impact Measurement Scales. *Journal of Rheumatology, 16*, 1105–1109.

Weinert, C. (1987). A social support measure: PRQ85. *Nursing Research, 36*, 273–277.

Weinert, C. (1988). Measuring social support: Revision and further development of the personal resource questionnaire. In C. Waltz & O. Strickland, (Eds.), *Measurement of nursing outcomes, volume one: Measuring client outcomes* (pp. 309–327). New York: Springer Publishing Co.

Weiss, R. (1969). The fund of sociability. *Trans-Action, 6*(9), 36–43.

[14]

Promoting a Learned Self-Help Response to Chronic Illness

Carrie Jo Braden

Anderson (1990) attributes the development of the self-care/self-help movement to the combined effects of the economic system, the power system controlling health care institutions, and our society's ideological system, which incorporates the values of productivity and self-management. Nurses have developed interventions that empower people to more fully participate in their health care. However, the ability of nurses to carry out these interventions depends on policy decisions in which costs weigh heavily. Therefore, nursing research is needed to demonstrate the cost-effectiveness of self-care/self-help promoting programs.

A health service is cost-effective if it is worth the expenditure of the resources required to deliver the service (Warner & Luce, 1982). Two kinds of outcomes are necessary for cost-effectiveness analysis: the dollar amounts for financial outlay and the health effects or outcomes (Russell, 1987). Russell (1987) includes the nonmonetary variables of desirable direct outcomes, desirable indirect outcomes, and undesirable outcomes in net effectiveness. The nonmonetary part of cost effectiveness analysis thus represents many variables of interest to nurses who are designing, implementing, and evaluating self-management programs. The nonmonetary variables addressed in this chapter are quality of life, self-care, and self-help.

Our study of learned response to chronic illness experience began with the clinical observation that the actual severity of the illness appeared unrelated to a person's ability to remain involved in valued life activities. Some persons having a great deal of debility from their illnesses routinely worked, raised children, participated in social and community activities, and took part in recreation. Others with similar or less debility withdrew from life and let others care for them. These clinical observations are consistent with Browne, Arpin, Corey, Fitch, and Gafni's (1990) recent finding that psychosocial adjustment, defined as the capacity to live with chronic illness with a minimum loss of valued vocational, domestic, and social roles, was the strongest correlate of health care service utilization. Their study of 215 chronically ill individuals from oncology, rheumatology, and gastroenterology clinics in Toronto found a statistically significant association between total annual health costs per patient and the patient's level of adjustment. The higher the adjustment, the lower the cost.

The Self-Help Model was generated to describe the dynamics of learned response to chronic illness (Braden, 1990a, 1990b). The model is based on the assumption that adjustment is a learned rather than an inherited capacity or personality trait. The model recognizes the resilience of people by describing how a repertory of enabling skills helps individuals meet the situational and cognitive challenges of illness. The model is consistent with Rosenbaum's (1990) hypothesis that while exposure to disruptive forces interrupts smooth execution of a desired behavior, self-management of internal events through enabling skills minimizes the undesirable interfering effects of the disruptive forces.

The Self-Help Model (see Figure 14.1) consists of seven major variables. Perceived severity of illness, which operates as a stimulus for learning, is at Stage One. Severity of illness is defined as one's perceived level of affliction as a result of chronic disease course characteristics. The Stage Two variables of uncertainty and dependence are major adversities that are part

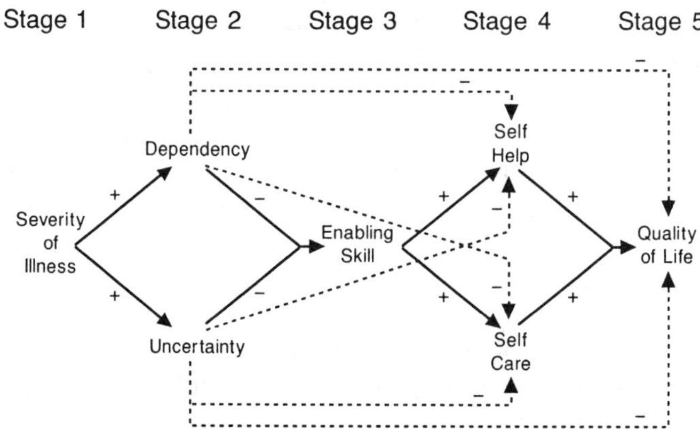

FIGURE 14.1. Self–Help Model.

of the chronic illness experience. Uncertainty is defined as inability to determine meaning within the chronic illness situation (Mishel, 1988). It can occur, for example, when one is unable to use cues from the illness, such as symptoms, to predict what will happen in the future in terms of illness outcomes. Many chronic conditions have symptoms that wax and wane and do not seem to be clearly tied to the progress of the disease. Dependence is defined as one's perceived level of reliance on others to perform daily living activities. The particular daily living activities that are often connected to persons' perceptions of being dependent on others are the functional outcomes discussed by McBride in Chapter 2 of this volume; they include eating, toileting, personal grooming, and mobility. Enabling skill, the mediator of these aversive aspects of chronic illness, is at Stage Three in the model. Enabling skill is defined as one's perceived ability to manage adversity. Stages Four and Five consist of the desired outcomes of self-help, self-care, and quality of life. Self-help is defined as one's perceived level of adult role performance—that is, being able to do the things one finds important in life, the things that define who one is. McBride describes these functional outcomes as having to do with grocery shopping, participating in social activities, recreational activities, etc. Self-care is defined as the level of direct action behaviors for prevention or alleviation of treatment side effects or of preventable complications of illness. Quality of life is defined as one's level of satisfaction with one's current situation.

In the Self-Help Model, perceived severity of illness is a variable that increases exposure to the aversive aspects of chronic illness. Hence, as perceived illness severity increases, so do the level of uncertainty about the illness and the level of dependence. These two adversities are negatively related to enabling skill: as adversities increase, one's enabling skills are eroded; they decrease. Enabling skills include problem solving, cognitive reframing, and belief in self. These are the kinds of personal resources that McBride identifies as pivotal for maintaining optimism. If sufficient enabling skills are present, uncertainty and dependence will not undermine self-help, self-care, and quality of life. Thus, if persons are able to problem solve and, in particular, to generate alternatives, if they are able to cognitively reframe events or use non-negative thinking, and if they believe they are capable persons, they will be able to overcome the effects of the uncertainties in the illness experience as well as the effects of circumstances that promote dependence. They will then be able to continue participating in desired role behaviors, to do things they consider important, and to maintain their life quality. The studies reported here, therefore, focused on interventions to maintain or increase enabling skill.

STUDY 1

The purpose of the first study (Braden, 1989) was to determine if there were differences between people who participated in self-help programs and those who did not choose to participate, and to determine if the proposed self-help model was supported by data collected from the two groups. The study retrospectively examined 396 subjects having diagnoses of rheumatoid arthritis or other arthritis-related conditions. Data were collected through mailed questionnaires to 500 persons who had participated in programs offered by an arthritis center (200 of these questionnaires were returned), and through completion of an identical questionnaire by 196 people contacted at three different health fairs. Two hundred and thirty subjects had attended some type of self-management program—for example, the Arthritis Self-Help Course sponsored by and distributed through the Arthritis Foundation; 138 subjects had not attended a program (28 did not indicate whether or not they had attended a program). Significant differences between the two groups were found in learned response [$T^2 = .05$; $F(7,360) = 2.4, p < .02$]. Discriminant function analysis indicated that group differences were due to differences in perceived severity of illness, dependence, uncertainty, enabling skill, and self-help.

The Self-Help Model relationships were also tested within each group using regression procedures. Despite differences between the groups on the levels of the variables, the linkages or relationship patterns between the variables specified by the Self-Help Model were essentially the same for both groups.

This type of retrospective study cannot provide an evaluation of a self-management program's effectiveness, but it did demonstrate that the variables and relationships in the Self-Help Model were the same whether or not learning was facilitated by participation in self-management programs.

In both groups, enabling skills as measured by Rosenbaum's (1980) Self-Control Schedule (SCS) mediated the effects of uncertainty and dependence on self-help, self-care, and life quality. Among those who had not attended a self-management program, uncertainty and dependence reduced the level of enabling skills. The diagnosis of systemic lupus erythematosus (SLE) also reduced the level of enabling skills among those who had not attended a self-management program. For those persons who had attended a self-management program, uncertainty did not significantly reduce enabling skill. Only dependence undermined their enabling skills. While these results appeared promising, this first study raised questions about whether those who choose to attend self-management programs have a lower level of illness severity than those who do not attend and about what the potential role of self-management interventions is and what the characteristics are of those who may be helped by such a resource.

STUDY 2

A second set of studies, using a pre-experimental design, evaluated the effectiveness of a Systemic Lupus Erythematosus (SLE) Self-Help Course designed to enhance problem solving, cognitive reframing, and belief in self, and to decrease uncertainty and depression (Braden, 1991, 1992). With the support of health professionals the course was designed by a group of laypersons having a diagnosis of SLE (Braden, Brodt-Weinberg, McGlone, Depka, & Pretter, 1987). The course includes seven 2-hour classes organized into activities addressing different aspects of living with a chronic condition. Several activities are designed to strengthen problem-solving skills, to foster the ability to cognitively reframe events and do non-negative thinking, and to increase participants' belief in themselves. Other class activities foster specific self-care strategies and provide information about SLE. A teacher's manual contains a protocol for carrying out each activity and the amount of time each activity should take (Arthritis Foundation, 1987). Course leaders are persons with SLE and health professionals, who form teaching teams after participating in a Leaders' Training Session (McGlone, Tnetter, & Depka, 1990). The course is distributed by the Arthritis Foundation and has been offered at more than 17 sites across the country.

A convenience sample of 291 subjects who had a diagnosis of SLE and who participated in the self-help course provided data at three points in time: T_1, prior to initiation of the course; T_2, 7 weeks later, immediately after the course was completed; and T_3, 2 months following completion of the course. Somewhat different variables were used in the Self-Help Model for this study since the persons who developed the course said that their level of limitation, or how much their disease interfered with the ability to carry out daily living activities, was more applicable to them than dependence or reliance on other people. The course designers also were more interested in looking at self-worth as an outcome than at self-help and self-care. In addition, they were interested in using self-efficacy—or belief in one's ability to perform specific activities—as a mediator along with enabling skill. Finally, they wanted to look at depression because depression had made it more difficult for them to learn how to live with their chronic condition. Depression was thus a negative mediator, that is, one that interfered with the learning process.

The study questionnaire was developed by laypersons having a diagnosis of SLE and health professionals who had participated in the course development. Limitation, one's perceived level of inability to do things for oneself, was measured by a single item having a score range from 1 to 4. The higher the score, the greater the limitation. Uncertainty, one's perceived amount of ambiguity about treatment effectiveness, was measured by three items using a visual analogue (VAS) response format. Items addressed were certainty about the ability to use self-care techniques, effectiveness of lupus medications to improve SLE, and the ability to decrease pain or stiffness. Scores could range from 0 to 300, with higher scores indicating less certainty (greater uncertainty). Depression, one's level of despondency, was measured by four items using a VAS response format. Scores could range from 0 to 400, with higher scores indicating greater depression. Enabling skill, one's perceived level of ability to manage adversity, was measured by six items drawn from Rosenbaum's (1990) Self-Control Schedule. A VAS response format was used. Scores could range from 0 to 600 with higher scores indicating greater enabling skill. Self-efficacy, the strength of one's conviction that one can do what is necessary to control a primary SLE-related symptom, was measured by a single item using a VAS response format. The score could range from 0 to 100 with higher scores indicating greater self-efficacy. Self-worth, one's level of positive feelings about one's own being, was measured by ten items with a VAS response format. Scores could range from 0 to 1000, with higher scores indicating greater feelings of self-worth. Quality of life, or perceived level of satisfaction with one's personal situation, was measured by three items drawn from Campbell, Converse, & Roger's (1976) 10-item semantic differential scale, the Inventory of Well-Being (IWB). Scores could range from 0 to 300, with higher scores indicating better quality of life.

A repeated measures MANOVA was used to determine if participants in the course changed significantly in any of the Self-Help Model variables over time. Subjects improved significantly on the set of variables ($F(14,2800) = 603, p < .001$). Follow-up ANOVAs examining each variable separately revealed significant increases ($p \leq .001$) in enabling skills, self-efficacy, and self-worth, and decreases in uncertainty and depression. Table 14.1 provides the means for the variables that changed significantly over time.

While this pre-experimental study did not have a control group and therefore the changes cannot be firmly attributed to the SLE course, the findings were encouraging and therefore an additional study was designed to measure the effectiveness of a self-help class for women receiving treatment for breast cancer (discussed later in this chapter). Also, further analysis was done to examine the differences over time in Self-Help Model variables for two groups of the SLE Course participants—those having high depression scores (≥ 272) at baseline and those having low depression scores (≤ 77) at baseline (Braden, 1992). The purpose was to determine whether those who were depressed could effectively use a

Table 14.1 Mean Changes Over Time in SLE Course Participants (n = 291)

Variables	Means over time[a]		
	T_1	T_2	T_3
Uncertainty	127.5	96.7	99.7
Depression	175.4	146.8	154.4
Enabling skill	395.3	419.3	431.8
Self-efficacy	39.3	53.1	56.4
Self-worth	632.5	680.4	667.9

[a]T_1 = prior to initiation of course; T_2 = immediately after course was completed; T_3 = 2 months following completion of course.

self-management promoting intervention offered in a class format. It was expected that persons who were depressed at entry into the course—but not so depressed that they could not use such a resource—would be helped most by the course because they had most to gain. Thirty-seven subjects had high depression scores at the time of entry into the course and 35 subjects had low depression scores. Repeated measures MANOVA was used to see if the two groups differed on the Self-Help Model variables at the three points in time. The depressed group did have lower mean scores on enabling skill, self-efficacy and self-worth and higher mean scores on uncertainty at baseline [$F(1,70) = 8.3, p = .01$]. Over time both groups made significant gains in enabling skill, self-efficacy, and self-worth [$F(18,1264) = 8.9, p = .001$]. In addition, the depressed group also significantly decreased in uncertainty and increased in quality of life over time. These findings suggest that the course was indeed beneficial for those who were depressed but had sufficient incentive to attend. Table 14.2 gives the mean scores on variables that changed significantly over time for the two groups.

STUDY 3

A third study was done to see if the amount of time spent on a particular in-class activity in the SLE Self-Help Course was associated with the amount of change over time in the outcome of the activity (Braden, McGlone, & Pennington, 1993). The sample included participants in the course over a 4-year period, from 1987 to 1990. Three hundred and thirteen subjects provided data for this study. A dose-response table (see Figure 14.2) was generated to look at the associations, between the amount of time spent on class activities and perceived limitations, depression, enabling

TABLE 14.2 Mean Scores Over Time of SLE Class Participants with High and Low Depression Scores

	Means over time[a]		
	T_1	T_2	T_3
High Depressed Group (n = 37)			
Uncertainty	159.1	118.6	127.0
Enabling skill	330.8	375.0	388.8
Self-efficacy	28.9	54.1	47.7
Self-worth	461.4	570.8	499.6
Life quality	108.7	157.6	135.9
Low Depressed Group (n = 35)			
Enabling skill	441.0	454.4	484.4
Self-efficacy	54.6	60.0	67.6
Self-worth	808.5	822.7	851.9

[a]T_1 = prior to initiation of course; T_2 = immediately after course was completed; T_3 = 2 months following completion of course.

skills, and the self-care behaviors of use of heat, rest, exercise, and relaxation. The amount of time spent in class was associated with change over time in the perception of limitations, depression, enabling skill and engaging in rest, relaxation, heat, and exercise activities. As Figure 14.2 shows, less than 10 minutes of class time was spent on limitations and on the self-care activities of use of heat and rest. There were no significant changes in these variables. However, more than an hour was devoted to depression and enabling skill, and to the self-care behaviors of relaxation and exercise, and there were significant changes in these variables. The findings support the efficacy of the course as an intervention for persons with SLE.

STUDY 4

A current study is testing self-help promoting interventions with women receiving treatment for breast cancer. As in the SLE studies, this project focuses on enhancing problem solving, cognitive reframing, and belief in self. In addition, the project focuses on management of uncertainty as another means of facilitating a learned self-help response to this chronic illness experience. The Self-Help Intervention Project (SHIP) has a control group and random assignment to the intervention groups. There are five different sets of interventions being tested. One is a self-help course made up of six weekly 2-hour sessions; the others are an independent study program that uses the content from the classes, a nurse-client telephone contact focused on uncertainty management, the nurse-client contact used in

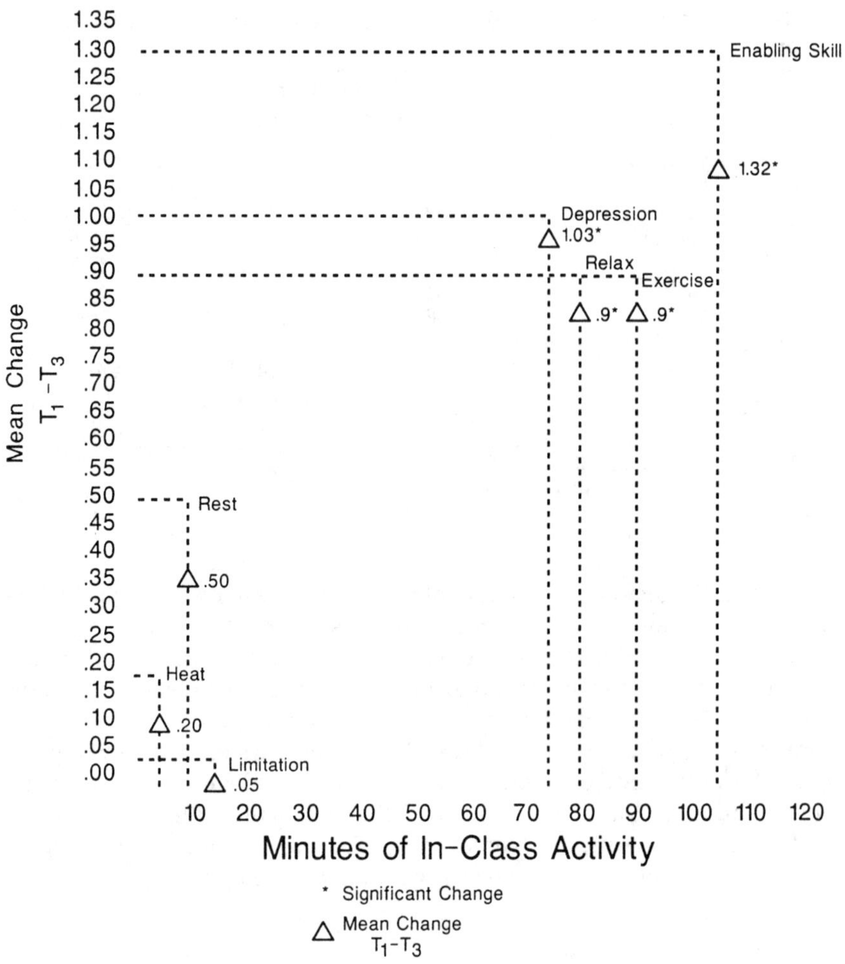

FIGURE 14.2. Relationship between treatment strength and response for self-care behaviors (heat, rest, relaxation, and exercise) and psychosocial concerns (limitations, depression, and enabling skill).

combination with the class, and the nurse-client contact used in combination with the independent study. Over 120 women will provide data at five points in time. The total time covered by the study extends to 9 months after the intervention. The 6-week interventions are offered beginning approximately 3 weeks into the women's adjunctive treatment regime. The analyses will address differences in the intervention groups over time and compare them to the control group, and will include a cost-effectiveness analysis that examines both monetary and nonmonetary aspects. Preliminary findings are available only for the independent study intervention and the combination of independent study and a nurse-client contact.

About half of the women assigned to the independent study group did not complete the lessons. When the independent study intervention was paired with the nurse-client contact intervention, more women completed the lessons. Those who completed the lessons, that is, those who actually received the treatment, differed significantly from the control group in cancer knowledge and other self-help model variables after completing the intervention.

Preliminary analyses have also revealed that the older women (mean age of 71 years) differed from the younger women (mean age of 50 years) on marital status and living arrangements, with older women being more often widows and living alone. The older group was also less ethnically diverse, which is consistent with the literature suggesting that minority women do not seek attention for breast cancer until later in the disease process, if at all. Fewer older women had discovered their cancer through breast self-exam; more were diagnosed through routine mammogram. Older women experienced more prompt physician follow-up than younger women, but received less aggressive treatment despite the fact that they did not differ from younger women on stage, node status, metastases, or recurrence. The older and younger groups also differed at baseline on self-help model variables. The interventions were effective for older women. Data on older women have also indicated the number and kinds of self-help class activities that are rated as very helpful. Such information is being used to modify the intervention for older women.

DISCUSSION

The studies to date support the mediating role of enabling skills in reducing the impact of chronic illness adversities on self-help, self-care, and quality of life. The findings also suggest that self-help classes designed to enhance enabling skills work for a variety of chronic illness populations. The findings further suggest that those in greatest need benefit most from self-help promoting interventions. Thus, the studies to date show the importance of nonmonetary aspects of cost effectiveness. Desirable direct outcomes of interventions include increases in enabling skill as a mediator for self-help, self-care, and quality of life outcomes. Desirable indirect outcomes include various uses of the self-help class intervention for a variety of persons, including those who may be depressed by their chronic illness. Undesirable outcomes have yet to be identified. Given the data showing a positive impact of self-help promoting interventions on self-care, self-help, and quality of life, clinicians can now justify incorporating in their practice strategies that enhance problem solving and cognitive reframing skills and that increase a sense of personal worth or mastery. The SLE (Lupus) Self-Help Course is available through the Arthritis Foundation and can serve as a prototype for self-help courses for other chronic conditions. For example, there is a Multiple Sclerosis Self-Help Course (McGlone et al., 1984) that uses many of the same activities to enhance enabling skills that are included in the SLE (Lupus) Self-Help Course.

In summary, data on the nonmonetary aspects of cost effectiveness of self-care/self-help promoting programs are now available to nurses who want to incorporate such activities in their work. There are also emerging data about the monetary aspects of such interventions (Brown, Arpin, Corey, Fitch, & Gafni, 1990). There are prototype self-help promoting programs available. There are programs of nursing research that can provide the tools and methods essential for evaluation of self-care/self-help promoting interventions. Finally, there are persons with chronic illness diagnoses who desire help in maintaining their functional status and quality of life.

ACKNOWLEDGMENT

These studies were supported by grants from NRSA 423976, University of Arizona Small Grant award, NCNR R29 NR01696, NCI R01 CA48450.

REFERENCES

Anderson, J. M. (1990). Home care management in chronic illness and the self-care movement: An analysis of ideologies and economic processes influencing policy decisions. *Advances in Nursing Science, 12,* 71–83.

Arthritis Foundation. (1987). *Systemic Lupus Erythematosus Self-Help Course. Program guidelines and procedures manual.* Atlanta, GA: Author.

Braden, C. J. (1989, March). *Modeling learned response to chronic illness.* Paper presented at the International Conference on Community Nursing 1989. World Health Organization, 's-Herrogenbosch, The Netherlands.

Braden, C. J. (1990a). Learned self-help response to chronic illness experience: A test of the alternative learning theories. *Scholarly Inquiry for Nursing Practice: An International Journal, 4,* 23–40.

Braden, C. J. (1990b). A test of the self-help model: Learned response to chronic illness experience. *Nursing Research, 39,* 42–47.

Braden, C. J. (1991). Patterns of change over time in learned response to chronic illness among participants in a Systemic Lupus Erythematosus (SLE) Self-Help Course. *Arthritis Care and Research, 4,* 158–167.

Braden, C. J. (1992). Description of learned response to chronic illness experience: Depressed vs. nondepressed SLE (Lupus) Self-Help Class participants. *Public Health Nursing, 9,* 103–108.

Braden, C. J., Brodt-Weinberg, R., McGlone, K., Depka, L, & Pretter, S. (1987). *Systemic Lupus Erythematosus (SLE) Self-Help Course, Leader's Manual.* Atlanta, GA: Arthritis Foundation.

Braden, C. J., McGlone, K., & Pennington, F. (1993). Specific psychosocial and behavior outcomes from the SLE Self-Help Course. *Health Education Quarterly, 20,* 29–41.

Browne, G. B., Arpin, K., Corey, P., Fitch, M., & Gafni, A. (1990). Individual correlates of health service utilization and the cost of poor adjustment of chronic illness. *Medical Care, 28,* 43–58.

Campbell, A., Converse, P., & Rogers, W. (1976). *The quality of American life.* New York: Sage.

McGlone, K., Atherton, A., Brodt-Weinberg, R., Minella, M., Sodano, B., Wintrick, J. (1984). *Multiple sclerosis self-help course: Leader's guide.* Tucson, AZ: Southwest Arthritis Center.

McGlone, Tnetter, S., & Depka, L. (1990). *SLE Self-Help Course trainer's guide.* Atlanta, GA: Arthritis Foundation.

Mishel, M. H. (1988). Uncertainty in illness. *Image: Journal of Nursing Scholarship, 20,* 225–232.

Rosenbaum, M. (1980). A schedule for assessing self-control behaviors: Preliminary findings. *Behavior Therapy, 11,* 109–121.

Rosenbaum, M. (1990). *Learned resourcefulness: On coping skills, self-control and adaptive behavior.* New York: Springer Publishing Co.

Russell, L. B. (1987). Cost-effectiveness analysis in setting priorities for prevention: Promises and problems. In J. A. Meyer & M. E. Lewin (Eds.), *Charting the future of health care.* Washington, DC: American Enterprise Institute for Public Policy Research.

Warner, K. E., & Luce, B. R. (1982). *Cost-benefit and cost-effectiveness analysis in health care.* Ann Arbor, MI: Health Administration Press.

[15]

Uncertainty Management for Women Receiving Treatment for Breast Cancer

Judith McHenry, Carol Allen, Merle H. Mishel, and Carrie Jo Braden

Uncertainty, defined by Mishel (1988) as the inability to determine the meaning of illness-related events, is a well documented experience of women receiving treatment for breast cancer (Bloom et al., 1987; Dodd, 1988; Fallowfield, 1990; Thomas, 1978; Yasko, 1990). These women often express uncertainty about the meaning of treatment side effects. Also, they may not understand what symptoms indicate or what to expect from treatment, if, indeed, they know the treatment alternatives and understand them. They are unsure of the consequences of their illness and treatment and unsure how to manage life while receiving treatment. They frequently express anxiety about the possibility of recurrence or disease extension (Bloom, 1991; Penman et al., 1987; Siminoff, Fetting, & Abeloff, 1989; Vinokur, Threatt, Vinokur-Kaplan, & Satariano, 1990). This study was designed to describe the particular types of uncertainties experienced by women receiving treatment for breast cancer and to evaluate a nurse case manager intervention designed to help them manage uncertainty.

METHOD

The evaluation of the nurse case manager intervention was part of an ongoing project, "Nursing Interventions Promoting a Self-Help Response to Cancer." Subjects were women aged 18 years and older who were literate in English and currently receiving treatment for breast cancer. They were referred by a tertiary cancer center, private practice offices, and health maintenance organization clinics in a Southwestern state. Women who agreed to participate in the study were randomly assigned to the nurse case manager intervention group or to a control group.

The uncertainty management intervention was based on Mishel's uncertainty in illness theory (1988), which hypothesizes the relationships among antecedents to uncertainty and thus suggests interventions that might reduce or prevent uncertainty. The intervention included one or more telephone contacts per week for 6 weeks. Women were invited to call as often as they wished during the treatment period. However, most contacts were initiated by the nurse case manager.

The case manager used a standard Assessment/Appraisal/Intervention Guide displayed on a computer screen for easy reference during the phone conversation with each woman. Data pertinent to the individual woman were entered directly onto one portion of the guide to form a retrievable data set that could be recalled to the screen at the next phone call and used as a basis for reassessment, to make a determination of resolved uncertainties, and to identify new areas of uncertainty.

The Assessment/Appraisal/Intervention guide begins with assessment of uncertainty, using a list of potential problems affecting women with breast cancer, developed on the basis of information from focus groups, clinical practice, and research. This problem list is in six main categories: cancer diagnosis, treatment concerns, responses to treatment, living with cancer, self-care, and living with associated issues, for example, employment concerns. The assessment component of each phone contact addresses common types of uncertainty in these areas: the meaning of an event is unclear; the woman is lacking information needed for the management of an event; events are inconsistent or fluctuating in intensity, duration, frequency, etc.; unfamiliar events require management; outcomes of events are unknown; events occur beyond expectations in terms of intensity or any other parameter; or management of the event is conflictual with no easy resolution. For example, the meaning of shooting pains following mastectomy is sometimes not clear, and the experience of fatigue is often perceived as longer and more intense than anticipated. Women frequently express uncertainty about their ability to manage problems such as nausea or the discomfort of hot flashes.

During the telephone interview, the nurse case manager makes a diagnosis of the problem and specifies the type of uncertainty pertaining to that problem. For example, if the nurse determines that the woman is having pain, the nurse explores whether the perceived uncertainty concerns the meaning or management of the pain, or perhaps comes from confusion regarding the duration of the pain. Statements indicating uncertainty include these: "I didn't expect..., I guess it's okay..., I don't understand..., Is it normal..., What should I do about..., Sometimes I wonder..., I'm not sure..., Where can I get..., It keeps changing..., The doctor says it's okay, but..., Who should I call...?"

The existence of negative certainty is also assessed from the woman's commentary about a problem. In this case, there is an expressed expectation that the problem will have a negative outcome, the course of the situation is perceived as definitely worsening, or the actual trajectory is perceived as predictably downward.

Next, the woman's appraisal of the uncertainty is assessed. She may be evaluated as perceiving low, moderate, or high danger based upon specified criteria that ascend in severity as the perceived danger level rises. Sometimes the uncertainty is appraised as representing an opportunity for some type of positive gain. The criteria for these designations are provided in a secondary appraisal guide. On the basis of the information obtained using the assessment and appraisal guides, the case manager selects the interventions appropriate for the content of the uncertainty as well as for the appraisal of the uncertainty.

The interventions are organized around five goals:

1. to strengthen an existing structure and reinforce an opportunity appraisal through interventions that reinforce decisions and self-care behaviors, and support existing coping and buffering strategies;
2. to promote cognitive structure formation through providing information, structuring expectations, and normalizing the experience;
3. to reduce negative certainty in instances when a perception of negative outcome may be inappropriate or incorrect;
4. to regulate emotional response through encouragement of ventilation of feelings or selective use of humor;
5. to manage continual uncertainty through interventions to enhance personal control, to encourage probabilistic thinking by generating multiple options, or to reframe uncertainty into a normal situation for everyone.

As noted above, in this study the case manager entered both the assessment/appraisal portion of the interview and the interventions provided onto each woman's computer record. All information was available on the screen via a d-Base program presenting appropriate screens and providing summary reports either for individual subjects or for groups of subjects.

Data were collected at three points in time: T1, at baseline, prior to initiation of the intervention; T2, within 2 weeks after completion of the intervention; and T3, 3 months following completion of the intervention.

The outcomes measured were self-help, self-care, life quality, positive and negative affective state or mood, enabling skills, and uncertainty. Self-help, or perceived level of involvement in carrying out adult role activities, was measured by a 20-item Inventory of Adult Role Behavior (IARB) (Braden, 1986). The IARB includes items adopted from Given's (1984) Effect Scale, which measures social psychological health states of ambulatory chronically ill patients, and investigator-developed items measuring the degree to which individuals are involved in leisure time roles, social activity roles, and family roles. A visual analogue scale (VAS), a 100 mm. line anchored at each end by oppositional descriptors, provides for a range of scores from 0 to 2000 cm. The higher the IARB score, the greater the involvement in adult role functions. The standardized Cronbach's alpha was .92 in data collected from 196 subjects at baseline. Criterion-related validity and construct validity have been supported across several populations.

Self-care, or the amount of direct coping actions engaged in to prevent or alleviate side effects or preventable complications of treatment and to maintain healthy life patterns, was measured by two scales, The Inventory of Adult Self-Care (IASC) (Braden, 1986) and the Self-Care Inventory (SCI) (Pardine, Napoli, & Dytell, 1983). The IASC measures the degree to which an individual is involved in self-care. It is an 8-item visual analogue scale containing statements about participating in self-care activities. Subjects rate the degree to which each statement is true about them. Scores range from 0 to 800. The higher the score, the greater the involvement in self-care. The SCI is a 30-item Likert scale which rates from 1 to 4 the frequency with which the subject has engaged in health care behaviors during the past week. Scores range from 0 to 120. The higher the score, the greater the involvement in self-care. Both scales have internal consistency reliability above the ≥ .70 criterion set by Nunnally (1978). Criterion-related validity and construct validity were established in the pilot study for this project.

Life quality, the perceived degree of overall satisfaction with life, was measured by the 8-item Inventory of Well-Being (IWB) (Campbell, Converse, & Rogers, 1976). The 10-item IWB was adapted from its original semantic differential form to a visual analogue response format. The scale includes words and phrases describing how an individual feels about his or her present life. The scale is scored in a positive direction for well-being, and scores range from 0 to 1000. Cronbach's alpha was .91 for the IWB in the analysis of the project sample ($n = 196$).

Positive and negative affective states, the dominant dimensions of emotional experience as reflected by mood states, were measured by the Positive and Negative Affect Scales (PANAS) developed by Watson, Clark, and Tellegen (1988). The PANAS consists of ten words that a subject chooses to describe feelings and emotions that the individual might have regarding his/her illness. Five words represent positive affect and five words represent negative affect. Both positive and negative affects are scored in a positive direction to indicate the degree to which an individual has that feeling. Affect is scored from 0 to 50. These scales have been shown to be highly consistent, largely without correlations between positive and negative affect, and stable at appropriate levels over a 2-month period under usual life circumstances. In the current study, Cronbach's alpha was .85 for positive affect and .90 for negative affect, in the data on 196 subjects. Normative data and factorial and external evidence of convergent and discriminant validity for the scales have been reported (Watson, Clark, & Tellegen, 1988).

Enabling skills represent the ability to eliminate or modify the effects of disruptive factors inherent in adverse situations—in this case, the impact of the cancer and treatment. The Self Control Schedule (SCS) by Rosenbaum (1983) was used to measure enabling skills. The SCS is a 36-item visual analogue scale; the scoring is 0–3600. The higher the score, the higher the level of enabling skills. There are reported estimates of reliability and validity (Rosenbaum, 1983), and the instrument has strong support for construct validity through predictive modeling (Braden, 1986). Cronbach's alpha from the pilot study was .89.

Uncertainty, as defined earlier, was measured by the Mishel Uncertainty in Illness Scale (MUIS) (Mishel, 1988). The 33-item MUIS is in a visual analogue format. The items are scored in a positive direction for uncertainty in illness. Scores range from 0 to 3300. The MUIS has construct validity and reliability across multiple illness populations (Mishel & Braden, 1988).

RESULTS

One hundred and one women received the nurse case manager intervention. One of these failed to complete the 6 weeks of the intervention and eight others failed to complete the three sets of data collection instruments. The average age of the 92 subjects in the final sample was 57.6 years. Most subjects had Stage I or II disease and were receiving two types of treatment—for example, chemotherapy and radiation, radiation and hormone, hormone and chemotherapy. The number of nurse contacts ranged from 1 to 11; the average was 5.3 per subject. The amount of time spent on the phone per subject ranged from 5 minutes to 52.5 minutes. The average amount of time spent was 19.9 minutes.

The most frequently expressed problems were in the area of "responses to treatment" and included fatigue, pain, and hot flashes. "Treatment concerns" were a second area of problems that were commonly identified; these included outcomes from treatment, questions about the treatment plan, and treatment efficacy. A third category of problems identified pertained to "caring for self," including problems in implementing self-care behaviors, communicating needs to health care providers, and managing appearance (see Table 15.1).

The uncertainty expressed most frequently came from the perception that management of the identified problem was unsure or unknown or the woman lacked information about it. The second most common source of uncertainty was difficulty in understanding the meaning of the problem, which was perceived as being unclear, unknown, or uncertain.

As noted earlier, problem identification and uncertainty appraisal were followed by a secondary appraisal, to evaluate the woman's perception of the danger in her uncertainty. The highest percentage (49%) of the appraisals reflected moderate danger; smaller percentages (35.4%) saw low danger, high danger (10.6%), or opportunity (5%). These findings are important because an appraisal of moderate danger signifies that a subject is concerned enough about the problem to desire and accept information, and sufficiently motivated to make necessary change, both of which are important for planning and delivery of interventions. As noted earlier, intervention choices were based not only on the content of the uncertainty-related problem, but also on the woman's secondary appraisal.

The nurse case manager interventions used most frequently included those promoting a cognitive structure or schema with respect to the problem, providing information, clarifying or normalizing the problem, and promoting assertive communication with health care providers or significant others. For example, for a reported symptom of fatigue, if the subject

TABLE 15.1 Most Frequently Reported Uncertainty Problems

Uncertainty category	Specific uncertainty problem[a]	Frequency reported
1. Responses to treatment		280
	a. fatigue	40
	b. pain	25
	c. hot flashes	22
2. Treatment concerns		119
	a. outcomes from treatment	31
	b. treatment plan	20
	c. treatment efficacy	13
3. Caring for self		80
	a. implementing self-care	19
	b. communicating needs to health care providers	14
	c. managing appearance	13

[a]Only the three most frequently reported problems are presented in the table.

lacked information and understanding of the fatigue, the nurse provided information to help her understand why she was fatigued and provided information as to whether the fatigue was normal under the circumstances, and how to best manage the fatigue. This information provided the subject with a mental picture (cognitive schema) to deal with the fatigue. Other commonly used interventions included those to reinforce an existing structure or understanding of the identified problem; they included validating the subject's view of her situation, validating self-care behaviors, and reinforcing decisions about problems.

DISCUSSION

The finding that nearly all women participated in the intervention (only 1 of 101 women withdrew from the case manager intervention group) indicates that women valued the contact with the nurse case manager. The average amount of time spent in a given contact was 20 minutes. This finding provides an estimate of the time required for a clinical nurse to provide psychobehavioral support, as defined by the five intervention goals described previously, to women with breast cancer. This is the kind of information needed prior to incorporating a telephone case management service as a part of adjunctive therapy for women with breast cancer. In addition, the existence of a d-Base program for accessing individual information and updating a record with further assessments, as well as tracking and noting the outcomes of specific nursing interventions, is an important aspect of the intervention. Used in a service setting, such a system could facilitate monitoring of an optimum number of women. Thus, although work needs to be done to document the effectiveness of the intervention, these preliminary indications provide support for its potential as a practical intervention.

ACKNOWLEDGMENT

Support for this study was provided by a National Cancer Institute grant #1 R01 CA48450, "Nursing Interventions Promoting a Self Help Response to Cancer."

REFERENCES

Bloom, J. R. (1991). Quality of life after cancer. A policy perspective. *Cancer, 67*, 855–859.

Bloom, J. R., Cook, M., Flamer, D. P., Fotopoulis, S., Gates, C., Holland, J. C., Muenz, L. R., Murawski, B., Penman, D., Ross, R. D. (1987). Psychological response to mastectomy. *Cancer, 59*, 189–196.

Braden, C. J. (1986). *Self-help as a learned response to chronic illness experience: A test of four alternative theories.* Unpublished doctoral dissertation. The University of Arizona, Tucson, AZ.

Campbell, A., Converse, P., & Rogers, W. (1976). *The quality of American life.* New York: Russell Sage Foundation.

Dodd, M. J. (1988). Patterns of self-care in patients with breast cancer. *Western Journal of Nursing Research, 10,* 7–24.

Fallowfield, L. J. (1990). Psychosocial adjustment after treatment for early breast cancer. *Oncology, 4*(4), 89–96.

Given, C. W. (1984). Measuring the social psychological health status of ambulatory chronically ill patients: Hypertension and diabetes as tracer conditions. *Journal of Community Health, 9,* 179–195.

Mishel, M. H. (1988). Uncertainty in illness. *Image: Journal of Nursing Scholarship, 20,* 225–232.

Mishel, M. H., & Braden, C. J. (1988, April). *Measurement of antecedents of uncertainty in the Mishel uncertainty in illness model: Pilot study.* Paper presented at the Stress, Coping Processes and Health Outcomes: Future Directions for Theory Development and Research Conference; co-sponsored by University of Rochester School of Nursing and Epsilon XI Chapter of Sigma Theta Tau, Rochester, NY.

Nunnally, J. C. (1978). *Psychometric theory* (2nd ed.). New York: McGraw-Hill.

Pardine, P., Napoli, A., & Dytell, R. (1983, August). *Health-behavior change mediating the stress-illness relationship.* Paper presented at the Ninety-First Annual Convention of the American Psychological Association, Anaheim, CA.

Penman, D., Bloom, J. R., Fotopoulis, S., Cab, R., Vargese, A., & Speigel, D. (1987). The impact of mastectomy on self-concept and social function: A combined cross-sectional and longitudinal study with comparison groups. In S. Stellman (Ed.), *Women and health* (pp. 101–130). New York: Haworth Press.

Rosenbaum, M. (1983). Learned resourcefulness as a behavioral repertoire for the self-regulation of internal events: Issues and speculations. In M. Rosenbaum, C. Franks, & Y. Jaffee (Eds.), *Perspectives on behavior therapy in the eighties* (pp. 54–73). NY: Springer Publishing Co.

Siminoff, L. A., Fetting, J. H., & Abeloff, M. D. (1989). Doctor-patient communication about breast cancer adjuvant therapy. *Journal of Clinical Oncology, 7,* 1192–1200.

Thomas, S.G. (1978). Breast cancer: The psychosocial issues. *Cancer Nursing, 1*(1), 53–60.

Vinokur, A. D., Threatt, B. A., Vinokur-Kaplan, D., & Satariano, W. (1990). The process of recovery from breast cancer for younger and older patients. *Cancer, 65,* 1242–1254.

Watson, D., Clark, L., & Tellegen, A. (1988). Development and validation of brief measures of positive and negative affect: The PANAS scales. *Journal of Personal & Social Psychology, 34,* 1063–1070.

Yasko, J. M. (1990). Women with breast cancer: Living with a chronic illness. *Innovations in Oncology Nursing, VI,* 1, 16 & 17.

[16]

Quantitative Progressive Exercise Rehabilitation (QPER): Rehabilitation of Patients with Osteoarthritis

Nadine M. Fisher and David R. Pendergast

Many musculoskeletal diseases lead to functional limitations and, ultimately, loss of independence. Osteoarthritis (OA) of the knee is particularly disabling since the knee is necessary for such activities as walking, climbing stairs, and rising from a chair. Physical function as well as muscle strength and aerobic power are reduced in patients with OA symptoms (e.g., crepitus, decreased range of motion, pain, deformity, and instability) (Beals et al., 1985; Harkcom, Lampman, Banwell, & Castor, 1985; Hsieh, Didenko, Schumacher, & Torg, 1987; Lankhorst, Van de Stadt, & Van der Korst, 1985; Minor, Hewett, Webel, Anderson, & Kay, 1989; Nordesjö, Nordgren, Wigren, & Kolstad, 1983).

Reductions in physiological muscle function (strength, endurance, and contraction speed) have been shown to occur as a function of aging (Fisher, Pendergast, & Calkins, 1990). These reductions are greater in patients with OA of the knee (Fisher, Gresham, & Pendergast, 1992; Fisher, Pendergast, Gresham, & Calkins, 1991). While cardiovascular function is important, muscle function is the limiting factor for normal physical functioning (Pendergast, Fisher, & Calkins, in press); therefore, maintaining muscle function should be a priority. This is particularly important in OA of the knee, since the thigh musculature (i.e., quadriceps and hamstrings) supports and stabilizes the knee joint during movement. This flowchart is shown in Figure 16.1.

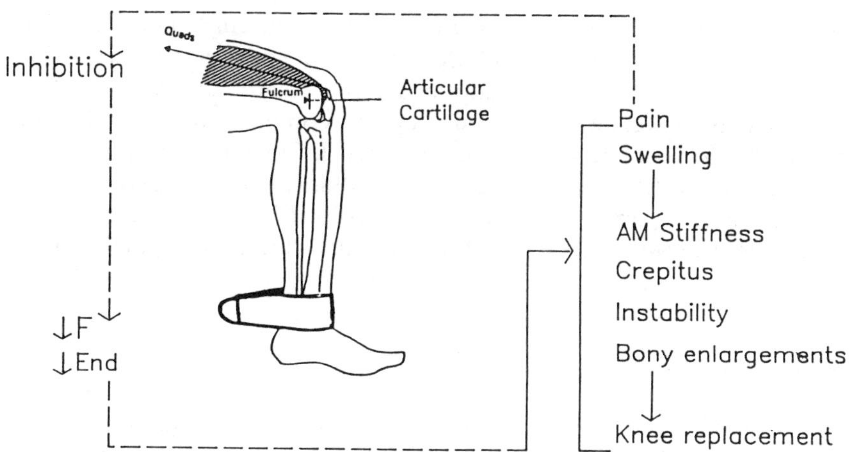

FIGURE 16.1. Hypothetical flowchart for sequences of events that occur in patients with OA of the knees. The goal is to reverse the arrows (dotted line). Inhibition indicates neuromuscular inhibition (F = force and End = endurance).

The initial symptoms of knee OA—pain and swelling—lead to morning stiffness, crepitus, instability, bony enlargements, and deterioration of the articular cartilage. The end result may be a knee replacement. As the pain and swelling increase, the patient becomes less active. There is neurological inhibition of the musculature, which results in a decrease in muscle function (less force generation, less endurance, and lower contraction speed). As the musculature becomes weaker, the patient may experience more pain and swelling and become even less active. The goal is to reverse this process by decreasing inhibition, thus increasing motor unit recruitment and muscle function, and thereby increasing or maintaining functional performance (i.e., walking and other activities of daily living).

It is well documented that exercise is a beneficial treatment. Unfortunately, the benefits obtained may not be those needed most. For example, aerobic exercise programs for arthritis patients have not demonstrated increases in functional performance or muscle function (Beals et al., 1985; Lankhorst et al., 1985; Minor et al., 1989). One study of progressive resistance exercises showed reductions in pain and increased function (Chamberlain, Care, & Harfield, 1982), but the results were not measured quantitatively. We have developed a muscle rehabilitation program based on quantitative assessment of the changes in physiological muscle function (strength, endurance, and contraction speed) that occur not only in the elderly, but also in those with OA of the knee. In our program, titled Quantitative Progressive Exercise Rehabilitation (QPER), all physiological functions as well as functional performance are measured quantitatively. From the data obtained, highly specialized exercises are prescribed in a specific progression to rehabilitate the supporting musculature of the knee. In a previous study we showed that this exercise program was effective for nursing home residents (75% increase in muscle function), many of whom suffered from OA (Fisher, Pendergast, & Calkins, 1991). This chapter describes the QPER program for patients with OA of the knee and reports a study demonstrating the effects of QPER on muscle function and functional performance.

METHOD

Fifteen men with radiographically documented OA of at least one knee volunteered for the study (Fisher et al., 1991). The patients received a medical history and resting ECG. Muscle function and functional performance were quantitatively measured on a specially designed exercise bench initially, and then after 2 and 4 months of the QPER program.

A diagram of the exercise bench used for QPER is shown in Figure 16.2. A standard weight bench was adapted for the program. It was raised up higher from the floor and the seat and seat back were widened in order to accommodate the elderly and those with functional limitations. Special features of the bench include a variable seat position (A) that makes it possible to alter hip angles (increase muscle length); a weight stack (B) with the ability to increase resistance in 0.25 kg increments; a variable knee extension arm with a potentiometer (C), used to alter knee angles (vary muscle length) and measure contraction speed and range of motion; and a force transducer (D) to measure isometric strength and endurance.

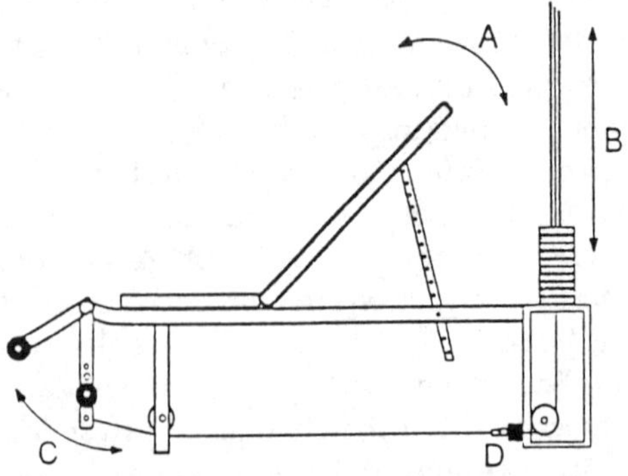

FIGURE 16.2. Schematic diagram of the exercise bench (A = variable hip angle, B = weight stack, C = variable knee angle, and D = force transducer).

Quantitative Assessment Protocols

Muscle function In the QPER program, muscle strength, endurance, and contraction speed are measured on each leg separately since the degree of OA and, therefore, disability may differ. For these subjects with OA of the knee, we isolated the quadriceps muscle group since it supports the knee and its primary action is to extend the knee. All muscle function measurements were performed on the exercise bench described above. By varying the knee and hip angles on the bench, it is possible to both measure and train the muscle at different muscle lengths. This is important since many functional activities (e.g., walking, climbing stairs, and rising from a chair) require the muscle to generate the appropriate force at different muscle lengths throughout the range of motion. Previously we have shown that reductions in muscle function are greater at longer muscle lengths than at shorter lengths (Fisher et al., 1990; Fisher et al., 1991).

In the QPER program muscle length is measured with a tape measure, from the anterior inferior iliac spine to the tibial tuberosity. Thigh muscle volume is calculated from various circumferences corrected for subcutaneous fat (Jones & Pearson, 1969). These variables are measured to assess changes in maximal muscle length and to determine if there is muscle hypertrophy as a result of QPER.

A force transducer, reading out to a recorder or computer, is used to measure the maximal isometric force of knee extension at three knee angles (45°, 90°, and 120°) and four hip angles (90°, 60°, 30°, and 0°). The different combinations allow for measurements at 12 different muscle lengths. Two trials are performed with each leg in each position.

Muscle endurance, the area under the fatigue curve, is calculated from the force transducer data. Subjects maintain a maximal isometric contraction for 90 seconds or until the patient reports fatigue or inability to continue (care is taken so that the patient does not perform a Valsalva maneuver). In the study reported here the measurements were performed one time at all knee angles, but at only two hip angles (60° and 30°).

The potentiometer on the knee extension arm of the bench allows for measurement of the maximal contraction speed of muscle (angular velocity) by knee extension. These data were collected at all hip angles and by placing increasing resistance on the bench (0, 1, 2, 3, and 4.5 kg).

All of these measurements are necessary to assess changes in muscle function with QPER. Strength and endurance of handgrip (a control group of muscles) were also measured to determine if changes occurred in unaffected joints, without QPER.

Functional performance In the QPER program, several tools are used to evaluate functional performance. Walking time is measured over 50 feet with a stopwatch. The Jette Functional Status Index (Jette, 1980), a self-report questionnaire, is used to assess the degree of dependence, difficulty, and pain while performing 18 different activities of daily living. A baseline clinical evaluation is used to assess the ability to walk, rise from a chair, and climb stairs. An interviewer watches the patient perform these activities, then reports on any deviations, level of pain, or patient comments. An interviewer-conducted functional assessment questionnaire is used to evaluate the degree of morning stiffness; problems or pain when walking, climbing stairs, or rising from a chair; and occurrence of an acute flare-up.

QPER Protocol

A detailed description of the QPER protocol is given in Table 16.1. The program requires patients to exercise three times per week (~1 hour each session) for 16 weeks. Generally one exercise technician is able to supervise up to four patients at once. Subjects' medical treatments and medications are not altered.

Maximal isometric contractions by knee extension (quadriceps) are performed at all muscle lengths (12) with each leg separately. Subjects alternate legs for each contraction. This allows for adequate recovery between contractions and builds a flexibility component into the program by requiring the muscle to sustain a specific muscle length (stretch). At each muscle length, all repetitions of isotonic range-of-motion knee extension contractions are performed first with one leg, then the other. The program is adjusted depending on the patient's progress.

TABLE 16.1 Four-Month QPER Protocol for OA of the Knees

Week		Exercise
1		Initial test
2,3	(A)	Maximal isometric contractions (3x for 5 sec. at all hip and knee angles) for quadriceps.
	(B)	Slow isotonic range of motion contractions (3x with no resistance) for quadriceps.
4–8	(A)	Maximal isometric contractions (3x for 5 sec.)
	(B)	Isotonic contractions with resistance (3x at all hip angles). Resistances begin at 10% of the subject's initially tested maximum and increase 10% each week, up to 50% of max. All resistances are lifted rapidly.
9		Mid test
10–16	(A)	Continued maximal isometric contractions (5x for 9 sec.).
	(B)	Continued rapid isotonic contractions with resistance (5x), up to 50% max.
	(C)	Endurance contractions for quadriceps. Subjects sustain maximal isometric contraction for 90 seconds or until fatigue.
17		Posttest

The testing protocols are completed over 3 days so as not to completely fatigue the patient or exacerbate any symptoms. The training protocol features isometric contractions as the first exercise and these continue throughout the program because they increase motor unit recruitment and strength faster than any other activity. Since the knee joint does not move, there is no pain involved. We begin with slow isotonic contractions, in order to maintain range of motion and reduce any swelling in the knees. The progression to rapid isotonic contractions with resistance, in Week 4, requires prescribing the appropriate resistance for each leg at each hip angle from the initial test results. Resistances begin at 10% of maximum and increase each week by 10%, up to 50%. The test results at the halfway point of the program allow for fine tuning of the exercises, as the rate of progress can be determined and used in subsequent weeks' prescriptions. Endurance contractions (sustaining a maximal isometric contraction for 90 seconds at different muscle lengths) are added to the second half of the program. Isotonic contractions are performed rapidly in order to train the muscle to quickly contract when called upon. This has special implications for balance and falls.

RESULTS

Typically, 90% of patients complete the QPER program. Further, only 10% of the dropouts discontinue because of complications related to their arthritis condition. None of the subjects who finished 4 months of QPER had any exacerbation of symptoms. The session attendance rate is typically about 80%.

Data from the study reported here support the effectiveness of the QPER program. Selected muscle function results are shown in Figure 16.3. The maximal isometric quadriceps strength, as a function of increasing muscle length, is shown in Figure 16.3A. These data were averaged for all knee angles. Pre-QPER strength was significantly less (33%) than for asymptomatic subjects of the same age [$F(1,19) = 41.94, p < .05$]. After QPER, there were large increases in strength at all muscle lengths, averaging 35%. Although the improvements were statistically significant only at 60° [$F(1,20) = 4.69, p < .05$] and 30° [$F(1,20) = 4.49, p < .05$], the improvements at 90° (shortest muscle length) and especially at 0° (longest muscle length) are very important clinically. High levels of strength need to be maintained at these positions, especially the longest muscle lengths, since most functional activities are performed at these lengths. As strength declines at these lengths, the ability to do activities declines, ultimately affecting functional independence.

Muscle rehabilitation also brought a measurable, though nonsignificant, increase in muscle length. This is shown in Figure 16.3B. Both pre- and

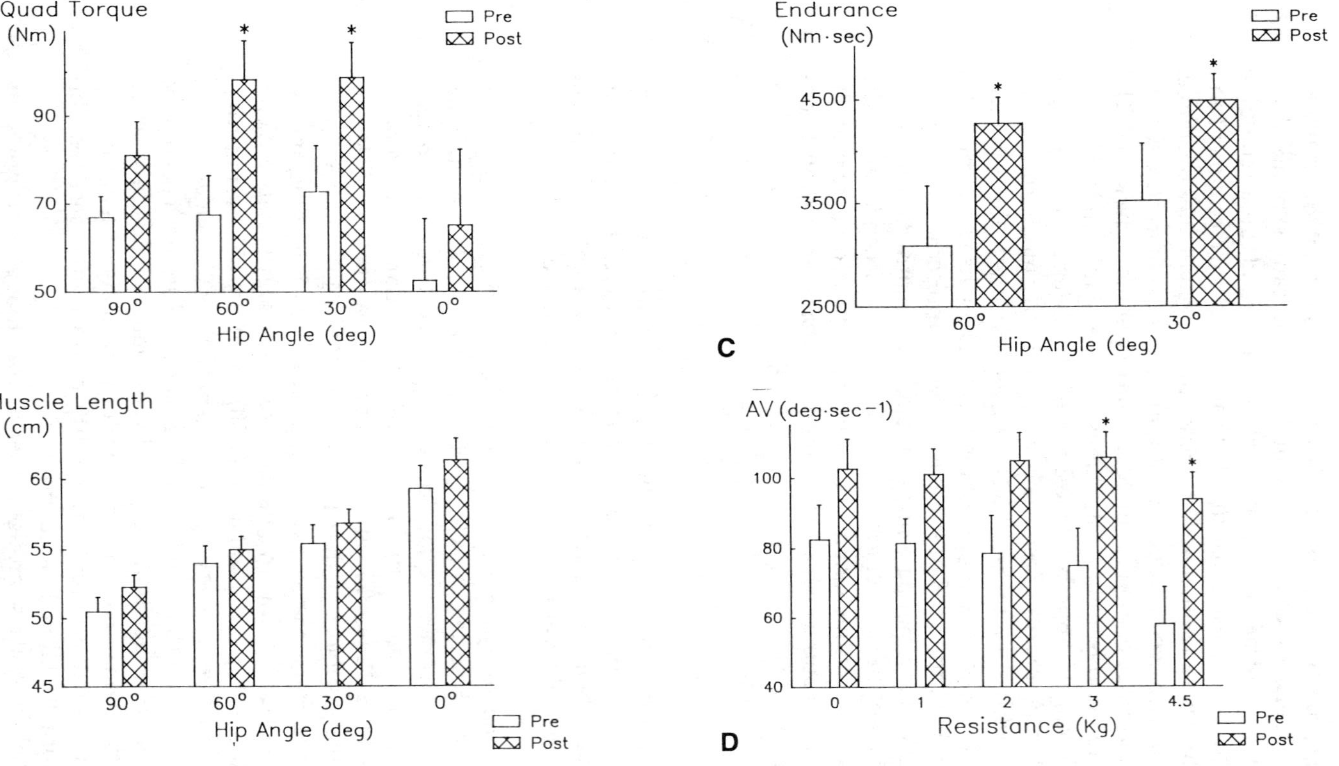

FIGURE 16.3 **A**: Means ± SDs for maximal isometric strength of knee extension, represented by quadriceps torque (Nm), plotted as a function of hip angle (muscle length) for pre (open bars) and post (cross-hatched bars) QPER. **B**: Means ± SDs for muscle length (cm) plotted as a function of hip angle for pre (open bars) and post (cross-hatched bars) QPER. **C**: Means ± SDs for maximal isometric quadriceps endurance (Nm · sec) plotted as a function of hip angle for pre (open bars) and post (cross-hatched bars) QPER. **D**: Means ± SDs for angular velocity (degrees · sec^{-1}) plotted as a function of increasing resistance (kg) for pre (open bars) and post (cross-hatched bars) QPER. The * indicates a significant difference from pre to post ($p < .05$).

post-rehabilitation, muscle length increased with increasing hip angle. Although the magnitude of change was relatively small, it did demonstrate the capacity of the OR patients' muscle to maintain a stretch. This is important since 73% of the patients were provided relief from "night cramps."

The effect of QPER on maximal isometric quadriceps endurance (area under the fatigue curve) is shown in Figure 16.3C. This figure represents an average of all knee angles. The pre-QPER endurance was significantly less than for age-matched controls [$F(1,18) = 8.43, p < .05$]. After muscle rehabilitation, the average increase in endurance was 35%; significant increases were found at all muscle lengths [$F(1,20) = 4.73, p < .05$; $F(1,20) = 4.41, p < .05$].

Data on the speed of muscle contraction, or angular velocity, are plotted in Figure 16.3D as a function of increasing resistance. Before the QPER program, the speed was significantly less among experimental subjects than among the age-matched asymptomatic controls [$F(1,19) = 107.91, p < .05$]. After QPER, angular velocity increased at all resistances; these increases were significant for the 2 heaviest resistances [$F(1,20) = 4.54, p < .05$; $F(1,20) = 8.82, p < .05$]. The average increase was 50%.

Measurements of thigh muscle volume indicated no change after QPER. There were also no changes in handgrip strength or endurance. This is not surprising since these muscles were not trained.

All functional performance measurements indicated significant improvements following 4 months of QPER. One variable, the Jette Functional Status Index, is shown in Figure 16.4. The greatest impacts on functional

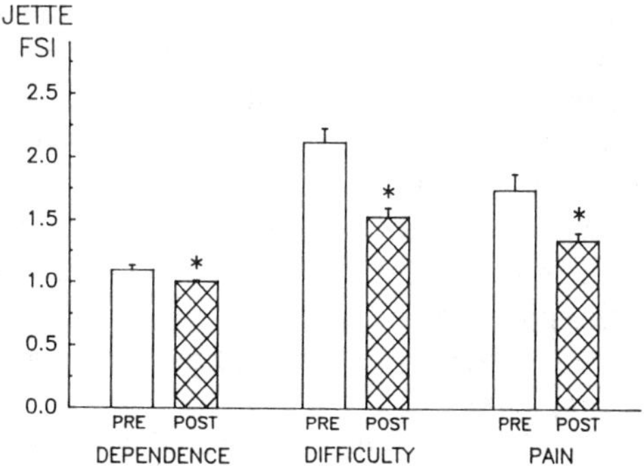

FIGURE 16.4. Jette Functional Status Index. Means ± SDs for degrees of dependence, difficulty, and pain for various activities of daily living pre (open bars) and post (cross-hatched bars) QPER. The * indicates a significant difference from pre to post ($p < .05$).

performance statistically, and from the patient's point of view, were the decreases in the difficulty (30%) [$F(1,19) = 19.4, p < .05$] and pain (40%) [$F(1,19) = 7.93, p < .05$] of performing activities of daily living. The decrease in dependence was also statistically significant [$F(1,19) = 5.48, p < .05$].

To summarize, QPER produced significant improvements in muscle function (strength, endurance, and contraction speed) and functional performance. There also was a high correlation between muscle function and functional performance. The quantitative evidence demonstrates the effectiveness of the program. Anecdotal evidence from the patients points to the practical effectiveness of the program. Representative patient comments included these: they could kneel at church now (no pain); get in and out of a boat easier; carry things up and down stairs without feeling that their knees would buckle; walk 9 holes of golf with no pain and 18 holes with only mild discomfort; stand on one leg in the shower; put pants, shoes, and socks on easier (easier to bend knees—no pain); walk straighter and farther; and climb up and down stairs normally now, not just one stair at a time (no pain). Also, they found it was not necessary to pull on a handrail as much and it was easier to get out of low chairs; they had no more cramps at night and not as much stiffness in the morning or after sitting for a long time; and lastly, they had better balance.

DISCUSSION

The treatment for OA usually consists of rest, exercise, and/or medication, and eventually surgery. A typical exercise program may include joint range-of-motion activities, isometrics, and progressive resistive isotonics. Unfortunately, there is little quantitative data, particularly on functional capacity, demonstrating that these types of programs are beneficial. One study did find improvements in joint range of motion, strength, and endurance; however, qualitative measurement techniques were used, so the amount of improvement could not be determined (Chamberlain et al., 1982). Other types of programs, such as range of motion or aerobics, may show changes in aerobic power or walking time, but changes in strength, endurance, or functional performance have not been demonstrated. The patients in our program showed much greater improvements in muscle function and functional performance than those in more traditional programs.

QPER for patients with OA of the knee was developed as a result of considering the following:

1. the basic physiological changes that occur with aging;
2. further changes that occur in the neuromuscular and musculoskeletal systems as a result of OA;

3. the pathology of the disease;
4. the methods of treatment;
5. the indications and contraindications for exercise;
6. the proper quantitative measurements;
7. the proper progression and intensity of exercise;
8. the cost-effectiveness and ease of implementation;
9. the palatability of the program to the patient.

All of these points must be blended together to have a safe, low-risk program that is conservative, yet aggressive enough to produce maximal benefits for the patient.

Clinical Implications of QPER

The QPER strategy can be used in clinical practice quite easily. The basis is quantification. Accurately measured baseline data give the investigator not only the cornerstone on which to build an intervention program, but the basis for assessing the success or failure of the intervention. Also, quantitative measurement can be used to determine if an intervention is even necessary or whether a patient is at risk of losing independence. The cost of quantifying function is obviously higher than qualitative assessment. With some planning and imagination, however, equipment costs may be kept low. This type of program is cost-effective in that an exercise technician can supervise up to four patients at one time, unlike one-to-one physical therapy.

Our program can also be conducted over 2- or 3-month periods, with slight alterations to keep the program from becoming too aggressive and causing injury. These shorter programs show slightly less improvement than the 4-month QPER. Currently we are incorporating the hamstring muscle group (knee flexion) in QPER, since the hamstrings also support the knee. A logical next step would be a QPER program to improve all-around fitness for patients with OA of the knee, with exercises to improve first muscle function, then cardiovascular function.

The short-term effectiveness of QPER has been clearly demonstrated; however, it is the long-term benefits that are clinically important. Our data show that the effects of QPER remain for at least 8 months after rehabilitation. There is also some indication that this program has a positive impact on cardiovascular function. We are currently following patients for as long as 1 to 2 years post-QPER. In those patients who have continued to function at a higher level, we find continued benefits.

Adjustments can be made to the QPER program so that it is more applicable to other clinical areas. Besides arthritic (OA and RA) and orthopedic conditions, the QPER program may be rearranged for neuromuscular, musculoskeletal, and cardiac diseases, for athletic injuries, and for general conditioning purposes in the well elderly and nursing home populations.

ACKNOWLEDGMENTS

The authors would like to acknowledge the technical support of Mary Lou Wilson and Jennifer O'Connell. This study was partially supported by the Department of Veterans' Affairs Medical Center, Batavia, NY, and the National Institute on Disability and Rehabilitation Research.

REFERENCES

Beals, C. A., Lampman, R. M., Banwell, B. F., Braunstein, E. M., Albers, J. W., & Castor, C. W. (1985). Measurement of exercise tolerance in patients with rheumatoid arthritis and osteoarthritis. *Journal of Rheumatology, 12,* 458–461.

Chamberlain, M. A., Care, G., & Harfield, B. (1982). Physiotherapy in osteoarthritis of the knees. A controlled trial of hospital versus home exercises. *International Rehabilitation Medicine, 4,* 101–106.

Fisher, N. M., Gresham, G. E., & Pendergast, D. R. (1992). *Effects of a quantitative progressive rehabilitation program applied unilaterally to the osteoarthritic knee.* Manuscript submitted for publication.

Fisher, N. M., Pendergast, D. R., & Calkins, E. (1990). Maximal isometric torque of knee extension as a function of muscle length in subjects of advancing age. *Archives of Physical Medicine and Rehabilitation, 71,* 729–734.

Fisher, N. M., Pendergast, D. R., & Calkins, E. (1991). Muscle rehabilitation in impaired elderly nursing home residents. *Archives of Physical Medicine and Rehabilitation, 72,* 181–185.

Fisher, N. M., Pendergast, D. R., Gresham, G. E., & Calkins, E. (1991). Muscle rehabilitation: Its effect on muscular and functional performance of patients with knee osteoarthritis. *Archives of Physical Medicine and Rehabilitation, 72,* 367–374.

Harkcom, T. M., Lampman, R. M., Banwell, B. F., & Castor, C. W. (1985). Therapeutic value of graded aerobic exercise training in rheumatoid arthritis. *Arthritis and Rheumatism, 28,* 32–39.

Hsieh, L. F., Didenko, B., Schumacher, H. R., Jr., & Torg, J. S. (1987). Isokinetic and isometric testing of knee musculature in patients with rheumatoid arthritis with mild knee involvement. *Archives of Physical Medicine and Rehabilitation, 68,* 294–297.

Jette, A. M. (1980). Functional status index: Reliability of a chronic disease evaluation instrument. *Archives of Physical Medicine and Rehabilitation, 61,* 395–401.

Jones, P. R. M., & Pearson, G. (1969). Anthropometric determination of leg fat and muscle plus bone volumes in young male and female adults. *Journal of Physiology (Lond), 204,* 63P–66P.

Lankhorst, G. J., Van de Stadt, R. J., & Van der Korst, J. K. (1985). The relationships of functional capacity, pain, and isometric and isokinetic torque in osteoarthritis of the knee. *Scandinavian Journal of Rehabilitation Medicine, 17,* 167–172.

Minor, M. A., Hewett, J. E., Webel, R. R., Anderson, S. K., & Kay, D. R. (1989). Effica-

cy of physical conditioning exercise in patients with rheumatoid arthritis and osteoarthritis. *Arthritis and Rheumatism, 32*, 1396–1405.
Nordesjö, L-O., Nordgren, B., Wigren, A., & Kolstad, K. (1983). Isometric strength and endurance in patients with severe rheumatoid arthritis or osteoarthritis in the knee joints. *Scandinavian Journal of Rehabilitation Medicine, 12*, 152–156.
Pendergast, D. R., Fisher, N. M., & Calkins, E. (in press). Cardiovascular, neuromuscular, and metabolic alterations with age leading to frailty. *Journal of Gerontology: Biological Sciences.*

[17]

Exercise Testing and Training in Physically Disabled Subjects with Coronary Artery Disease

Barbara J. Fletcher and Lilian M. Vassallo

Diseases of the heart and blood vessels are responsible for more deaths, illnesses, and loss of work hours in the United States than any other single cause. Standard medical care after non-fatal cardiac events often includes cardiac rehabilitation, which involves education, diet intervention, and exercise. Since sedentary life-style is now labeled a major risk factor for coronary artery disease (CAD) (Fletcher et al., 1992), exercise is considered an important component of treatment for patients with CAD. A certain percentage of patients with significant CAD also have cerebrovascular disease and/or peripheral vascular disease, resulting in physical impairments, stroke, or amputation. There is reason to believe that these individuals would also benefit from cardiac rehabilitation, but they usually do not participate because of their physical impairments. In fact, these impairments do not prevent exercise, but few data exist on the benefits of exercise training for patients with CAD and an accompanying physical disability (PD).

The study described here was designed to assess the efficacy of exercise testing and training for PD/CAD subjects.

METHOD

The primary objective of the study, which is ongoing, is to evaluate the cardiovascular benefits to PD/CAD subjects participating in an exercise training program. Secondary objectives are to evaluate a commercially available device that modifies a wheelchair into a stationary wheelchair ergometer for cardiovascular training, and to determine whether a home exercise program combined with a low cholesterol, low saturated fat diet for PD/CAD subjects results in improved body composition, blood lipids, psychological well-being, functional activities, and return to work potential.

To date, 47 PD/CAD males aged 72 years or less have been randomized to routine care at home or to a medically prescribed home exercise program for 6 months (see Figure 17.1).Only male subjects are included in the study because the primary objective involves obtaining the echocardiogram at peak exercise. This requires rapid and precise maneuvers and can best be performed without the delay or hindrance of breast tissue.

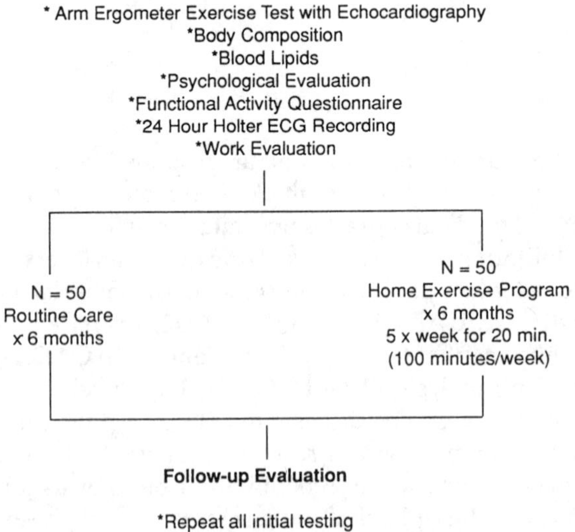

FIGURE 17.1. Project design.

In order to assure that the experimental and control groups are similar, subjects are stratified according to (1) left ventricular ejection fraction (EF) ≥50% vs <50%, (2) cerebrovascular accident, and (3) amputation. Subjects are randomized within strata to the Home Exercise Group or the Routine Care Group.

The home exercise group uses a wheelchair ramp that enables the wheelchair to become a stationary wheelchair ergometer (see Figure 17.2). Both groups are counseled and requested to follow a low cholesterol, fat controlled diet according to the American Heart Association guidelines. Both undergo evaluations at baseline (E1) and 6 months (E2) for comparison. Each evaluation consists of an arm ergometer exercise test with echocardiography (see Figures 17.3 and 17.4), a 24-hour Holter ECG recording, assessment of body composition, blood lipids, dietary intake, psychological profile, functional activity, and work capacity.

Exercise Training Protocol

All subjects randomized to home exercise are given a wheelchair ramp and telephone ECG recording device. These subjects are instructed to exercise using their wheelchair and ramp (wheelchair and rollers) (see Figure 17.2) as a stationary wheelchair ergometer. Subjects move the wheels of the wheelchair against the resistance force created by the rollers. This method provides an easy and inexpensive way for disabled subjects to exercise in their home. However, the actual power output remains unknown. Subjects are asked to exercise five times per week for a duration of 20 minutes each day, or 100 minutes each week, resulting in a 50% to 75% target heart rate range. Subjects telephone one ECG for heart rate and rhythm to the center immediately after training each week for evaluation of safety, intensity, and frequency of exercise. Exercise compliance is defined by categories: high compliance (≥ 50 min/week) and low compliance (< 50 min/week). Subjects randomized to routine care are told to continue their daily activities as instructed by their private physician.

Measures

Improvement in cardiovascular function is measured by improvement in the exercise testing determinants and in the left ventricular ejection fraction (EF) as determined by echocardiography before and at peak of the exercise test. To determine the EF (see Figure 17.3), the M-mode echo is used, providing a cross section of the parasternal long axis view, then the short axis view. The M-mode is recorded through the left ventricle at the papillary muscle level past the mitral valve. The exercise test consists of an arm ergometer exercise test (see Figure 17.4) continuously monitored by 12 lead

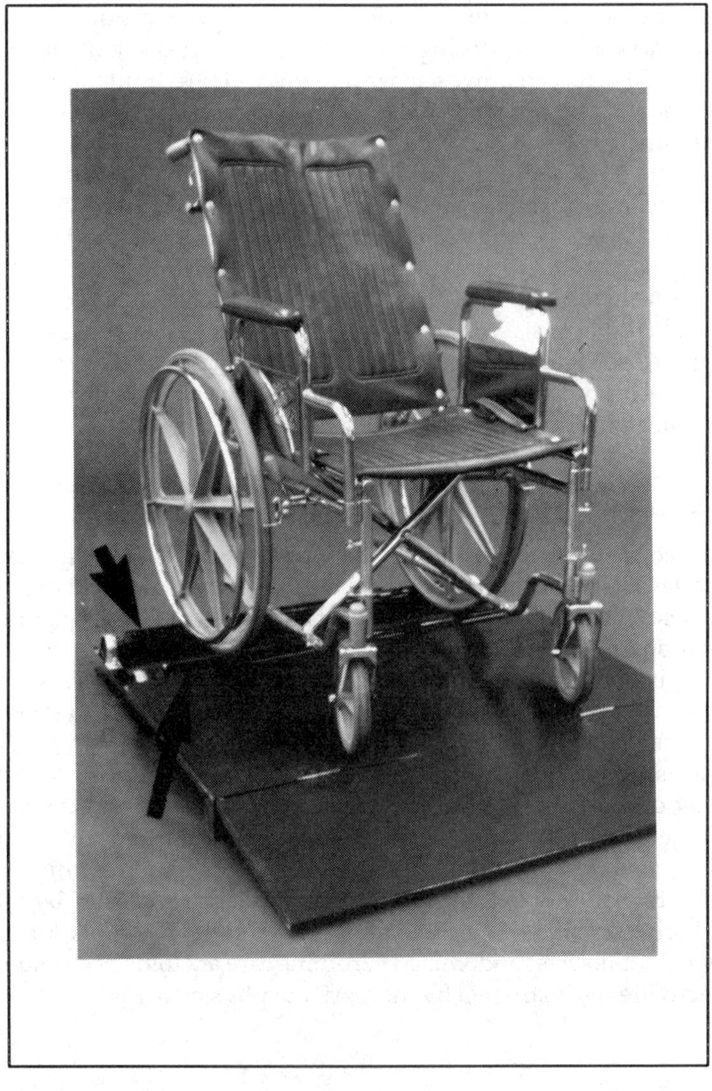

FIGURE 17.2. Stationary wheelchair ergometer. Standard wheelchair positioned on ramp with two horizontal rollers (see arrows). Ramp rollers cradle large wheel of chair in stationary position which enables subject to "wheel in place."

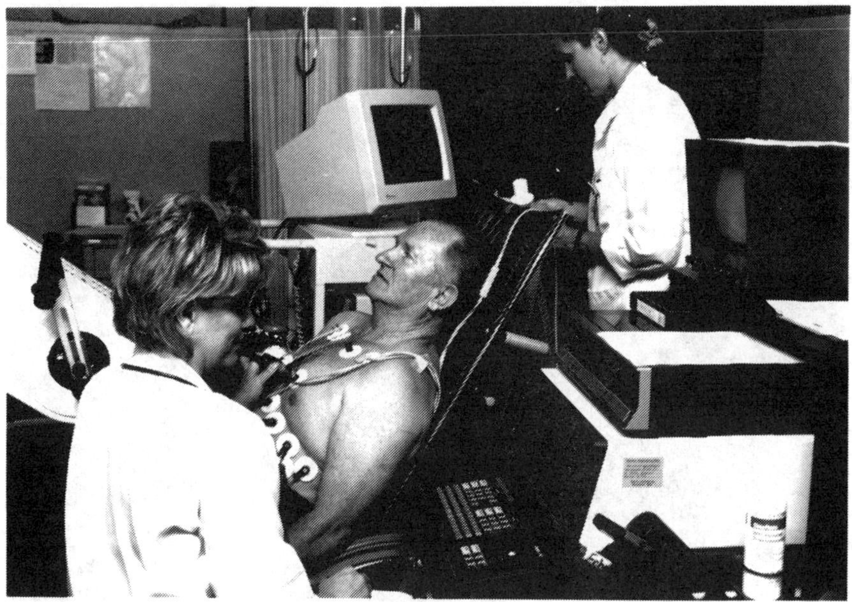

FIGURE 17.3. Physically disabled subject undergoing pre-exercise arm ergometer test echocardiogram. Sonographer obtaining echocardiogram by holding echo transducer on chest of subject (seen in left foreground). Subject is reclined to 120°. Exercise physiologist preparing gas collection tubing for oxygen consumption analyses seen in right background.

ECG to detect heart rate, arrhythmias, and ECG changes of myocardial ischemia.

The exercise test is performed in increments of 3-minute stages. Each stage consists of 2 minutes of exercise followed by 1 minute of rest. Blood pressure is evaluated before exercise and immediately after the 2-minute exercise portion of each stage. Stage One begins with a resistance of 20 watts, and this resistance is increased 10 watts at each subsequent stage. The revolutions per minute (rpm) remain constant at 50 rpms throughout the test. Oxygen consumption is recorded throughout the test using Medical Graphics equipment and breath-by-breath analysis. The exercise test is terminated at 85% of predicted maximal heart rate or at the point of fatigue. Post-exercise ECG, blood pressure, and echocardiographic (ECHO) measures are analyzed for 6 minutes.

A wheelchair with a reclining back and removed arms is used for the exercise test (see Figures 17.3 and 17.4). Initially the subject is placed at 120° to obtain the baseline ECHO. The subject is then positioned at a 90° angle

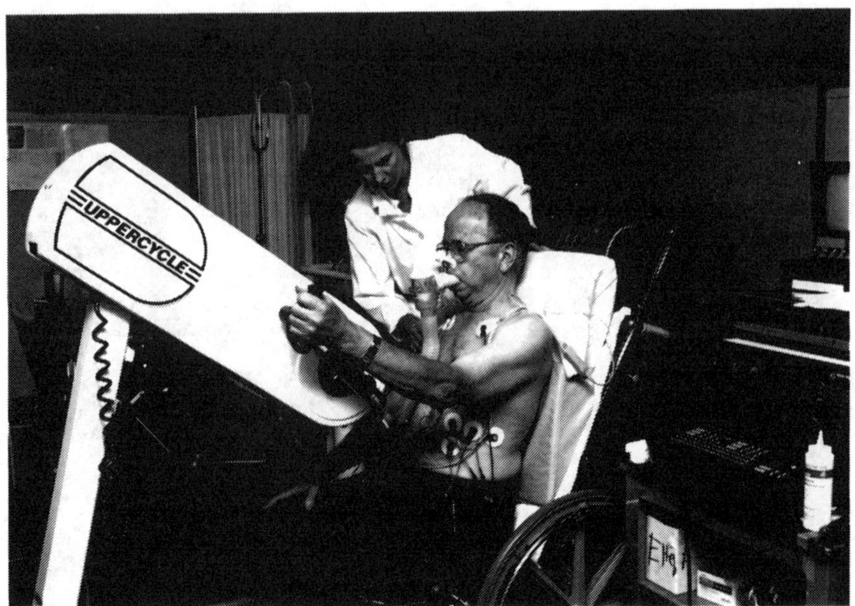

FIGURE 17.4. Physically disabled subject undergoing arm erogmeter exercise test with continuous analyses of expired gases (oxygen consumption). (Subject with cerebrovascular accident resulting in paralysis of right arm.) ECG leads are attached to subject's chest for continuous ECG monitoring. Exercise physiologist in background. Subject positioned at 90° angle during exercise test performed with left arm only.

for the exercise test. At the termination of the exercise test, the subject resumes a 120° position and the post-exercise ECHO is obtained.

Blood lipid profile consists of fasting total cholesterol, HDL cholesterol, and triglycerides, with calculated LDL cholesterol. Body composition is analyzed using the sum of three skinfolds in order to assess the amount of body fat relative to body muscle mass. After completing a 24-hour dietary intake, all subjects are instructed on the American Heart Association Step I, low cholesterol, low saturated fat diet. This dietary information is analyzed by Nutrition III software for average daily intake of fat, cholesterol, and calories.

Four instruments for psychological evaluation are used in the project. The first three are given both to the patient and to the significant other, typically the spouse. The Beck Depression Inventory (Beck, Ward, Mendelson, Mock, & Erbaugh, 1961) is a 21-item instrument in which the subject reports on mood state, sleep, appetite, and self-esteem. The Affects Balance Scale (Derogatis, 1980) is a 40-item inventory that measures positive affects of joy, contentment, vigor, and affection and negative affects of anxiety, depression, guilt, and hostility. The overall score reflects the balance between positive and negative affects. The McMasters Family Assessment Device (FAD) (Epstein, Baldwin, & Bishop, 1983) is a 53-item self-report questionnaire that assesses the perception of family role and relationship style. The scale measures different aspects of family functions such as problem solving, communication, affective responsiveness, involvement, behavior control and general functioning. The Millon Behavior Health Inventory (MBHI) (Millon, Green, & Meagher, 1979) is a 150-item questionnaire that assesses coping style and styles of interpersonal relating that pertain to the patient's medical condition. This instrument was specifically designed to be used with medical patients and therefore it is not given to the significant other.

PD/CAD patients are also asked to complete or update a functional restoration questionnaire at baseline and at the 6-month evaluation. The functional restoration questionnaire was developed by the Emory University Health Enhancement Center staff; it is based on theory and compiled from previous questionnaires. The questionnaire was approved by a panel of cardiologists and occupational therapists for use in the Emory University Health Enhancement Center Cardiac Rehabilitation Program. To date the instrument has not been used with PD/CAD subjects. It is being included in the present study to evaluate the usefulness of the tool for this population.

A work evaluation is done for each patient by the Occupational Therapy Department using the Baltimore Therapeutic Evaluation (BTE). The four strength tests performed are ladder climb, medium crank, hand turn, and hand grip/finger pinch. The objective of this evaluation is not to determine whether the subject has returned to work but whether there is potential for returning to work. A 24-hour Holter ECG recording is activated prior to BTE assessment so that heart rates and arrhythmias can be compared with those recorded throughout the 24-hour period.

PRELIMINARY RESULTS

Preliminary results are presented here for the initial 47 of the 100 subjects; these 47 have completed both the baseline evaluation (E1) and the evaluation of the 6-month exercise program (E2). Twenty-two of the 47 subjects were in the home exercise group, and 25 were in the routine care group. Fifty-one percent of the exercise group reached high exercise compliance while 49% were considered in the low exercise compliance range. During testing, length of exercise time until fatigue or 85% of maximal heart rate, workload achieved, peak exercise heart rate, blood pressure, and maximal oxygen consumption remained similar in both groups (see Table 17.1). Af-

TABLE 17.1 Hemodynamic Variables at Baseline (E1) and After 6 Months of the Exercise Program (E2)

	Home exercise (n = 22)				Routine care (n = 25)			
	E1		E2		E1		E2	
Variable	*M*	*SD*	*M*	*SD*	*M*	*SD*	*M*	*SD*
Exercise time (min)	11.4	4.9	12.8	5.2	9.5	5.8	11.5	6.1
Workload (watts)	50.4	20.0	57.4	21.0	45.7	10.7	53.3	19.0
Peak HR (beats/min)	116.4	21.4	112.9	19.3	109.7	22.7	107.8	18.6
Peak SBP (mm Hg)	164.8	30.7	162.7	32.4	168.7	25.5	171.0	20.5
Peak DBP (mm Hg)	88.1	13.0	91.8	14.9	89.9	15.6	88.0	12.2
VO_2 max (ml/kg/min)	12.3	3.6	11.5	3.2	11.0	3.2	11.2	3.1
Ventricular ectopy (PVC/24hr)	44.0	125.0	34.8[a]	102.7	52.3	118.8	71.6	117.8
Peak LV fractional shortening (%)[b]	27.5	8.7	35.2[c]	4.7	30.4	8.2	30.0	10.0
Peak ejection fraction (%)[b]	51.4	10.4	61.3[a]	6.6	51.5	19.2	56.3	13.9

[a] $p < .07$ compared with routine care group (ANOVA).
[b] $n = 12$ in each group.
[c] $p < .05$ compared with routine care group.

ter the exercise training, echocardiographic peak exercise LV fractional shortening was significantly better in the home exercise group than in the routine care group; peak EF tended to increase at E2 in home exercise, although not significantly at this time (see Table 17.1). High grade ventricular ectopy recorded on 24-hour ECG tended to be less in the exercise group at E2 than in the routine care group.

The home exercise group also significantly improved their dietary habits (see Table 17.2), lessening their percentage of fat intake and their intake of total milligrams of cholesterol. Intake of dietary fat and cholesterol did not change in the routine care group. Percent body fat did not change in either group. Blood lipid analysis did not significantly differ from baseline except that there was improvement in HDL cholesterol in both groups (see Table 17.2).

Functional activity questionnaire scores improved in both groups, but there was no significant difference between the groups. There were also no significant differences in the psychological scores of the subjects in the two groups. However, caregivers of the home exercise group appeared more depressed than caregivers of the routine care group.

Preliminary data indicate that exercise testing and training are safe for this population. Home exercise training appears to improve exercise capacity, lessen high grade ventricular ectopy, improve cardiac fractional shortening, and improve dietary compliance.

TABLE 17.2 Non-Hemodynamic Variables at Baseline (E1) and After 6 Months of the Exercise Program (E2)

	Home exercise			Routine care		
		E1	E2		E1	E2
Variable	*n*	*M*	*M*	*n*	*M*	*M*
Intake of fat (%/day)	16	35.0	30.1[a]	19	33.3	31.0
Intake of cholesterol (mg/day)	16	326.0	268.7[b]	19	285.5	275.1
Body fat (%)	22	22.3	22.5	25	23.5	23.6
Total cholesterol (mg/dl)	15	206.3	212.4	17	197.4	210.0
HDL cholesterol (mg/dl)	15	32.1	39.9[c]	17	35.9	42.1[c]
Affects Balance score[e]	9	1.4	0.9	9	1.1	1.3[d]
Beck Depression Inventory score	9	5.7	7.2	9	7.1	5.6[d]

[a] $p < .01$ compared with E1 home exercise group.
[b] $p < .05$ compared with E1 home exercise group.
[c] $p < .001$ compared with E1 (paired *t* test).
[d] $p < .04$ compared with home exercise caregivers (ANOVA).
[e] Psychological scores of caregivers.

DISCUSSION

It is widely accepted that endurance training produces significant increases in functional capacity (Adams et al., 1981). Blumenthal and colleagues (1991), who worked with a group of older men and women in regular aerobic exercise, observed improvements of 10% to 15% in cardiopulmonary training after 4 months of exercise. Subjects who maintained the exercise for 14 months achieved an average increase in peak maximal oxygen consumption (VO_2) of 18%. Other authors have reported similar results (Adams et al., 1981; Canonie et al., 1991; Hagberg et al., 1989). Some authors have also studied the effects of exercise on functional capacity in physically disabled subjects. Davis, Shephard, and Leenen (1987) evaluated change in VO_2 in male paraplegics after upper-body endurance training and found that peak VO_2 during arm ergometry significantly increased for the exercise group following 8 weeks (19%) and 16 weeks (31%) of training. Men physically disabled from spinal cord injury (Davis, Plyley, & Shephard, 1991) who had long-duration arm crank training significantly augmented their peak VO_2 after 8, 16, and 24 weeks of exercise. None of these studies, however, included subjects with CAD. The main bases of the enhanced cardiopulmonary performance seemed to be an increase in maximal arterio-venous oxygen difference, secondary to increased extraction of oxygen by the working muscles, and an increase in cardiac output due entirely to an increase in stroke volume (Adams et al., 1981). In our study, there was no significant difference in VO_2 max between the exercise and non-exercise groups. This may be partly explained by physical disability since, after stroke, some people cannot hold the mouthpiece in an airtight position.

Hagberg et al. (1989) compared the effects of 6 months of resistance training with the effects of endurance exercise training in elderly subjects and observed that maximal heart rate, systolic, and diastolic blood pressure did not differ significantly between the groups. These results support our data, but it is interesting to note that some authors (Canonie et al., 1991; Hagberg et al., 1989) have found that heart rate, diastolic, and mean blood pressure decrease significantly at rest in subjects who have had endurance training.

Several investigators (Adams et al., 1981; Keul, Dickhuth, Simon, & Lehmann, 1981) have demonstrated by ECHO studies that dynamic and isometric training produce different cardiac adaptations. As a result of isometric exertion, there is an increase in left ventricular wall thickness at the expense of the volume and end diastolic diameter. After dynamic exertion, there is a small increase in ventricular wall thickness and a marked increase in the dimensions of the cardiac chambers. The EF is increased in endurance training whereas isometric training causes a moderate decrease. The fractional shortening is not altered at rest in either group, but if cardiac performance is assessed after acute exercise in endurance trained subjects, significant immediate post-exercise reductions in end-systolic diameter and increases in fractional shortening and velocity of circumferential fiber shortening are observed (Brown et al., 1991). We noted that peak echocardiographic exercise fractional shortening significantly improved in the home exercise group after endurance training.

No studies have evaluated arrhythmias in trained and nontrained subjects with PD/CAD. Wolf, Stern, Kieselstein, Chenzbraun, and Tzivoni (1991), however, evaluated the 24-hour ECG Holter recording of elderly cerebrovascular accident patients during activities and rehabilitation. Seventy-one percent of the subjects had a history of CAD prior to their cerebrovascular accident. ECG findings were mainly ventricular and atrial arrhythmias; only a few patients showed ischemic ST changes. We found high grade ventricular ectopy in both the exercise and routine care groups, but this arrhythmia tended to lessen in the home exercise group after training.

Studies of body composition and exercise training in young and middle-age people have revealed that during early phases of exercise training body fat is lost while gains occur in lean body mass. At later stages of training, lean body mass changes very little and changes in body fat begin to be reflected by decreases in body weight (Pollock, Wilmore, & Fox, 1984). Studies of the effects of endurance and resistance exercise training on body composition in elderly subjects (Canonie et al., 1991; Hagberg et al., 1989) have shown no significant changes in body weight or lean body mass, but the sum of 7 skinfolds decreased significantly after 26 weeks of training. Our data support these studies in part. It seems that there may be a minimum frequency, duration, and intensity of training necessary to achieve significant alterations in body composition (Pollock et al., 1984). Six months may be too short for a PD/CAD population and the home exercise protocol may need to be increased in duration and frequency.

Higher HDL cholesterol concentrations have been almost invariably reported after endurance training (Pay, Hardman, Jones, & Hudson, 1992). Blumenthal et al. (1991) found a reduction in total and low-density lipoprotein cholesterol in older subjects between 4 and 8 months, and significant increases in high-density lipoprotein cholesterol after 14 months of exercise. In our study, the home exercise group improved dietary habits, reducing the percentage of fat intake and the total milligrams of cholesterol. We observed an increase in HDL-cholesterol in both groups; this may be explained in part by the energy required for routine daily activities in physically disabled subjects.

Many authors have commented on the sense of increased well-being associated with regular physical activity. Possible explanations include diversion and relaxation, social reinforcement and improved self-sufficiency, a decreased secretion of catecholamines, and increased endorphins. The self-concept of the body is potentially vulnerable to many of the stresses of aging, retirement, bereavement, institutionalization, declining physical capabilities, and major diseases such as myocardial infarction (Shepard, 1987). It has been suggested that endurance exercise provides a regular "release of tension" that reduces anxiety. The decrease in anxiety and depression may result in the "feeling good" sensation noted after exercise training. Exercise training also provides an intrinsically rewarding sense of mastery and control and therefore leads to enhanced self-concept. The aspect of self-concept that seems reinforced most by exercise training is that which pertains to one's own body and ability. Of course, if the individual is made to feel inadequate as the result of exercise training, there may be a negative effect on self-concept (Shepard, 1987).

Shepard (1991) feels that the ability of exercise to elevate mood, relieve anxiety, and improve self-image depends greatly upon initial status, with benefit more likely if the person is substantially disturbed at the outset.

Many types of disabled subjects thus seem well qualified to benefit from exercise. Nevertheless, the benefits of regular exercise depend on the ability of the disabled subject to meet the expectations of the program and his family; a training regime perceived as too demanding may have a negative impact upon body image and mood state. In our study we have not found significant differences in psychological scores between the exercise and routine care groups, but the greater depression seen in caregivers of the home exercise group is of concern. It is possible that caregivers perceive the home exercise protocol to be too demanding.

Some authors (Shepard, 1991) have correlated hours of physical inactivity (such as passive watching of television) with depression in disabled subjects; those disabled subjects who were productive showed effective social and intellectual functioning, with a high level of self-esteem. It is important to target the portion of the disabled who are employable but remain unemployed. PD/CAD subjects must be offered ways to increase their strength and endurance, and thus to increase their ability to cope with daily existence—which may include barriers to transportation and the physical demands of an occupation. The preliminary results described here support endurance training in the PD/CAD population for enhancement of their daily accomplishments. More research is needed, however, to determine the type of program that will produce ideal benefits.

ACKNOWLEDGMENT

The authors are grateful to the National Institute of Disability and Rehabilitation Research, U.S. Department of Education Grant # H133A80052 for the support of this study.

REFERENCES

Adams, T., Yanowitz, F., Fisher, A., Ridges, J., Lovell, K., & Pryor, A. (1981). Noninvasive evaluation of exercise training in college aged men. *Circulation, 64*, 958–965.

Beck, A., Ward, C., Mendelson, M., Mock, J., & Erbaugh, J. (1961). An inventory for measuring depression. *Archives of General Psychiatry, 4*, 561–571.

Blumenthal, J., Emery, C., Madden, D., Coleman, R., Riddle, W., Schniebolk, S., Cobb, F., Sullivan, M., & Higginbotham, M. (1991). Effects of exercise training on cardiorespiratory function in men and women > 60 years of age. *American Journal of Cardiology, 67*, 633–639.

Brown, S., Thompson, W., Bean, M., Wood, L., Nayak, K., & Goff, J. (1991). The relationship of early versus two-minute recovery echocardiographic values following maximal effort resistance exercise. *International Journal of Sports Medicine, 12,* 241–245.

Canonie, C., Graves, J., Pollock, M., Phillips, M., Sumners, C., & Hagberg, J. (1991). Effect of exercise training on blood pressure in 70 to 79 year old men and women. *Medicine and Science in Sports and Exercise, 23,* 505–511.

Davis, G., Shephard, R., & Leenen, F. (1987). Cardiac effects of short term arm crank training in paraplegics: Echocardiographic evidence. *European Journal of Applied Physiology, 56,* 90–96.

Davis G., Plyley, M. & Shephard, R. (1991). Gains of cardiorespiratory fitness with arm-crank training in spinally disabled men. *Canadian Journal of Sport Sciences, 16,* 6472.

Derogatis, I. (1980). *Affect balance scale.* Ridgewood, MD: Clinical Psychometric Research, Inc.

Epstein, N., Baldwin, L., & Bishop, D. (1983). The McMaster Family Assessment Device. *Journal of Marital and Family Therapy, 9,* 171–180.

Fletcher, G., Blair, S., Blumenthal, J., Caspersen, C., Chaitman, B., Epstein, S., Falls, H., Froelicher, S., Froelicher, V., & Pina, I. (1992). American Heart Association medical/scientific statement on exercise. *Circulation, 86,* 340–344.

Hagberg, J., Graves, J., Limacher, M., Woods, D., Legget, S., Canonie, C., Fruber, J., & Pollock, M. (1989). Cardiovascular responses of 70–79 year old men and women to exercise training. *Journal of Applied Physiology, 66,* 2589–2594.

Keul, J., Dickhuth, H., Simon, G., & Lehmann, M. (1981). Effect of static and dynamic exercise on heart volume, contractility and left ventricular dimensions. *Circulation Research, 48,* 1162–1170.

Millon, T., Green, C., & Meagher, R. (1979). The MBHI: A new inventory for the psychodiagnostician in medical settings. *Professional Psychology, 10,* 529–539.

Pay, H. E., Hardman, G., Jones, F., & Hudson, A. (1992). The acute effects of low intensity exercise on plasma lipids in endurance-trained and untrained young adults. *European Journal of Applied Physiology, 64,* 182–186.

Pollock, M., Wilmore, J., & Fox, S. (1984). *Exercises in health and disease.* Philadelphia, PA: Saunders.

Shepard, J. (1991). Benefits of sport and physical activity for the disabled: Implications for the individual and for society. *Scandinavian Journal of Rehabilitation Medicine, 23,* 51–59.

Shepard, R. (1987). *Physical activity and aging* (2nd ed.). Rockville, MD: Aspen.

Wolf, E., Stern, L., Kieselstein, M., Chenzbraun, A., & Tzivoni, D. (1991). Holter monitoring in the evaluation and rehabilitation of post-cerebrovascular accident patients. *International Disability Studies, 13,* 134–137.

[18]

Exercise Training for Frail Rural Elderly: A Pilot Study

Carol C. Hogue and Sharon M. Cullinan

Four of every five Americans who live to be 65 years old have one or more chronic illnesses (U. S. Senate Special Committee on Aging, 1989). Thus, coping with chronic illness is part of the daily experience of older adults. Chronic illness and the treatment of chronic illness interact with features of biological aging and inactivity to place older adults at high risk of functional decline. This functional decline has recently been labeled frailty (Weindruch, Hadley, & Ory, 1991) or preclinical disability (Fried, Herdman, Kuhn, Rubin, & Turano, 1991). Probable relationships between biological aging, disease, inactivity, and impairment, frailty, and disability, as well as factors leading to inactivity, are represented in Figure 18.1, The Web of Causation for Frailty and Disability. Frailty makes it difficult to maintain psychological well-being, perform social roles, and care for oneself at home (Brody, 1989). Theoretically, frailty can be reversed by reducing chronic illness, by preventing biological aging declines, or by reducing inactivity. In reality, once people reach old age, the most promising of those interventions is the third: Stated positively, our best hope lies in increased activity.

Increasing activity for elderly persons is difficult because many who are old today grew up believing exercise was harmful, many have never learned to exercise, and many are so deconditioned or frail that they have neither the muscle strength nor the functional aerobic capacity to exercise effectively. Rural elderly are at a particular disadvantage because they tend not to have skilled exercise professionals available to help them.

Exercise training has been shown to improve attributes such as skeletal muscle strength and cardiopulmonary endurance in older people (Anians-

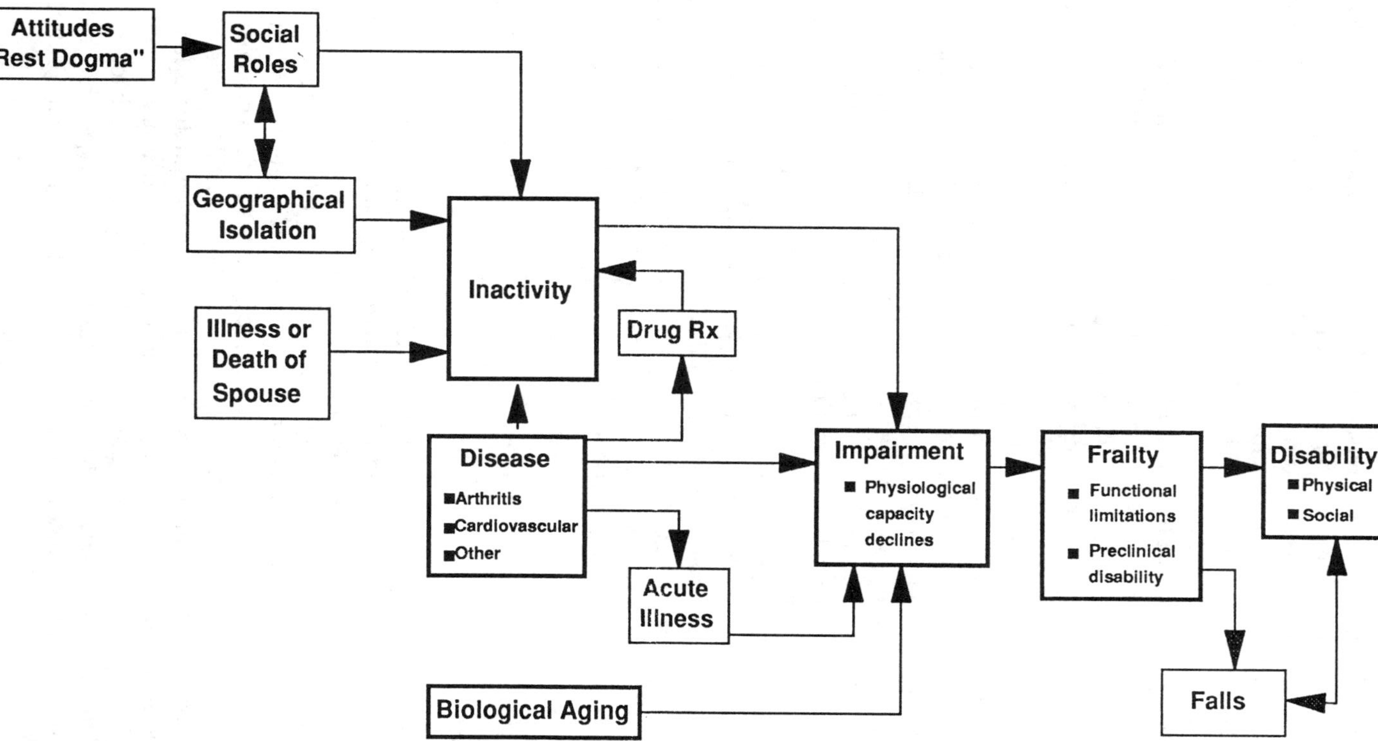

FIGURE 18.1 The Web of Causation for frailty and disability.

son & Gustafson, 1981; Frontera, Meredith, O'Reilly, Knuttgen, & Evans, 1988; Seals, Hagberg, Hurley, Ehsani, & Holloszy, 1984), but it is unclear whether the training improves function and health status. It is also unclear whether older persons with chronic illness will maintain their physical activity and exercise after the conclusion of a supervised program. Because training effects disappear within 4 weeks (Fiatarone et al., 1990), long-term exercise is crucial.

We report here the results of a pilot study in which we examined the feasibility and effectiveness of a 12-week training program for frail elderly residing in a rural community. The purpose of the study was to collect process and outcome data to strengthen sampling, interventions, and data collection for randomized controlled studies to follow. Specific study aims were 1) to demonstrate the feasibility of exercise testing and training of frail elderly; 2) to adapt survey research instruments for rural elderly; 3) to show improvements in subjects' muscle strength, flexibility, and functional aerobic capacity; and 4) to build community support for research in this area. We also wanted to show effects on health status and function of our subjects at the conclusion of the training and 3.5 months later. Finally, we wanted to demonstrate that the testing and training could be effectively carried out by a nurse clinician whose experience included home health nursing for adults with chronic illness but who had no prior training in exercise physiology, in physical therapy, or in psychoeducational interventions. Following the suggestion of Shepard (1990), we included in the pilot an elderly lay person we called the "peer exercise facilitator." The peer exercise facilitator was a role model for the exercisers; she also made home visits to each subject's support person.

METHOD

Design

The pilot was a one-group, prospective study with repeated measures design. The study was conducted with a convenience sample of 15 elderly residents of a rural county in Eastern North Carolina in which the largest town has 8,000 residents. All measurements and the interventions for 13 subjects were conducted in a senior center; 2 subjects received their training in the home of one of them. Our sample included males and females who were at least 62 years old, who were sedentary or frail, who had the consent of their physician to participate, and who nominated a family member or friend willing to support their exercise. Sedentary behavior was defined as not exercising vigorously more than twice a week for more than 20 minutes. However, to be eligible for the study, subjects had to be able to walk at least 15 feet without a walking aid, and to ascend and descend at least three stairs. A brief cognitive screen, the Blessed-Katzman Orientation-Memory-Concentration test, "the Short Blessed" (Katzman, Brown, & Fuld, 1983), was used to exclude persons with severe cognitive impairment. Other screening criteria excluded persons who were obviously unsafe for testing and training (for example, with systolic or diastolic blood pressure greater than 200/100), or who were unlikely to benefit because of the presence of conditions such as lumbar stenosis or multiple sclerosis.

Intervention

The goals of the intervention were to improve health status by increasing lower extremity joint flexibility, muscle strength, balance, general endurance, and physical functioning; and to encourage long-term maintenance of physical activity. The intervention consisted of three components: physical training, psychoeducational training, and social support. It was tailored to individuals; that is, each participant had an exercise prescription generated from baseline data collection. The intervention was delivered three times a week, for 12 weeks, for 2 hours at a time. Transportation to the senior center was provided for all who needed it.

The physical training was circuit-interval training which included progressive, light resistance exercise, calisthenics to exercise all major muscle groups, and vigorous activity building to 40%–70% estimated peak VO_2. Circuit training refers to a series of exercise activities, usually at different stations. The series is repeated several times and provides opportunities for individualization within a group setting. Interval training involves alternating an exercise interval with a rest interval. The training was considered progressive because the vigorous activity periods increased until they were continuous or nearly continuous; 40%–70% estimated peak VO_2 refers to the intensity of the aerobic component. Estimated peak VO_2 is the greatest amount of oxygen a person can use while performing dynamic exercise involving a large part of total muscle mass (Fletcher, Froelicher, Hartley, Haskell, & Pollock, 1991). The estimated VO_2 peak was derived from each individual's heart rate response to submaximal, graded exercise tests given at baseline. Individual target heart rate zones were then generated from the baseline exercise test, using the formula of Karvonen (Karvonen, Kentala, & Mustala, 1958).[1]

The psychoeducational strategies included instruction and experience in problem solving (D'Zurilla, 1986; Kanfer & Goldstein, 1991), goal setting (Dishman, 1988; Meichenbaum & Turk, 1987) and relapse prevention (Marlatt & Gordon, 1985; Meichenbaum & Turk, 1987). Information about health and self-care was included in each training session. Topics included foot care, home safety, vision care, and nutrition.

Social strategies were of two kinds: support from the group, including the leader, and support for participation from a family member or friend. The family member or friend, the "support person," was visited by the peer exercise facilitator in the first couple of weeks of the study and at the conclusion of the supervised training program. In the first visit, the benefits and rigors of the training program were described to the support person. This person was also given two or three suggestions about how to support without nagging and was asked to encourage the participant to attend classes and to increase activity and exercise. At the second visit, the same approach was taken to encourage exercise maintenance after the supervised program ended.

Measurement

Physiologic, psychologic, and functional evaluations were performed prior to and twice following the intervention: immediately and 3.5 months later. The intervention process was observed at each session and at the conclusion of the supervised exercise training. Observations were recorded in diary format and included data collected through direct observation of performance, measures of physiologic variables and function, and participant responses to survey research instruments administered by an interviewer. Physiologic measures were blood pressure and heart rate. Functional measures included estimated VO_2 peak and time on step test, both indicators of aerobic capacity; pounds lifted by lower and upper extremities, indicators of muscle strength; walking speed, a measure of gait; and a one-legged stand and steps off a "balance beam" placed on the floor (Kauffman, 1990), clinical measures of balance. Psychological measures included morale measured by the Philadelphia Geriatric Center Morale Scale (Lawton, 1975), and self-esteem measured by Rosenberg's instrument (Rosenberg, 1965). The Yale Physical Activity Scale (DiPietro, Caspersen, Ostfeld, & Nadel, 1990) was administered to identify frequency and intensity of household, recreational, and exercise activity. Process measures included participation rates and satisfaction with the program. We used multiple, redundant measures for several variables to help us choose the best instruments and measurement strategies for the larger study to follow. For example, we conducted three graded exercise tests at each of the three testing periods: bicycle ergometry, a step test adapted for elderly subjects (Amundson, DeVahl, & Ellingham, 1989), and the chair step test (Smith & Gilligan, 1983).

Snow's Inventory of Functional Tests (SIFT), was used to measure function. The SIFT integrates tasks that are intermediate in complexity between basic neuromuscular abilities such as strength and flexibility (indicators of impairment) and performance of social roles such as activities of daily living (ADLs) and instrumental activities of daily living (IADLs) (indicators of disability). These performance-based measures of function yield scores that are used to rank an individual's function over a range of performance levels from 1 to 3. An example of a SIFT item is "squats," a graded task to assess strength, balance, and coordination at the end ranges of hip, low back, knee, and ankle musculature. The three grades or levels of the task, in increasing order of difficulty, are to sit down and rise from an armless chair, a 12" stool, and the floor (Snow, Hogue, & Cullinan, 1993).

The Sickness Impact Profile (SIP) (Bergner, Bobbitt, Carter, & Gilson, 1981) was used to assess health status. The Sickness Impact Profile is a behaviorally based, comprehensive multidimensional measure of health status with strong evidence of reliability and validity in adult samples, including elderly persons (Bergner et al., 1981). The SIP is intended to describe the impact of illness on a person's behavior. Twelve domains or categories of functioning are assessed and reported individually, or summed to yield two scores, physical and psychosocial, or one total SIP score. The SIP domains include ambulation, mobility, body care and movement, social interaction, alertness behavior, emotional behavior, communication, sleep and rest, eating, work, home management, and recreation and pastimes. The SIP can be self-administered or interviewer-administered. We elected interview administration because the literature reports higher reliability for interviewer administration (Rothman, Hedrick, & Innui, 1989).

At follow-up a relatively unstructured interview was conducted with each subject prior to administration of the standard measures and direct observation of performance. The purpose of the interview was to increase our knowledge of how much activity and exercise people were getting, and to strengthen our understanding of the barriers to and facilitators of their exercise.

RESULTS

Of the 15 subjects who began the study, 87% were female and 60% African American. Their average age was 73 years; the range, 62–80. Subjects had 5–12 years of education; the median educational level was 8 years. All subjects had chronic illness, muscle weakness, poor aerobic capacity, and poor flexibility. Most had arthritis (79%) and/or hypertension (71%), 2 had diabetes, 2 had strokes, several had myocardial infarctions, 1 had early Parkinson's Disease, several had joint replacements, and several reported a lower extremity fracture from 1 to 10 years prior to the study. Participants were very skeptical about their ability to complete the program.

One subject dropped out early in the program and was not replaced. As 14 of 15 subjects completed the program, the participation rate was 93.3%. Among the 14 subjects who completed the program, attendance was 90.6%.

Subjects improved in aerobic capacity, measured on bike ergometer from baseline to posttest, from 15.3 to 19.3 ml/Kg/minute, with a slight drop to 19.0 at follow-up; this improvement was both statistically and clinically significant [$t(7) = 3.68, p < .01$]. Peak VO_2 was converted to METS, a multiple of the actual resting metabolic rate. The improvement of 4.4 to 5.5 METS (with virtually no decline at follow-up) means that at baseline the average participant, functioning at maximal aerobic capacity, could make a bed; at follow-up, the average participant could also be an active gardener. Time on step test, another measure of functional aerobic capacity, increased from 6.3 minutes to 8.2 minutes [$t(9) = 2.62, p < .05$], with a decline to 7.5 minutes at follow-up [$t(9) = 1.92$, n.s.]. Walking speed improved: a 30-foot walk with a turn was performed in 20.6 seconds at baseline, 17.3 seconds immediately after the program, and 12.5 seconds at follow-up (see Table 18.1). We believe the additional improvement at follow-up, however, was an artifact caused by different instructions to subjects about walking fast.

The total score and both psychosocial and physical scores on the SIP improved significantly from baseline to follow-up [$t(13) = 4.39, p < .001$; $t(13) = 3.66, p < .001$; and $t(13) = 2.47, p < .05$, respectively]. The improvements in SIP scores suggest that increasing strength and endurance enabled subjects to be more active despite their chronic illness.

Physical activity, assessed by the Yale Physical Activity Scale (DiPietro, Casperson, Ostfeld, & Nadel, 1990) increased from 20.0 hours per week at baseline to 27.9 hours at posttest, with a decline to 22.1 at follow-up. The improvement from baseline to posttest was statistically significant [$t(13) = 3.11, p < .01$]. This was expected since subjects included the 6 hours of exercise class in the total activity assessed at posttest. Since most subjects planned to exercise only 3 hours per week independently, a decline in reported activity was expected at follow-up.

Scores on Rosenberg's Self-Esteem Scale (Rosenberg, 1965) improved from 31.7 to 34.9 [$t(13) = 3.10, p < .01$], then declined slightly to 33.2 at follow-up.

On the basis of the unstructured interview at follow-up, we rated the intensity, frequency, and duration of exercise, and the intensity and frequency of physical activity, on a scale from 1 to 3. The highest possible score was 15. Participants' scores ranged from 7 to 14. Six of the 13 subjects interviewed at follow-up had become moderate to vigorous exercisers, exercising at least 15–30 minutes 2–3 times each week.

TABLE 18.1 Means and Standard Deviations of Selected Variables at Baseline, Immediate Posttest, and 3.5 Months after Exercise Intervention

	Baseline		Posttest		Follow-up	
Variable	Mean	S.D.	Mean	S.D.	Mean	S.D.
VO_2 peak ml/kg/min cycle ergometry	15.3	3.7	19.3	2.2	19.0	2.2
METS	4.4	—	5.5	—	5.4	—
Time on step test (min)	6.3	1.7	8.2	2.0	7.5	1.6
Ambulation time (30 ft, turn) sec	20.6	17.9	17.3	12.1	12.5	5.8
Left hip flexion tasks (# completed: 0–3 potential range)	1.6	0.8	1.8	0.8	1.7	0.9
Left arm tasks (# completed: 0–8 potential range)	6.6	1.7	7.4	1.2	7.3	0.9
Yale Physical Activity score (hrs/wk)	20.0	9.8	27.9	8.1	22.1	6.9
Self esteem (4–44 range, high score high esteem)	31.7	5.4	34.9	4.1	33.2	4.9
Sickness Impact Profile[a]						
Total (potential range 0–100, low score better health status)	20.5	1.5	12.5	1.2	9.6	1.0
Physical category score	12.8	0.8	9.9	1.5	6.0	10.0
Psychosocial category score	23.0	2.0	15.8	1.6	11.6	1.1

[a]These scaled percent scores are summed within categories and for the total. The total percent is not the sum of the psychosocial and physical scores.

DISCUSSION

The study sample was small and there was no control group, but the results are promising. The pilot suggests that exercise training for the elderly can be done in a small group. Further, bike ergometry is clearly feasible and is preferable to the step test or chair step test as a graded exercise test in a population that often experiences arthritic changes in lower extremity joints. No change in hip or knee range of motion is needed to complete a bicycle ergometry test. However, step and chair step tests require increasing range of motion as subjects progress through the four levels. This pilot also indicates that people with little education can learn new concepts such as problem solving and goal setting. The social experience of the group is important, and the support person adds reinforcement. We recommend, however, that the transition to home/independent exercise begin earlier, last longer, and increase in strength.

NOTES

1. 220 - Age - resting heart rate (RHR) = heart rate reserve (HRR)
   HRR x .70 + RHR = upper limit of exercise heart rate
   HRR x .40 + RHR = lower limit of exercise heart rate

REFERENCES

Amundson, L. R., DeVahl, J. M., & Ellingham, C. T. (1989). Evaluation of a group exercise program for elderly women. *Physical Therapy, 69*, 475–483.

Aniansson, A., & Gustafson, E. (1981). Physical training in elderly men with special reference to quadriceps muscle strength and morphology. *Clinical Physiology, 1*, 87–98.

Bergner, M., Bobbitt, R. A., Carter, W. B., & Gilson, B. S. (1981). The Sickness Impact Profile: Development and final revision of a health status measure. *Medical Care, 19*, 787–805.

Brody, J. A. (1989). Toward quantifying the health of the elderly. *American Journal of Public Health, 79*, 685–686.

DiPietro, L., Casperson, C., Ostfeld, A., & Nadel, E. (1990). Comparison of physical activity surveys for older adults. *Medicine and Science in Sports and Exercise, 22*, S29.

Dishman, R. K. (Ed.). (1988). *Exercise adherence. Its impact on public health*. Champaign, IL: Human Kinetics Books.

D'Zurilla, T. J. (1986). *Problem-solving therapy: A social competence approach to clinical intervention*. New York: Springer Publishing Co.

Fiatarone, M. A., Marks, E. C., Ryan, N. D., Meredith, C. N., Lipsitz, L. A., & Evans, W. J. (1990). High-intensity strength training in nonagenarians. *Journal of the American Medical Association, 263*, 3029–3034.

Fletcher, G. E., Froelicher, V. F., Hartley, H., Haskell, W. L., & Pollock, M. L. (1991). *Exercise standards*. Dallas, TX: American Heart Association.

Fried, L., Herdman, S. J., Kuhn, K. E., Rubin, G., & Turano, K. (1991). Preclinical disability: Hypotheses about the bottom of the iceberg. *Journal of Aging and Health, 3*, 285–300.

Frontera, W. R., Meredith, C. N., O'Reilly, K. P., Knuttgen, H. G., & Evans, W. J. (1988). Strength conditioning in older men: Skeletal muscle hypertrophy and improved function. *Journal of Applied Physiology, 64*, 1038–1044.

Kanfer, F. H., & Goldstein, A. P. (1991). *Helping people change: A textbook of methods* (4th ed). Elmsford, NY: Pergamon Press.

Karvonen, M., Kentala, K., & Mustala, O. (1958). The effects of training on heart rate: A longitudinal study. *Annales Medicinae Experimentatus et Biologie Fenniae, 35*, 307–315.

Katzman, R., Brown, T., & Fuld, P. (1983) Validation of a short orientation-memory-concentration test of cognitive impairment. *American Journal of Psychiatry, 140*, 734–739.

Kauffman, T. (1990). Impact of aging-related musculoskeletal and postural changes on falls. *Topics in Geriatric Rehabilitation, 5*, 34–43.

Lawton, M. P. (1975). The Philadelphia Geriatric Morale Scale: A revision. *Journal of Gerontology, 30*, 85–89.

Marlatt, G. A., & Gordon, J. R. (Eds.). (1985). *Relapse prevention*. New York: Guilford.

Meichenbaum, D., & Turk, D. C. (1987). *Facilitating treatment adherence: A practitioner's guide*. New York: Plenum.

Rosenberg, R. (1965). *Society and the adolescent self-image*. Princeton: Princeton University Press.

Rothman, M. L., Hedrick, S., & Innui, T. (1989). The Sickness Impact Profile as a measure of the health status of noncognitively impaired nursing home residents. *Medical Care, 27*, S157–S167.

Seals, D. R., Hagberg, J. M., Hurley, B. F., Ehsani, A. A., & Holloszy, J. O. (1984). Endurance training in older men and women. I. Cardiovascular responses to exercise. *Journal of Applied Physiology: Respiratory, Environmental and Exercise Physiology, 57*, 1024–1029.

Shepard, R. J. (1990). The scientific basis of exercise prescribing for the very old. *Journal of the American Geriatrics Society, 38*, 62–70.

Smith, E. L., & Gilligan, C. (1983). Physical activity prescription for the older adult. *The Physician and Sports Medicine, 11*, 91–101.

Snow, T., Hogue, C. C., & Cullinan, S. M. (1993). *The Snow Inventory of Functional Tests (SIFT)*. Unpublished instrument.

U. S. Senate Special Committee on Aging. (1989). *Aging America, 1988: Trends and projections*. Serial No. 101–E, Washington, DC: U.S. Government Printing Office.

Weindruch, R., Hadley, E. C., & Ory, M. G. (Eds.). (1991). *Reducing frailty and falls in older persons*. Springfield, IL: Charles C. Thomas.

[19]

Family Caregivers of Severely Head-Injured Adults in the Community Setting

Joanne V. Hickey

Every year in the United States approximately 500,000 individuals, primarily between the ages of 16 and 35, sustain traumatic head injuries serious enough to require hospitalization. Of that number 70,000 experience head injuries severe enough to preclude return to independent living and about 290,000 experience symptoms that interfere with activities of daily living (DeJong, Batavia, & Williams, 1990). Deficits include severe physical, cognitive, personality, communicative, psychosocial, and behavioral dysfunction. The rehabilitation needs of this population are extensive, and recovery takes months to years.

Family and the family environment play an important role in the long-term outcomes for head-injured persons (Bond, 1975; Mauss-Clum & Ryan, 1981). Studies suggest that families of ill persons generally function less well than families in which all members are healthy (Dimond & Jones, 1983; Marinelli & Dell Orto, 1984). Furthermore, the more severe and long lasting the illness, the greater the potential for family disruption and stress. Lezak (1978) suggested that the problems and stresses endured by the family are usually experienced most poignantly by the family member who is the primary caregiver.

There is a paucity of research on caregivers of head injured persons (HIPs), especially within the community setting. Most caregiver research has focused on caregivers of Alzheimer's disease patients, but these studies are not generalizable to HIP caregivers, who tend to be younger, have different responsibilities and needs, and are at different developmental stages. The purpose of this study, therefore, was to describe the characteristics of primary family caregivers of head injured adults, including levels of anxiety and depression in these caregivers, and to examine family function and support among this caregiver group.

Moos's (1984) model of coping with the crisis of physical illness guided the study. Moos identifies three sets of determinants that account for an individual's cognitive appraisal of a serious physical injury and, ultimately the coping strategies the individual uses to adapt to the illness. The three sets of determinants are background and personal factors, illness-related factors, and physical and social environmental factors. Background and personal factors include age, gender, socioeconomic status, cognitive and emotional maturity, ego strength and self-confidence, philosophical or religious beliefs, and prior illness and coping experiences. Illness-related factors include the type and location of symptoms and whether they are painful, disfiguring, or in a body region vested with special importance, such as the brain. Physical and social environmental factors include the physical living arrangements as well as family cohesiveness and support and social involvement and support. Further, Moos suggests that family and friends are affected by the injury and will encounter many of the same or closely related adaptive tasks and use the same types of coping skills.

METHOD

In order to identify caregiver characteristics, family function and responses to the caregiver role, a questionnaire developed by the investigator and standardized instruments were completed by a sample of primary family caregivers.

Setting and Sample

The setting for this study was the home environment of the primary family caregivers of HIPs located in all regions of the United States, including urban and rural areas. The criteria for participation were as follows:

1. ability to read and speak English;
2. age 18 years or over;
3. severely head-injured family member injured between the ages of 17 and 44 and in the posthospital phase of recovery;
4. primary responsibility for the care or for coordination of care of the HIP;
5. consent to participate.

Subjects were recruited through local chapters of the National Head Injury Foundation, referrals from caregivers and health professionals, and an advertisement placed in the National Head Injury Foundation Newsletter. Subjects who met the study criteria were sent a study packet, cover letter, and stamped self-addressed envelope. The cover letter explained the study and assured anonymity. Return of the completed questionnaire was considered consent to participate.

Data Collection

Five self-administered instruments were used to collect data: the Caregiver Data Sheet (CDS); the Barthel Index (BI); the Family Relationships Inventory (FRI); the Beck Depression Inventory (BDI); and the State-Trait Anxiety Inventory (STAI). The CDS is 25-item questionnaire developed by the researcher to collect data on three major areas in Moos' model: the caregiver's demographic and personal characteristics, the caregiver's social environment, and illness variables. Questions are asked, for example, about the caregiver's age and experience with serious illness; living arrangements and support group attendance; satisfaction with free time; and degree of behavioral/cognitive deficits in the head injured family member. The CDS was piloted on five caregivers and adjustments were made based on a review of their responses and comments.

The BI (modified by Granger, Albrecht, & Hamilton, 1979) measures current level of dependence/independence in ADLs and mobility on a scale of 0–100. Numerical values are assigned for each category of activity and the values are added together to make a total score. The total score indexes dependence in five categories as total, very severe, marked, moderate, and minimal/no dependence; 0–20 represents total dependence, 21–40 very severe dependence, 41–60 marked dependence, 61–80 moderate dependence, and 81–100 represents minimal to no dependence. Interrater reliability is .95. Examples of items include these:

- Dress upper body: can do by self (5); can do with help (3); cannot do at all (0).
- Get in/out of chair: can do by self (15); can do with help (7); cannot do (0).

The three subscales of the Family Environment Scale which form the Family Relationship Inventory (Moos & Moos, 1986) were used to collect data on family function: cohesion, or the degree to which family members are helpful and supportive to each other; expressiveness, or the extent to which family members are encouraged to act openly and to express their feelings directly; and conflict, the extent to which open anger, aggression, and hostile situations exist. In addition, the three subscales are combined to produce a measure of perceived family support called the Family Relationship Inventory (FRI). To calculate the overall FRI, the direction of scoring is reversed on the conflict scale and that score is added to the scores on the cohesion and expressiveness scale. A higher score reflects better family relationships. There are nine items on each of these three subscales. Subjects read nine statements and respond with "true" or "false." Items include:

- Cohesion: "Family really help and support one another" True/False.
- Expressiveness: "Family members often keep their feelings to themselves" True/False.
- Conflict: "We fight a lot in our family" True/False.

The internal consistency for these three subscales ranges from .69 to .78. Test-retest reliabilities are .73 to .86 for a 2-month interval between administrations. Internal consistency for the FRI is reported as .89. The subscales are considered stable but reflect changes in family milieu and discriminate between normal and distressed families.

The BDI (Beck, 1978) is a 21-item self-report instrument used to measure the presence and degree of depression. Four statements form each item. The respondent is asked to read these and choose the one which best describes how he/she feels at the moment. Items are scored thus: I do not feel sad or unhappy (0); I feel sad (1); I am sad all the time and I can't snap out of it (2); I am so sad that I can't snap out of it (3). The overall score is determined by adding the weighted scores for each of the 21 items. A score of 0–9 is considered within the normal range, 10–15 is mild depression; 16–19 mild–moderate depression; 20–29 moderate–severe depression; and 30–63 severe depression. Split-half reliability has been reported as .86 and Spearman-Brown as .93.

State anxiety was measured using the state portion of the STAI (Speilberger, Gorsuch, Lushene, Vagg, & Jacobs, 1983). The respondent is asked to rate his or her current feelings about 20 items, thus: I feel anxious: almost never = 1; sometimes = 2; often = 3; almost always = 4. Scores are summed and range from a minimum of 20 to a maximum of 80; the higher the score, the greater the anxiety. Internal consistency is reported as .93.

RESULTS

Data were collected over a period of 6 months; 85 of the 110 questionnaires mailed were returned. Seventy-nine percent of the caregivers were female and 21% male. Their age range was 25–78 years with a mean of 49 years. Forty-two percent had completed high school, and 42% were college graduates. Their median income was $30,000 – $39,999. Seventy-four percent were married; 75% had very little or no previous experience with illness caregiving. The mean time spent in the caregiver role was 28.6 months.

Most of the head-injured persons cared for (75%) were the children of the caregivers. The HIPs' ages ranged from 19 to 46 years (Mean [*M*] = 28.4 years). Family units varied greatly. The most frequent groupings were caregiver, spouse and HIP (32%), and caregiver, children and HIP (27%). Most caregivers (74%) reported that the HIP lived at home with them. Twenty-eight percent of the caregivers had no helpers, and 41% had one helper; 88% of the primary caregivers assumed 50% or more of caregiving. A third never attended support groups, 38% occasionally attended, and 29% attended often. A majority of caregivers (56%) were unsatisfied or very unsatisfied with the amount of free time they had.

The time since the head injury varied from 3 to 69 months (M = 35.5 months). The age of the HIP at time of injury ranged from 17–43 years (M = 25.5 years). Most of the injuries (73%) were caused by motor vehicle accidents. The period of unconsciousness ranged from 2 to 998 days (M = 115 days). The length of time before continuous day-to-day memory was regained ranged from 2 to 500 days (M = 337 days). After hospitalization, 74% were in a rehabilitation facility, with stays ranging from 0.5 to 24 months (M = 5.5 months).

When caregivers were asked to identify outpatient and community resources used by the HIP, the most frequently cited services were physical therapy (69%), occupational therapy (57%), speech therapy (52%), vocational rehabilitation (38%), psychologists (27%), and visiting nurses (19%). Only 2.4% reported use of respite care. The following HIP deficits and problems were reported: memory (67%); concentration (60%); stress tolerance (56%); judgment (53%); inability to learn from experience (49%); impulsiveness (40%); restlessness (39%); disinterest in life (38%); emotional outbursts (37%); child-like behavior (35%); argumentativeness (34%); demanding behavior (32%); and over-talkativeness (28%).

Fifty-one percent of the HIPs scored 100 on the Barthel Index which represents total independence in ADLs. The scores ranged, however, from 0 to 100 (M = 74.89) (see Table 19.1).

Scores on the three subscales of the Family Environment Scale were as follows: Cohesion ranged from 0 to 9 (M = 6.85). Normative data indicate a mean of 6.61 for a normal family and 5.05 for a distressed family. Expressiveness ranged from 0 to 9 (M = 5.54). The mean is 5.45 for a normal family and 4.60 for a distressed family. Conflict ranged from 0 to 9 (M = 2.45). The mean for a normal family is 3.31 and for a distressed family, 4.28. The score for the combined Family Relationship Inventory, a measure of family support, ranged from 4 to 26 (M = 18.2). No normative data are available for the FRI, but a normative score of 17.75 was calculated by adding the means for the three subscales of the FRI (reversing the conflict score).

Scores on the Beck Depression Inventory ranged from 0 to 24 (M = 8.40). Using guidelines for interpretation of scores, 58% of these caregivers scored within the normal range, 29% had mild depression, 8% had mild to moderate depression, and 4% had severe depression.

Scores on the State Anxiety Scale ranged from 20 to 64 with a mean of 38. Normative data have been calculated for a number of different samples; the norm closest to this sample was for female working adults and was

TABLE 19.1 Means and Ranges for Study Variables

Scale[a]	Possible range	Observed range	Mean
Barthel Index of Independence	0–100	0–100	74.89
Family Relationship Inventory			
Cohesion	0–9	0–9	6.85
Expressiveness	0–9	0–9	5.54
Conflict	0–9	0–9	2.45
Total	0–27	4–26	18.20
Beck Depression Inventory	0–63	0–24	8.40
State Trait Anxiety	0–80	20–64	38.00

[a]For each scale, higher scores reflect more of the characteristic (e.g., greater anxiety).

35.2. The difference in these means was significant [t (84) = 2.21, $p < .05$] indicating greater anxiety in these caregivers.

Scores on all FRI scales were significantly related to depression and anxiety scores (see Table 19.2). As the amount of cohesion, expressiveness, and family support decreased, anxiety and depression increased. As conflict within the family increased, both anxiety and depression also increased.

When selected caregiver variables were correlated with anxiety, lower income ($r = -.30, p < .01$), fewer helpers ($r = -.27, p < .01$), and dissatisfaction with leisure time ($r = -.45, p < .001$) were found to be correlated with increased anxiety. Lower income ($r = -.32, p < .01$) and dissatisfaction with leisure time ($r = -.46, p < .001$) were related to increased depression.

TABLE 20.2. Correlations between FRI Scales and Depression and Anxiety

FRI Scale	Correlations with Depression	Anxiety
Cohesion	–0.32[a]	–0.32[b]
Expressiveness	–0.53[b]	–0.43[b]
Conflict	0.25[a]	0.30[a]
FRI total	–0.46[b]	–0.46[b]

[a]p < .01
[b]p < .001

Length of time since injury was not significantly related to scores on the FRI or its subscales. This may be attributable to the relatively good family function of those willing to participate in this study. There were also no significant relationships between length of time since injury and level of depression and anxiety in the caregiver, suggesting that the stress of the caregiver role continues over time. Likewise, there was not a significant relationship between Barthel scores and scores on the FRI or its subscales. This is consistent with the literature, which suggests that caregiver stress is greater with behavioral and cognitive impairments than with physical impairments.

DISCUSSION

Cost containment and the shift in emphasis in health care from an acuity model to a chronicity model have important ramifications for nurses. With the focus on the community as the setting for care, nurses will have a greater role in providing care to clients and their families. Some of those clients will be head-injured persons who survived trauma because of technological advances—at the price of ongoing physical and mental deficits. Knowledge gained about family caregivers of HIPs in this study will be helpful to nurses in recognizing HIP caregivers at high risk for the effects of long-term stress and burnout. In particular, family support and expressiveness are helpful indicators of family dynamics and can help identify which caregivers are at high risk for anxiety and depression. Caregivers may need help in recognizing the importance of openly discussing concerns with other family members as a way to ventilate feelings and problem solve. Expressiveness also produces an environment in which the caregivers can ask for what they need from other family members. Nurses who care for these patients and families should:

- teach caregivers how to take care of themselves, to prevent stress and maintain self;
- provide information to anticipate needs and provide education and support for HIP caregivers;
- monitor the caregiver for physical and emotional signs of stress;
- promote open discussion of feelings and collaborative problem solving among family members;
- encourage use of community resources for relief of caregiver responsibility and support.

REFERENCES

Beck, A. T. (1978). *Beck depression inventory.* Philadelphia: Center for Cognitive Therapy.

Bond, M. R. (1975). Assessment of the psychosocial outcome after severe head injury. In *Outcome of severe damage to the central nervous system* (pp. 141–157). Newark: CIBA Foundation Symposium.

DeJong, G., Batavia, A. I., & Williams, J. M. (1990). Who is responsible for the lifelong well-being of a person with a head injury? *Journal of Head Trauma Rehabilitation, 5*(1), 9–22.

Dimond, S., & Jones, S. (1983). *Chronic illness across the life span.* Norwalk, CN: Appleton-Century-Crofts.

Granger, C. V., Albrecht, G. L., & Hamilton, B. B. (1979). Outcome of comprehensive medical rehabilitation: Measurement by PULSES profile and the Barthel index. *Archives of Physical Medicine and Rehabilitation, 60,* 14–17.

Lezak, M. D. (1978). Living with the characterologically altered brain injured patient. *Journal of Clinical Psychology, 39,* 592–598.

Marinelli, R. P., & Dell Orto, A. E. (Eds.). (1984). *The psychological and social impact of physical disability,* (2nd ed). New York: Springer Publishing Co.

Mauss-Clum, N., & Ryan, M. (1981). Brain injury and the family. *Journal of Neurosurgical Nursing, 16,* 165–169.
Moos, R. H. (1984). *Coping with physical illness 2: New perspectives.* New York: Plenum.
Moos, R. H., & Moos, B. S. (1986). *Family environment scale manual.* Palo Alto, CA: Consulting Psychologists Press.
Spielberger, C., Gorsuch, R., Lushene, R., Vagg, P., & Jacobs, G. (1983). *Manual for the state-trait anxiety inventory: STAI (Form Y).* Palo Alto, CA: Consulting Psychologists Press.

[20]

Role Acquisition in Family Caregivers for Older People Who Have Been Discharged from the Hospital

Barbara J. Stewart, Patricia G. Archbold, Theresa A. Harvath, and Ngozi O. Nkongho

Family caregiving to frail older people is increasing in this society as the relative percentage and the actual number of older people increase. No one would dispute the fact that the family plays a pivotal role in the provision of long-term care services in the home (Brody, 1985; Horowitz, 1985; Stone, Cafferata, & Sangl, 1987). It is well known that for some family caregivers the experience brings extensive physical, emotional, and financial costs (Doty, 1984; George & Gwyther, 1986; Poulshock & Deimling, 1984). However, an aspect of family caregiving that has received little attention in the literature is family caregiver role acquisition, or the way in which family caregivers learn about various aspects of the role of caregiver.

Classic role theory suggests that the degree and quality of role acquisition mediate role strain (Burr, Leigh, Day, & Constantine, 1979; Cottrell, 1942; Mederer, 1980; Merton, 1968). We thought that an understanding of how caregivers acquire various aspects of the caregiving role might thus have important implications for nursing practice with families.

Traditionally, role acquisition has been viewed as a one-step process that occurred simultaneously with entrance into a new role; the emphasis was and skills needed to perform a specified role are learned both prior to and during role occupation (Thornton & Nardi, 1975). Analysis of data from one of our previous studies suggests that acquisition of the family caregiver role occurs primarily after entering into the role. For example, one caregiver indicated that she learned "by doing." Another said that his learning had been "gradual" — as his wife's abilities were lost. Thus in the caregiving role, post-entry role acquisition may play a greater part than pre-entry role acquisition.

We have identified several ways in which caregivers might learn their role. Two ways occur prior to entering the role. We call this pre-entry role acquisition, and it includes previous work experience and previous caregiving experience. Four other ways of learning the role of caregiver occur after entry into the role. We call this post-entry role acquisition, and it includes learning from health professionals, books or articles, friends or relatives, and trial and error. In a recent longitudinal study we conducted with family caregivers and care receivers, we were interested in sources of information that caregivers used in learning how to provide care, and how much caregivers learned from these sources about different aspects of caregiving. In this chapter, we look at whether caregivers used various sources of caregiving information during the first 6 weeks after the hospital discharge of the older care receiver. We also describe how much caregivers learned from these sources about the content of the caregiving role, which includes meeting the care receiver's physical and emotional needs, handling the stress of caregiving, and getting formal services that might help the care receiver.

METHOD

Sample

The study was conducted within a health maintenance organization in the Pacific Northwest, and used a sample of 103 family members who provided care to a person 65 years of age or older who had been discharged from the hospital. To qualify for the study, the older person had to require assistance in one or more of the following areas: (a) medications or injections; (b) bathing, shampooing, or dressing; (c) walking, shopping, or errands; or (d) household chores such as cleaning. Caregivers had to be 18 years of age or older and able to speak English. Data were collected from family caregivers 6 weeks after the discharge of the older family member.

Fifty-two percent of the caregivers were spouses. The average age of the caregiver was 64 years with an age range of 21 to 88 years. Caregivers were related to the older family member as wives (28%), husbands (24%), daughters (21%), sons (6%), daughters-in-law (10%), or others (11%). Most placed on anticipatory socialization, or the process of learning the role before entering it (Burr, 1972). However, some theorists view role acquisition as a developmental process involving several stages, where the knowledge

(75%) lived with the older person. Most of the caregivers were married (68%), most were female (68%), and most were white (98%). The average caregiver was a high school graduate. The median yearly income of the caregivers was $15,000–$24,999. The duration of caregiving in this sample ranged from 1 month to 24 years; the average length was 3.7 years.

Measures

Data were collected using the Family Caregiving Inventory (FCI) (Archbold & Stewart, 1986). The FCI is composed of two structured interview instruments—one for the caregiver and one for the care receiver (Archbold, Stewart, Greenlick, & Harvath, 1990); however, only data from the caregiver interview are presented here. The instrument contains two measures of role acquisition—the Source of Role Acquisition Scale and the Amount Learned Scale.

The Source of Role Acquisition Scale measures whether six pre- and post-entry sources of information about the caregiver role were used by the caregiver. The Amount Learned Scale contains items that ask caregivers how much they have learned from different information sources about four aspects of the caregiving role: how to take care of the care receiver's physical needs, how to take care of the care receiver's emotional needs, how to handle the stress of caregiving, and how to find out about and set up services for the care receiver.

Six other scales described by Archbold et al. (1990) were employed in the analyses reported here. They included the Amount of Direct Care Scale (38 items), Strain from Direct Care Scale (38 items), Strain from Worry Scale (10 items), Strain from Lack of Resources Scale (6 items), Strain from Increased Tension Scale (4 items), and Global Strain Scale (4 items).

RESULTS

Sources of Information

Item percentages provide an interesting picture of the sources of information used by caregivers. At 6 weeks after the care receiver's hospital discharge, 69% of caregivers reported that during the time they had been caregivers, they had talked with professionals such as doctors, nurses and social workers about how to give care to their family member; 59% reported that they had used a trial-and-error approach to see what would work in caring for their family member; 59% said that they had previously cared for another family member or friend who was ill; 53% had talked with friends or relatives; 37% had read books or articles about how to take care of their family member; and only 15% reported that they had had a job in which they took care of sick or disabled people before starting caregiving. About 10% of the caregivers reported using none of the four post-entry sources of information; 23% reported using one source, 17% reported using two sources, 30% reported using three sources, and 20% reported using all four sources.

Interpretation: Sources of Information

These results indicate that caregivers obtain information from multiple sources, but vary in the number of sources they use. We think that nurses can work with caregivers, building on knowledge the caregivers learned before entering the role as well as what they have learned after entering the role, to help caregivers think through ways to apply such information to their particular situation.

Amount Learned about Taking Care of Physical Needs

Findings about the amount caregivers learned reflect the varying utility of the six information sources. Based on mean scores, where a value of 4 represents *a lot*, 3 represents *some*, 2 represents *a little*, and a value of 1 represents *none*, on the average caregivers reported learning *some* about meeting the older person's physical needs from professionals (mean [M] = 3.06), trial and error ($M = 2.90$), previous work ($M = 2.80$), books or articles ($M = 2.76$), and previous caregiving experiences ($M = 2.68$). They reported learning only *a little* from friends or relatives ($M = 2.24$) about taking care of the care receiver's physical needs (see Table 20.1). Compared to the amount learned from friends or relatives, caregivers reported learning significantly more about taking care of the care receiver's physical needs from health professionals [$t(54) = 4.45, p < .01$], trial and error [$t(54) = 3.71, p < .01$], previous work [$t(14) = 2.29, p < .05$], books or articles [$t(37) = 2.28, p < .05$], and previous caregiving [$t(54) = 2.07, p < .05$]. The kinds of physical needs that caregivers managed included helping the care receiver with dressing, walking, and medications.

Interpretation: Learning about Physical Needs

The findings regarding where caregivers learned about managing the care receiver's physical needs support our notion that, immediately following a hospitalization, caregivers are likely to consult with health professionals about the physical care of their older family member. For many of the care receivers in our study, the hospitalization represented a dramatic change in functional status; thus it is not surprising that caregivers reported learning most about the care receiver's physical needs from health professionals. The small amount learned from friends or relatives may reflect lack of experience among this group with the types of physical problems experienced by posthospitalized older people. It may also reflect the relative availability of health services during this period of illness—an availability that decreases with decreasing acuity of the health problem.

TABLE 20.1 Amount Learned about How to Take Care of the Care Receiver's Physical Needs

Information source	*M*[a]	*SE*[b]	*N*[c]
Professionals	3.06	.12	71
Trial and error	2.90	.11	61
Previous work	2.80	.33	15
Books or articles	2.76	.18	38
Previous caregiving	2.68	.16	60
Friends or relatives	2.24	.14	55

[a]M = Mean on 4 point scale: 4 = a lot, 3 = some, 2 = a little, 1 = none.
[b]SE = Standard error of the mean.
[c]N = Number rating the information source.
Note: As shown in Tables 20.1, 20.2, 20.3, & 20.4, the means are based on different numbers (*N*s) of caregivers. This variation in sample size occurred because caregivers reported the amount learned only for those sources of information that they had used. Thus, caregivers had legitimate missing data on amount learned from a source of information if they had not used that source. This variation in *N*s makes it difficult to compare these means statistically, because neither a *t*–test for independent samples nor a *t*–test for paired data applies. For any pair of means, some caregivers had scores used in computing both means and other caregivers had scores used in computing only one of the means. To address the issue of whether the means were significantly different from one another, we applied the following rationale. We used the formula for a *t*–test for two independent samples, employing the separate variance estimate in the denominator, and used the smaller of the two sample sizes to estimate degrees of freedom (smaller $N-1$). We believe this is a conservative estimate of the significance of the difference between any two means. In general, the correlations between any two sources on amount learned were low positive values, with the middle 90% of the *r*s ranging from –.10 to .56, with a median *r* of .22. Had paired *t*–tests been appropriate, they might have resulted in slightly larger *t*–values because the denominator would have been made smaller due to the positive correlation.

Amount Learned about Taking Care of Emotional Needs

Overall, caregivers reported learning most about how to take care of the older person's emotional needs from previous work in which they took care of sick or disabled people ($M = 2.73$), from previous caregiving experience ($M = 2.62$), and from a trial-and-error approach ($M = 2.50$). Caregivers reported that they learned only *a little* about handling their family member's emotional needs from books or articles ($M = 2.24$), professionals such as doctors, nurses, and social workers ($M = 1.83$), and friends or relatives ($M = 1.80$) (see Table 20.2). Statistical comparisons of means indicate that,

TABLE 20.2 Amount Learned about How to Take Care of the Care Receiver's Emotional Needs

Information source	*M*[a]	*SE*[b]	*N*[c]
Previous work	2.73	.33	15
Previous caregiving	2.62	.15	61
Trial and error	2.50	.13	60
Books or articles	2.24	.18	38
Professionals	1.83	.12	70
Friends or relatives	1.80	.11	55

[a]M = Mean on 4 point scale: 4 = a lot, 3 = some, 2 = a little, 1 = none.
[b]SE = Standard error of the mean.
[c]N = Number rating the information source.

when it comes to learning about how to take care of the care receiver's emotional needs, experience seems to matter most. Previous work, previous caregiving, and trial-and-error approaches received significantly higher mean ratings than friends or relatives [$t(14) = 2.67, p < .05$; $t(54) = 4.41, p < .01$; and $t(54) = 4.11, p < .01$ respectively] and professionals [$t(14) = 2.56, p < .05$; $t(60) = 4.11, p < .01$; and $t(59) = 3.79, p < .01$; respectively].

Interpretation: Amount Learned About Taking Care of Emotional Needs

The results suggest to us that experience is an important ingredient in taking care of another's emotional needs. Managing difficult situations, often by trial-and-error, provides an opportunity for caregivers to grow in both knowledge and comfort. However, this conclusion must be interpreted in the light of the open-ended responses of caregivers to our questions about a trial-and-error approach. Based on their responses, we identified two distinctly different trial-and-error strategies. One was a thoughtful, problem-solving approach used to refine the care provided; the other was a kind of "flailing about," trying one thing after another, in a somewhat frantic manner. Thus, a trial-and-error approach may have limitations as well as benefits for caregivers.

We were a little surprised to see the relatively minor role that health professionals played in teaching caregivers about the care receiver's emotional needs. On reflection we realized that some of the emotional needs that caregivers find difficult to manage are related to cognitive and behavioral problems associated with dementia. Other emotional needs that are difficult to manage are the uncontrollable crying associated with strokes and the emotional ups and downs associated with recovery following a hospitalization. Dealing with these problems requires extended involvement with the family; but in our current health care system, with its emphasis on budgetary restraint, health professionals may have limited opportunities to address the emotional needs of the care receiver with the caregiver. Consequently, caregivers may be forced to seek alternative sources of information. We think this is an area where nurses could have a positive impact, and they need to challenge the current system. Nurses can also be creative in working within the restrictions of the system. For example, they may be able to couple assistance around emotional care issues with assistance on medical diagnoses or symptoms for which nursing care is reimbursed.

Amount Learned about Handling the Stress of Caregiving

Caregivers learned *some* to *a little* about handling the stress of caregiving from previous experience with caregiving ($M = 2.67$), trial and error ($M = 2.45$), and previous work in which they took care of sick or disabled people ($M = 2.43$). Caregivers indicated that they had learned only *a little* about how to handle the stress of caregiving from the other sources (books or articles $M = 1.97$; friends and relatives $M = 1.91$; and professionals, $M = 1.73$) (see Table 20.3). The importance of experience was highlighted once more by the significantly higher mean amount learned from previous caregiving and trial-and-error approaches than from health professionals [$t(60) = 4.89$, $p < .01$ and $t(59) = 4.07$, $p < .01$, respectively], from friends or relatives [$t(54) = 3.83$, $p < .01$ and $t(54) = 2.94$, $p < .01$, respectively], or from reading books and articles [$t(37) = 3.19$, $p < .01$ and $t(37) = 2.33$, $p < .05$, respectively].

Interpretation: Amount Learned about Handling the Stress of Caregiving

Again, it was interesting to find that most caregivers reported learning very little from health professionals about managing the stress of caregiving. We think this might be a result of the practitioner's focus on the care receiver's physical needs. However, given the vital role that caregivers

TABLE 20.3 Amount Learned about How to Handle the Stress of Caregiving

Information source	M^a	SE^b	N^c
Previous caregiving	2.67	.15	61
Trial and error	2.45	.13	60
Previous work	2.43	.33	14
Books or articles	1.97	.16	38
Friends or relatives	1.91	.13	55
Professionals	1.73	.12	70

[a]M = Mean on 4 point scale: 4 = a lot, 3 = some, 2 = a little, 1 = none.
[b]SE = Standard error of the mean.
[c]N = Number rating the information source.

TABLE 20.4 Amount Learned about How to Find Out About and Set Up Formal Services for the Care Receiver

Information source	M^a	SE^b	N^c
Professionals	2.88	.17	42
Books or articles	2.72	.17	25
Trial and error	2.40	.20	20
Friends or relatives	2.00	.14	38

[a]M = Mean on 4 point scale: 4 = a lot, 3 = some, 2 = a little, 1 = none.
[b]SE = Standard error of the mean.
[c]N = Number rating the information source.

play in the long-term care of older persons, we think it is important for nurses (as well as the health care system as a whole) to include the primary family caregiver, as well as other family support people, when targeting interventions for the care receiver.

Amount Learned about Setting up Services

On the average, caregivers reported learning *some* about how to find out about and set up formal services from professionals ($M = 2.88$), and from books or articles ($M = 2.72$). Caregivers reported learning *a little* about setting up formal services from trial and error ($M = 2.40$) and from friends or relatives ($M = 2.00$) (see Table 20.4). We did not ask about the amount learned about services from previous work or previous caregiving experiences. Caregivers learned significantly more about arranging services from professionals than from friends or relatives [$t(37) = 4.00, p < .01$] and from trial and error [$t(19) = 2.18, p < .05$]. Caregivers also learned significantly more about organizing services from reading books and articles than from friends or relatives [$t(24) = 3.27, p < .01$].

Interpretation: Amount Learned about Setting up Services

Again, it appears that following a hospitalization, health professionals may have the opportunity to assist family caregivers to find out about and set up services. Books, articles, and other reading material may also be helpful to caregivers as they explore the availability and use of services. The relatively high amount learned from professionals about setting up services and taking care of the care receiver's physical needs may reflect, in part, that caregivers have access to health care mainly through information-seeking about services and physical care. When nurses have contact with caregivers while providing services and physical care, they may want to use such opportunities to assess emotional care and stress.

Correlational Results

Six weeks after the care receiver's hospital discharge, caregivers who were doing more caregiving tasks also reported using significantly more of the four post-entry sources of information on how to provide care ($r = .34$, $p < .01$, N = 103). In addition, caregivers who reported higher levels of five aspects of caregiver role strain (strain from direct care, worry, lack of resources, increased tension, and global strain) also reported using more of these sources of information on how to provide care. The correlations of the five strain scales with the number of sources used ranged from .26 to .42 ($p < .01$, N = 103). However, there was no clear pattern of correlation between strain and amount learned. The correlations between the amount learned about the four aspects of caregiving and the role strain scales ranged from –.20 to .24, with a median correlation of .07.

Interpretation: Learning and Role Strain

The correlational results suggest that during times of increased caregiving activities and increased strain, caregivers are likely to seek help from a variety of sources. Although it was difficult to determine whether the help given at these times made a difference for the caregivers in our study, we think times of increased strain may represent windows of opportunity when families might be more receptive to new information. If nursing interventions could be delivered during these periods of high strain, they might be more relevant for families. In addition, because most caregivers are mature adults, effective methods for teaching adults may facilitate role acquisition and role maintenance. It is important for nurses to use the client's past experiences in developing interventions within a mutually respectful relationship.

It is a mistake to assume that caregivers who report using many sources of information to learn about caregiving are managing their role without too much strain; in fact, using more sources of information may be associated with higher strain. For example, a caregiver may tell a nurse that she has read a lot of books or talked with a lot of people about how to provide care. These statements should be considered as possible indicators of increased learning needs and greater stress in the caregiving situation.

DISCUSSION

Strategies for Enhancing Role Acquisition

Our findings about role acquisition and other findings from this study of 103 caregivers led to our most recent project called the PREP project. In this project we experimented with ways in which home health nurses, whom we referred to as PREP nurses, could enhance the caregiver's role acquisition. The nurses focused on increasing the caregiver's preparedness to manage the care receiver's physical and emotional needs, handle the stress of caregiving, find out about and set up services, and make caregiving more satisfying. Although we have not yet analyzed our quantitative data, we have clinical examples from our PREP project to illustrate how nurses worked with families to enhance role acquisition in these five areas.

One strategy used by the PREP nurses to increase the caregiver's preparedness to manage physical needs was to document the frequency and timing of the problem. For example, one caregiver reported having difficulty regulating her mother's bowels. The caregiver's anxiety regarding this problem was intense because her mother had been hospitalized recently for a bowel obstruction. The PREP nurse provided a form on which the family could document the frequency of bowel movements. This was a very effective tool for the caregiver. After just 1 week, she saw that in fact her mother had a regular pattern of constipation. This documentation made it possible to time an intervention to reduce the constipation. The caregiver also used the same form to improve her own regularity. This strategy of documenting the frequency and timing of behavior has been useful not only in detecting the pattern of the problem, but also in evaluating the success of the intervention strategy implemented.

One strategy used by PREP nurses to increase the caregiver's preparedness to manage emotional problems was to identify and reinforce activities that the caregiver did well. For example, one caregiver described how her husband, who had some cognitive impairment, became agitated in the evenings, asked repeatedly for his keys, and wanted to check the locks on doors and windows. Prior to his retirement this care receiver had been employed as a nighttime security guard. The caregiver interpreted his evening agitation to be related to his previous work pattern, but was uncertain whether she was reinforcing his agitation by helping him "secure the premises" at night. The PREP nurse supported the caregiver's interpretation of the behavior and helped her develop a variety of strategies that focused on dissipating her husband's anxiety and reassuring him of his safety. For example, they made it a nightly routine to walk around the perimeter of the house, checking the locks on the doors and windows, and they provided the care receiver with his own set of keys to carry in his pocket. This nightly ritual calmed him enough so that the family could proceed with the evening meal and bedtime routines. This strategy also helped to diminish the care receiver's anxiety when visiting the son or daughter's home.

A strategy used by PREP nurses to increase the caregiver's preparedness to manage the stress of caregiving was to help caregivers develop contingency plans for potential problems. For example, one of our families had a wedding planned that all members, including the care receiver, age 95, wanted to attend. The caregiver was worried that if her grandmother did not feel well enough to attend, she too would be unable to go. At the suggestion of the PREP nurse, the caregiver developed a contingency plan in the event that the care receiver did not feel well enough to attend the wedding when the day arrived. The caregiver interviewed a potential in-home respite volunteer who could be called on at the last minute to sit with the care receiver. She also composed a diary of daily caregiving events listing the details of care. She outlined specific ways in which to prepare and serve the meals, the schedule for naps, and the care receiver's favorite items of clothing. This diary would not only help the volunteer feel more relaxed with the care receiver, but would also reassure the caregiver that the daily pattern of care would not be interrupted by her absence.

A strategy used by PREP nurses to increase the caregiver's preparedness to set up services involved rehearsal and role playing. For example, in another PREP family, the care receiver had a 25-year history of rheumatoid arthritis (RA) and recently had had a total hip replacement. Following hospital discharge the woman experienced a painful flare-up of her arthritis. Although she wanted a referral to a rheumatologist, she was reluctant to ask her primary care provider because she was concerned that she might offend him. In addition, her husband, the caregiver, had some cognitive impairment and was unable to advocate for his wife. The PREP nurse rehearsed with the care receiver how she would ask her doctor for the referral, and helped her role play different scenarios. The care receiver's preparation helped her to advocate for her own needs and obtain the referral.

We also included interventions designed to enrich caregiving activities and make them more satisfying to the caregiver and the care receiver. For example, we might encourage a dyad to share a meal with special attention to place settings and ornamentation, or to participate in previously shared leisure activities. In one family, both mother and caregiving daughter had their own private interests. The times they chose to spend together were based on their mutual enjoyment of tending the garden. The mother had been able, in years past, to help with the weeding and harvesting as well as canning the vegetables. Now, because of her advanced age and diminished endurance, she could no longer do this. This was a source of frustration for the care receiver and of sadness for the caregiver. The PREP nurse observed the difficulty the care receiver might have in navigating the back yard when invited to tour it with the caregiver. The nurse then suggested that the caregiver make a container garden for the care receiver to tend while sitting at the patio table. The caregiver found a large shallow bowl in which the care receiver planted flower starts. It became a daily ritual to water, weed, tend, and nurture the flowers. The caregiver brought the container indoors when the season changed, so as to lengthen the care receiver's enjoyment of her garden. This strategy enhanced the time the family spent together and also helped to emphasize what the care receiver could do. By building on family strengths, we may also be sustaining optimism.

While these examples are from our experience in home health nursing, we think that the principles are equally applicable to the nursing of chronically ill people and their families in other settings.

ACKNOWLEDGMENTS

The study was conducted collaboratively at the School of Nursing, Oregon Health Sciences University, and the Center for Health Research, Kaiser Foundation Hospital. The results presented here are based on two research projects funded by grants from the National Center for Nursing Research (R01 NU/AG1140 and R01 NR 2088). Special thanks go to Jane Kirschling for her helpful comments on this chapter.

REFERENCES

Archbold, P. G., & Stewart, B. J. (1986). *Family caregiving inventory.* Unpublished instrument, Oregon Health Sciences University, Department of Family Nursing, Portland.

Archbold, P. G., Stewart, B. J., Greenlick, M. R., & Harvath, T. (1990). Mutuality and preparedness as predictors of caregiver role strain. *Research in Nursing & Health, 13,* 375–384.

Brody, E. M. (1985). Parent care as a normative family stress. *The Gerontologist, 25,* 19–29.

Burr, W. R. (1972). Role transitions: A reformulation of theory. *Journal of Marriage and the Family, 34,* 407–416.

Burr, W. R., Leigh, G. K., Day, R. D., & Constantine, J. (1979). Symbolic interaction and the family. In W. R. Burr, R. Hill, F. I. Nye, & I. L. Reiss (Eds.), *Contemporary theories about the family: Vol.* 2 (pp. 42–111). New York: Free Press.

Cottrell, L. S. (1942). The adjustment of the individual to his age and sex roles. *American Sociological Review, 7,* 617–620.

Doty, P. (1984). *Family care of the elderly: Is it declining? Can public policy promote it?* Working paper. Washington, DC: Office of Policy Analysis, Health Care Financing Administration.

George, L. K., & Gwyther, L. P. (1986). Caregiver well-being: A multidimensional examination of family caregivers of demented adults. *The Gerontologist, 26,* 253–259.

Horowitz, A. (1985). Family caregiving to the frail elderly. *Annual Review of Gerontology and Geriatrics, 5,* 194–246.

Mederer, H. J. (1980). *A theory of ease of role transitions in the acquisition of the parent caring role.* Paper presented at the Theory Construction Workshop of the National Council on Family Relations Annual Meeting, Portland, OR.

Merton, R. K. (1968). *Social theory and social structure*. Glencoe, IL: Free Press.
Poulshock, S. W., & Deimling, G. T. (1984). Families caring for elders in residence: Issues in the measurement of burden. *Journal of Gerontology, 39*, 230–239.
Stone, R., Cafferata, G. L., & Sangl, J. (1987). Caregivers of the frail elderly: A national profile. *The Gerontologist, 27*, 616–626.
Thornton, R., & Nardi, P. (1975). The dynamics of role acquisition. *The American Journal of Sociology, 80*, 870–885.

[21]

Chronic Sorrow: An Examination of Nursing Roles

Georgene G. Eakes, Mary L. Burke, Margaret A. Hainsworth, and Carolyn L. Lindgren

The term chronic sorrow was first coined by Olshansky (1962) to describe the recurring sadness that he observed in parents of mentally retarded children. Although the term quickly gained wide use in the professional literature, the phenomenon of chronic sorrow was not researched for almost 2 decades. Since 1980, however, several studies have pointed to the occurrence of chronic sorrow in parents of children with mental retardation (Wikler, Wasow, & Hatfield, 1981), parents of premature infants (Fraley, 1986), and parents of children with mixed physical and mental disabilities (Kratochvil & Devereux, 1988; Damrosch & Perry, 1989). Most recently, Burke (1989) identified chronic sorrow in mothers of children with spina bifida and redefined chronic sorrow as a pervasive sadness that is permanent, periodic, and progressive in nature.

The occurrence of chronic sorrow in populations other than parents of children with disabilities has not been explored. Yet confrontation with loss is an inevitable experience for individuals with long-term health problems and for the family members who care for them. The accompanying distress may be an obstacle to maintaining a sense of well-being and, further, may constitute an additional threat to health. With the increasing prevalence of chronicity among persons at all stages of life there comes a concomitant increase in the risk for the experience of chronic emotional pain among the ill and disabled and their family caregivers. Expansion of our understanding of chronic sorrow is an essential first step in developing effective nursing interventions for individuals experiencing this sorrow.

METHOD

The four pilot studies described here were designed to determine whether chronic sorrow existed in diverse populations of affected individuals and their caregivers, and to explore strategies for intervening with such persons. The individual pilot studies varied only in the populations sampled—infertile couples, individuals diagnosed with cancer, multiple sclerosis, and Parkinson's disease, and the Parkinson's disease spouse caregivers. A qualitative research approach was used to explore the occurrence of chronic sorrow in these populations. The studies also examined the characteristics of chronic sorrow in the samples and explored how nurses can assist individuals in coping with long-term emotional pain.

Subjects were 5 infertile couples, 10 individuals diagnosed with cancer, 10 individuals with multiple sclerosis, 6 individuals with Parkinson's disease, and 4 Parkinson's spouse caregivers. All subjects were at least 1 year postdiagnosis. Subjects came from the Northeastern, Midwestern, and Southeastern areas of the United States.

Data were collected using the Burke/Nursing Consortium for Research on Chronic Sorrow (NCRCS) Questionnaire (Affected Individual or Caregiver Version). This questionnaire is a modification of the instrument developed by Burke (1989) for use with mothers of children with spina bifida. It was based on an extensive review of the literature (Fraley, 1986; Olshansky, 1962; Wikler et al., 1981) and can be used in telephone or face-to-face interviews. Open-ended questions explore the feelings the individual experienced on first learning of his/her condition or that of the family member, and ask whether and when those or similar feelings have been re-experienced. Other questions focus on identification of factors perceived as helpful to individuals when they experienced these feelings.

Validity and reliability have been established on the original instrument. In the modified version, the content of the questions was not altered in any way; only limited changes were made so that the questions could be directed toward individuals with chronic or life-threatening conditions or toward their family caregivers.

Data were collected using face-to-face or telephone interviews. All interviews were tape-recorded. The data from the 40 subjects were analyzed independently by the authors and were then compared and common themes identified. Analysis included determination of the presence or absence of chronic sorrow, identification of the times when chronic sorrow recurred, exploration of the intensity of the sorrow experiences, and development of suggestions for nurses and other professionals providing care for persons with long-term health problems.

RESULTS

The presence or absence of chronic sorrow was determined by applying Burke's (1989) definition to subject responses to a series of questions exploring the recurrence of those feelings experienced when they first learned of their condition/situation. The findings suggest that chronic sorrow is very likely to occur in individuals with chronic health problems, across the life span. Eighty-three percent of the subjects were found to experience this phenomenon. Chronic sorrow was identified in 90% of the infertile couples, 90% of the individuals diagnosed with cancer, 80% of those with multiple sclerosis, 83% of those with Parkinson's disease, and 50% of their spouse caregivers. Interrater reliability among the independent ratings of the four researchers was 1.00.

Feelings associated with chronic sorrow included sadness, anger, frustration, fear, and helplessness. The data clearly indicate that these feelings occurred periodically over a protracted span of time. All of the characteristics of chronic sorrow are graphically portrayed in the following personal account by a woman who had completed treatment for breast cancer and had been disease-free for 3 years:

> Even right now discussing how I feel, I feel different. When I leave [the interview], I'll probably go cry because I feel like I'm on the verge of tears right now. After 3 years you think, "I've got it all under control," and I normally do. You put all these bricks around so that people can't look at you and see it and so that you can go on and you can function. When you start tearing them apart, you know, it's there. It's there.

Triggers to the recurrence of feelings associated with chronic sorrow were primarily management crises and comparisons with norms. For those with cancer, for example, management crises such as recurrence of the disease, routine tests and appointments, chemotherapy, and the presence of physical discomfort were the most common triggers. Milestones that brought comparisons with norms and triggered recurrent sorrow were classified as developmental, social, or personal. Chronic sorrow was most frequently triggered in infertile couples by events associated with normal family development. The birth of children to relatives or peers was especially painful for these subjects. Individuals with Parkinson's disease recognized a difference between themselves and social norms, and felt an element of stigma. Comparisons with personal norms were those in which subjects compared their present selves to their pre-illness states. These were most prevalent in subjects with multiple sclerosis, and the losses experienced included loss of career and inability to participate in previously enjoyed activities.

The intensity of feelings varied from individual to individual; in some subjects the sorrow tended to be progressive. This progressivity of feelings was particularly noted in the infertile couples.

Subjects identified a variety of nursing activities as being helpful to persons like themselves. The most frequently cited activities were categorized in the following nursing roles: empathetic presence (mentioned by 57.5% of subjects), caring professional (45%), competent professional (42.5%), and teacher/expert (32%). Nursing behaviors associated with the role of empathetic presence included listening, taking time, reassuring, making allowances for other problems, and recognizing the other's feelings. Evidence of the importance of this role is reflected in the following quote from a man with cancer:

> You have to be a pretty smart nurse to tell how much a person can handle. You need to find out what they already think and feel. Nobody's got time to do that, but it would be helpful if the nurse would sit down with you and let you talk about what you're feeling and help you get through it.

The role of caring professional was exemplified by nurses who were sensitive, respectful, nonjudgmental, accepting, tactful, patient, and compassionate. An eloquent description of these behaviors was provided by a woman with multiple sclerosis (MS). When asked what would be helpful to others like herself, she said:

> I would say not to lose patience with people and to remember that you're dealing with them [MS patients] as human beings who are not different from you other than, at the moment, they're different with whatever symptom happens to be going on at that time. So, I guess that's the most, the deepest level of caregiving that there is, that a nurse can do for an MS patient.

Nurses who were knowledgeable and proficient in providing care, who were responsible and accountable, and who provided continuity of care exhibited behaviors classified in the role of competent professional. The significance of this role is reflected in the comments made by the spouse caregiver of an individual with Parkinson's disease:

> Some of the nurses in the hospital or working in the nursing homes, when they get around to passing out medicine, that's when they do it. Parkinson's patients are supposed to get their medicines every 4 hours. If they don't get it in 4 hours, they're gone. Then it takes a while to bring them back.

Behaviors associated with the role of teacher/expert included provision of situation-specific information, practical tips for care, and teaching technical skills in a manner that was current, honest, and understandable. The following comment by the husband in one of the infertile couples illustrates the importance of these nursing behaviors:

> I think that in any major hospital, a large hospital that specializes in maternity, the Emergency Department should have a well informed nurse circulating to explain things and answer questions. A lack of information can cause stress. It even heightens your anxiety not knowing what is going on.

DISCUSSION

The presence of chronic or life-threatening situations causes a disruption of the anticipated life-style of affected individuals and their families. These four pilot studies suggest that this, in turn, may lead to the occurrence of chronic sorrow, that is, periodic recurrence of the intense feelings associated with loss and grief. The potential for progressivity of these feelings was also noted in these studies. Given the fact that 82.5% of the subjects interviewed evidenced chronic sorrow, we can conclude that such emotional responses are normal reactions to what may be termed abnormal situations. It is therefore important that nurses recognize chronic sorrow as an integral part of the experience of chronic conditions, both by affected individuals and family caregivers, and intervene in ways deemed helpful.

It is interesting to note that, for the diverse populations sampled in these studies, behaviors associated with the nursing roles of empathetic presence and caring professional were most frequently described as helpful. Both of these roles encompass actions that focus on meeting emotional needs through active listening, sensitivity, patience, and acceptance of feelings. The other nursing behaviors described as helpful by most of the subjects centered on demonstration of professional expertise. Provision of situation-specific information, proficiency in the provision of care, and skill in teaching were especially helpful. The fact that not all of these roles were cited by all of the subjects is indicative of the varying needs of those experiencing chronic sorrow and emphasizes the importance of individual needs assessment.

Nurses in all settings need to recognize that individuals dealing with chronic or life-threatening situations may experience chronic sorrow. Further, for some, these grief-related feelings may intensify over time. These studies indicate that nurses can assist those experiencing chronic sorrow by listening, allowing time for expression of feelings, and providing accurate information in a manner that can be understood. It is worthy of mention that the authors were able to identify specific strategies that were helpful simply by asking the study participants.

Of paramount importance in providing effective nursing interventions for those experiencing chronic sorrow is recognition of milestones and crises when these feelings are apt to recur. For the populations sampled in these studies, the most common precipitating factors were management crises and comparisons with norms. Nurses can use awareness of these vulnerable times to provide anticipatory guidance for those involved in chronic and/or life-threatening situations.

If chronic sorrow goes unrecognized or is viewed as pathological, this is likely to contribute to the pain of the chronic experience. The depth of this pain is reflected in a comment made by an infertile husband whose artificially inseminated wife was 6 months pregnant at the time he was interviewed: "*Nothing* will ever really erase the pain, the anguish we've endured these last 10 years." Conversely, when chronic sorrow is recognized as a normal phenomenon associated with chronicity, and when support is provided through appropriate nursing interventions, the outcome is likely to be increased comfort for both the individual and the family.

ACKNOWLEDGMENT

Partial funding for this study was received from the Rhode Island College Faculty Research Grants.

REFERENCES

Burke, M. L. (1989). *Chronic sorrow in mothers of school-age children with myelomeningocele disability.* Unpublished doctoral dissertation, Boston University.

Damrosch, S. P., & Perry, L. A. (1989). Self-reported adjustment, chronic sorrow, and coping of parents of children with Down's syndrome. *Nursing Research, 38,* 25–30.

Fraley, A. M. (1986). Chronic sorrow in parents of premature children. *Children's Health Care, 15,* 114–118.

Kratochvil, M. S., & Devereux, S. A. (1988). Counseling needs of parents of handicapped children. *Social Casework, 69,* 420–426.

Olshansky, S. (1962). Chronic sorrow: A response to having a mentally defective child. *Social Casework,* 43, 191–193.

Wikler, L. M., Wasow, M., & Hatfield, E. (1981). Chronic sorrow revisited: Parents vs. professional depiction of the adjustment of parents of mentally retarded children. *American Journal of Orthopsychiatry, 51,* 63–70.

Part III

CARING FOR CHRONICALLY ILL CHILDREN

[22]

Nurses' and Parents' Negotiation of Caregiving Roles for Medically Fragile Infants: Barriers and Bridges

Margaret Shandor Miles and Annette C. Frauman

Parents of medically fragile infants—infants with serious, long-term conditions—face a major challenge in coping with the child's illness and taking on the parental role (Goldberg, Morris, Simmons, Fowler, & Levison, 1990; Holaday, 1987; Office of Technology Assessment, 1987; Schraeder, 1980). These infants are critically ill and technologically dependent for many months during the first year of life. They experience long or repeated hospitalizations, often remaining for lengthy periods in intensive care units. The severity of the infants' health status reduces their ability to respond to parental attempts to develop a relationship; the equipment on or around the child and the child's treatments are additional barriers to parenting. In addition, parents often must take on the parental role in an environment—the intensive care unit (ICU)—which is highly stressful. In the ICU parents face an array of complicated health care equipment, large numbers of critically ill infants, other distressed parents, and a large number of staff with whom they must interact as they try to understand and cope with their child's illness.

Little is known about the experience of parenting the medically fragile infant. However, research with parents of preterm infants hospitalized in a neonatal ICU (NICU) suggests that the experience is highly stressful, especially for mothers (Able-Boone, Dokecki, & Smith, 1989; Affleck & Tennen,

1991; Brooten et al., 1988; Jones, 1982; Miles, 1989; Miles, Funk, & Kasper, 1991; Pederson, Bento, Chance, Evans, & Fox, 1987). Research on preterm infants further suggests that preterm birth and hospitalization of the infant may adversely affect the development of the parent–infant relationship, both while the infant is in the hospital (Beckwith & Cohen, 1978; Jeffcoate, Humphrey, & Lloyd, 1979; Minde, Whitelaw, Brown, & Fitzhardinge, 1983; Trause & Kramer, 1983), and over the longer term (Brown & Bakeman, 1978; Davis & Thoman, 1988; Easterbrooks, 1988; Goldberg, 1978; Goldberg, Brachfeld, & DiVitto, 1980).

From these studies of preterm infants it is clear that parents of medically fragile infants need individualized, extensive, ongoing support and guidance, both in coping with their child's illness and in taking on the parental role during their infant's extended stay in the hospital. Nurses, who are continually at the bedside, are an extremely important resource to these parents. A number of studies have found that parents viewed nurses as one of their most important sources of information about their child's illness and related care, and a major source of support in assuming their parental role (Able-Boone et al., 1989; Jones, 1982; Miles & Funk, 1987). Thus, the development of an effective nurse–parent relationship is essential. However, the development of this relationship can be complicated by a variety of factors (Able-Boone et al., 1989; Brown & Ritchie, 1990; Hayes & Knox, 1984; Marino, 1980; Stainton, 1992). Numerous opportunities exist for both barriers and bridges to develop.

Unfortunately, despite the importance of the nurse–parent relationship for parents of critically ill infants, almost no research has examined this relationship. Such research is particularly important with parents of infants who remain hospitalized and dependent on intensive nursing care for many months during the first year of life. Using data from a larger field research project focusing on parenting the medically fragile infant, this chapter examines the nurse–parent relationship from the perspective of both nurse and parent.

METHOD

The setting for the study comprised all the units providing care to infants and very young children in a tertiary care university hospital in the Southeast. The setting thus included the neonatal and pediatric ICUs, the intermediate care nursery, and two units caring for infants and toddlers.

Mothers of 15 medically fragile infants and toddlers constituted the parent sample. The children were considered "medically fragile" in that they all had a serious health problem that had left them medically unstable and necessitated technological support for long periods of time during infancy. In addition, the children had been hospitalized initially for at least 2 months and either remained in the hospital for many more months or were readmitted one or more times for an additional extended stay during the first year of life. Eleven of the children were prematures with serious sequelae such as bronchopulmonary dysplasia or short bowel syndrome. Four were full-term infants with serious congenital anomalies such as congenital heart disease or renal disease.

All the children were first admitted to the hospital at birth or within a few weeks of birth. However, because of the exploratory nature of the study, interviews were conducted with mothers who had had a wide range of experiences with their child's illness (i.e., differing age at onset, diagnosis, length of stay, primary unit on which hospitalized, and prognosis). Mothers also were at varying points in the child's illness trajectory when interviews were done (the time since first admission ranged from 6 months to 2 years; one child had died, and two children had been discharged). The age of the mothers ranged from 19 to 40. Mothers came from a wide range of socioeconomic, cultural, and ethnic backgrounds; six were African-American, one was Asian, and the remainder were Caucasian.

Subjects also included 15 nurses who worked on the units caring for these children; the sample included nurses working every shift and functioning in a variety of roles. They ranged in age from 24 to 56, their experience ranged from 9 months to 21 years, and they had been employed in the setting from 9 months to 16 years.

Parents were contacted on the units to tell them about the study's purpose; if they agreed to participate, they signed a consent form. Interviews were semi-structured and most were conducted on the hospital unit. Mothers were asked what it was like to be the mother of a very sick infant who had been hospitalized for many months. They also were asked about how and when they had assumed various aspects of their mothering role with their child. Probes focused on the factors that facilitated or hindered the development of their mothering role and on their perceptions of the nursing staff.

A semi-structured interview was also used with nursing staff. They were asked about their views of working with parents of medically fragile infants and about their experiences and perceptions of specific parents.

All interviews with mothers and nurses were tape-recorded. Both field notes and memos were also recorded to help establish a relationship between the data and evolving findings. Data were analyzed using the constant comparative method (Strauss & Corbin, 1990). Analysis was ongoing with data collection, and interviews were altered as themes were identified. The two investigators evaluated the transcribed interviews from nurses and mothers independently, using a process of open coding to identify themes related to the nurse-parent relationship from both perspectives. In further analyses, the investigators worked collaboratively to refine the themes and examine the interplay between the two perspectives.

RESULTS

Role Negotiation: A Key Element in the Nurse-Mother Relationship

Mothers and nurses both reported deep concern for the survival and well-being of the infant. They also shared a sense of responsibility toward the infant. One nurse noted, "I think she [the mother] knew that I wasn't trying to be his mother but that I would have a sense of concern for him that a mother would."

This shared concern and sense of responsibility led to an overlap in the roles of nurse and mother and to a need for negotiating their shared roles. One nurse noted that, "Parents are upset because nurses may be taking roles that they think are their roles." Another nurse noted friction "between whose role, who belongs to what role, . . . who [the nurse or the parent] knows what's best for that child." These role negotiations focused on care of the infant, including the usual infant care tasks and nurturing, as well as illness-related technological care.

Although nurses and mothers shared many responsibilities for the infant, the official roles were clearer for nurses than for mothers. This made the mothers unequal partners in role negotiations. Nurses had ongoing and total responsibility for the care and well-being of the infant. They were responsible for treatments, medications, and ongoing monitoring of symptoms. They also were responsible for seeing that normal infant care such as bathing, diapering, and feeding was done. In addition, nurses were concerned that the developmental and emotional needs of the infant were met. Most of these caregiving responsibilities would have belonged to the mother if the child had not been ill, but in the ICU the role of the mother was minimized: "We [the nurses] are making the decisions about when they eat, when they have this treatment. . . . This takes away the control parents usually have over their kids' lives."

Thus, in many ways the infant was in the "custody" of the nurse during the months he or she remained critically ill. As one mother noted, "Who is the surrogate mother, me or you, who is the real mother, me or you, because they [the nurses] did so many things for her when she was little that I didn't know how to do or was afraid to do because she was so tiny."

Mothers were assumed to have an important role with their infants, but their ability to implement that role was complicated by a number of barriers. Many barriers had to do with the fragile health status of the infant and the mothers' anxiety: "I touched her toes, that's all I could get hold of." In addition, the mothers had limited knowledge of the infant's health problems and related treatments, especially in the first weeks and months of their child's hospitalization. As one mother noted, "You want to do something for him and you want to figure out all the stuff he's hooked up to and how to work it." However, assuming most caregiving tasks required the permission and even the encouragement of the nurses: "You couldn't just go in there and pick her up and do what you wanted. You just came in and looked and that was it."

Because of the length of stay of these medically fragile infants, roles had to be constantly re-evaluated and altered. Over time, the infants were transferred from one unit to another, and each unit had a somewhat different philosophy of patient care and attitudes toward parents. Thus, parents had to negotiate their roles with numerous nurses on any particular unit and in different units.

Context of the Negotiations

The mother and nurse(s) had to negotiate and re-negotiate their roles in the context of their relationship with each other and their concern for the infant. These negotiations, however, were done in a situation that was both ambiguous and fluid, with lack of guidelines and direction in the formation of the relationship, ongoing negotiation, and evaluation of the relationship. As one nurse noted: "I wonder whether they want you to treat the child like it's yours or whether they don't want you to. . . and it's hard to say. . . . You don't want them to feel like you are going to take their place or anything." The mother of a toddler who had been hospitalized since birth noted the ambivalence she felt about the nurses' relationship with her child. She was pleased that her son had close ties with the staff because she could not visit often; yet at the same time, she felt replaced by the nurses when she did visit.

Negotiations made between one nurse and parent often were not recorded, with the result that a decision to provide care one way often was changed within the day by another provider who viewed the situation differently. One mother noted bitterly that the worst experience of her son's hospitalization occurred when an "older nurse, set in her ways," did not allow the mother to carry out her usual bedtime routine of holding her son during his tube feeding and placing him in his bed before leaving.

Fluidity, or rapid fluctuations, often occurred in a situation, with abrupt changes in an infant's health status and health care. Thus, sometimes parents were encouraged to participate in care one day, but this was impossible to do on the next visit because of the infant's altered condition. One mother described losing her ability to hold and give care to her son after he had emergency surgery: "It's just up and down the roller coaster because you can't always expect [things to be the same]. . . . There can always be something else."

Process Issues

For both mothers and nurses, a critical element in role negotiation was the development of trust in each other's competence. Sometimes there were tensions about a particular family: "There comes a cross purpose between the parents and nurses; each is evaluating the other's competence with the child." Nurses had to develop trust in the mothers' competence before they could feel secure in allowing them to give care and particularly to take actions that might directly affect the infant's well-being. One nurse said about a particular family: "I don't know how mentally competent they are. I just do not feel safe with them taking her home." As the nurses saw mothers' competence increase, they turned over ever more intensive caregiving opportunities—including illness-related caregiving—to parents, acting under the nurses' supervision. Parents who were not viewed as competent were not offered as many opportunities to give care.

The mothers also worked to establish trust in the caregiving provided by the nurses. They evaluated the competence of the nurses both individually and as a group. As one mother noted, "I'm watching them." Their need to evaluate the nurses' competence impelled the mothers to learn as much as they could so that they could check on staff more thoroughly; their recognition of the nurses' competence increased as the mothers' knowledge and sense of confidence and their own competence increased. Several mothers discussed watching how care was given, comparing care provided by different nurses, and questioning staff about their care. Essentially, they asked, "Are you doing things the way I want?" This questioning was perceived as particularly difficult by young staff nurses.

When an individual nurse was viewed as not competent enough, mothers stayed closer to the bedside, sending in others to watch and monitor care, and even requesting that a particular nurse not be assigned to their child. One nurse noted, "What I hear is [parents] requesting that somebody not take care of that child and maybe it's because they [the parents] aren't getting the support they need or somebody has been too rough with their child."

Individual Patterns in Maternal Role Negotiations

Despite the complications of role negotiation and related barriers, as these mothers became comfortable in the environment, learned more about their infant's responses and needs, and increased their confidence in caregiving, most of them took on some level of normal infant caregiving and gave attention to the infant's developmental and emotional needs. One summed it up thus: "Mainly I just wanted to be her mother so bad. I wanted to change her diaper and bathe her. I just wanted to be a mother."

The nurses facilitated parental involvement in normal caregiving. Most mothers reported that nurses helped them hold and care for their infant, despite the infant's fragile health status, and taught them about routine caregiving such as how to change a diaper on a sick infant, stimulate the infant's development, and communicate with the baby.

Eventually most mothers also assumed some involvement in illness-related caregiving. This required that mothers learn the specifics about the child's illness and treatments. One said, "This stuff is running into my son, I want to know what's going on and how to operate it." Eventually, one mother noted that she "took care of her daughter's tracheotomy as comfortably as changing her diaper."

Becoming involved in illness-related caregiving, however, involved more negotiation with the nursing staff. Although helping with the child's treatments and medical procedures often was encouraged and supported by the nurses, many mothers reported having to struggle to learn about illness-related care and to achieve involvement in this caregiving. A nurse noted that "the major weakness [of the situation] is their [parents'] lack of power. I think it's quite frequently our fault because we take the power away from them and we don't acknowledge their role as parents and their importance as parents. When we do that, we don't really give them any opportunity to do the things we really want them to do."

The patterns of maternal role negotiation differed among individual mothers. A few mothers described themselves as starting out with a strong sense of responsibility and concern about their infant. These mothers assumed that they had a role in the caregiving of their infant and immediately began to take on responsibility for the infant's care, with or without the permission of the nurses. One of these mothers noted that she established her presence at the infant's bedside so the staff would know she was the mother, and she let it be known what she would do for her son.

Most mothers in our study, however, initially assumed a more passive caregiving role. This was partly a result of their own need to recover in the early postpartum period and their stress related to the infant's health crisis; unfamiliarity with the intensive care environment; lack of knowledge about their infant's problems and needs; and the acuity of the infant's status. These mothers assumed whatever caregiving roles the nurses deemed appropriate. Some mothers were reluctant to assume even minor caregiving roles when offered the opportunity, out of fear of hurting the infant. One mother noted that when she was offered the opportunity to hold her child, she turned it down, saying, "I'm not going to hold her with all those tubes." For such mothers, loss of the maternal role with the infant was considered necessary to the survival and well-being of the infant, and their trust in the competence of the nurses was relatively high.

A few mothers never got beyond this passivity. They trusted the health care professionals and viewed them as the experts. These mothers wanted to take on the parenting role only when the infant came home. Several nurses noted this phenomenon in parents: "Parenting comes from the home . . . when they get the child home." Or: "The most commonly asked question is, when can I take him home?" A mother who was an infrequent visitor said, "Every time I would go up there, as soon as I got there, I would ask the nurse to let me take him home." This mother described the nurses as "letting her" do things for her son.

Control Issues

As the mothers' competence in caregiving increased, some gained more control over the care provided for their infants by nursing staff. One mother described her control over her daughter's care. She liked things done "her way"; if they were not done that way, she would not say anything at first but would "redo it [the care] my way" when the nurses left. Other mothers began to tell the nurses what they expected them to do and how they expected the care to be provided. One mother noted that she did this because she "wanted to be her mother so bad." A mother who was intent on seeing that her son got the kind of care she thought he needed placed lists by the bedside for new nurses caring for her son. This mother described her role with student nurses as a "trainer."

Struggles over control of parenting the infant sometimes ensued. One mother described her "struggle" to be an equal part of the team, and to provide normal infant care and illness-related care on her own as well as making decisions about the care nurses provided: "Everything was a struggle. . . . They sure are not going to take orders from a mother and I think there's a big control problem." A nurse described such mothers as "far more watchful. . . . They will pick up on everything. If. . . . they know a medication is due at 3:00 and it's 3:15, you'll be called on the carpet for that."

DISCUSSION

This study suggests that for parents of critically ill infants, establishment of the nurse–parent relationship is a dynamic process that unfolds over time; nurses and mothers often experience overlapping roles, and nurses can act as both facilitators and barriers to the assumption of the maternal caregiving role. Our findings are similar to those of Able-Boone, Dokecki, and Smith (1989), who found the ICU an intense environment in which parents felt burdened because of the limited roles allowed them in their child's care and caregivers acknowledged their control over parents.

The findings also are similar to those of Stainton (1992), who studied health care providers' and mothers' experiences in high-risk perinatal situations. She identified a phenomenon she termed "mismatched perceptions" between caregivers and mothers of high-risk newborns. In particular there was dissonance between the caregivers' continuous unrelenting focus on possible problems with the infant and the mothers' experience of intense concern about becoming parents. As in our study, Stainton found that both the nurse and the parent were protective of the high-risk infant, and nurses influenced mothers' accessibility to the infant. In addition, mothers perceived the nurses as "watching them" to evaluate their competence, causing the mothers to feel the nurses distrusted them.

Our study also found that the assumption of the maternal caregiving role with an infant differed depending on the mother. Many mothers started out passively. They may have been experiencing what Thorne and Robinson (1989) identified as "naive trust," waiting for health care providers to care for their child. It is important for nurses to understand this early parental response to a child's critical illness so that parents are not perceived as uninvolved or uncaring.

Our study suggests that difficulties in the nurse-parent relationship can lead to competition and a struggle for control of the child's care, or to erroneous assessments of parents. However, the findings also suggest that nurses are crucial in helping mothers share the parenting of their sick infant and, ultimately, take on the full parental role as the infant's condition stabilizes and improves. Parents in this study indicated that the nurses helped them overcome their fears and learn about their infant and his needs, and encouraged them to become more involved in care.

Thus, the trust established between nurse and parent is a keystone in the construction of parental role attainment with sick infants. Negotiating and renegotiating the relationship creates a bridge of communication between the nurse and parent, giving both parties opportunities to share feelings, needs, and desires.

In our study, ambiguity was a salient aspect of the context in which roles were negotiated between nurses and parents. Ambiguity in the development of the nurse–parent relationship is inherent in the system in which care is provided. Nurses often are hired as staff nurses in an ICU when they are very young and have little experience as pediatric nurses. Although training is provided for the technological care of the infant, little attention is given to preparing nurses to play a major role in working with distressed parents in the highly stressful ICU. At the same time, parents are suddenly thrust into the ICU environment with little or no experience in how to be the parent of a critically ill infant. Many of them are first time parents or young parents with few resources to help them in this highly complicated environment. Thus, both mothers and nurses are learning as they negotiate complex relationships.

The role negotiations between nurses and parents are a challenge for parents because of the large number of nurses with whom they must negotiate. This number includes, at the minimum, the primary nurse, nurses on various shifts who care for the infant, and the charge nurses. The behavior and expectations of this large group of nurses often vary greatly, creating confusion and mismatched expectations on both sides. Thus it is important to establish continuity of care through a primary nursing system or other method of staff assignment. Consistency in approaching parents can also be accomplished by clear nursing care plans focused on parents' needs, by ongoing assessment of parents, and by frequent nursing rounds, team meetings, or conferences focused on parents of long-term-stay infants.

Nurses in ICUs also have to establish relationships with a large number of highly stressed parents at any given time. Nurses are challenged to cope with a wide variety of parental values, beliefs, and behaviors. These nurses need ongoing consultation, counseling, and support to carry out their roles.

Our findings suggest that nurses need extensive inservice programs to prepare them for their important role in helping parents. They must have an understanding of parenting that includes the process of parental role attainment when an infant is critically ill, the meaning of infants to parents, the scope of the parental role with children, the needs of parents when a child is critically ill, and ways to work with highly stressed parents. As part of such inservice programs, nurses need assistance in becoming aware of their own values and beliefs about parenting, which may influence their assessments and approaches to parents.

Nurses and mothers are both concerned about the well-being of the critically ill infant, and they have important and complementary roles in caring for a critically ill infant. Role negotiation is essential for both nurses and parents in assuming their important roles with the infant. Nurses must become aware of the salience of this role-negotiation process with mothers and identify approaches that facilitate the development of the parental role with critically ill infants. Medically fragile infants belong to their parents, and a primary goal of nurses must be the parents' assumption of the nurturing role in preparation for the infant's discharge home.

REFERENCES

Able-Boone, H., Dokecki, P. R., & Smith, M. S. (1989). Parent and health care provider communication and decision making in the intensive care nursery. *Children's Health Care, 18*, 133–141.

Affleck, G., & Tennen, H. (1991). The effect of newborn intensive care on parents' psychological well-being. *Children's Health Care, 20*, 6–14.

Beckwith, L., & Cohen, S. E. (1978). Preterm birth: Hazardous obstetrical and postnatal events as related to caregiver-infant behavior. *Infant Behavior and Development, 1*, 403–411.

Brooten, D., Gennaro, S., Brown, L. P., Butts, P., Givons, A. L., Bakewell-Sachs, S., & Kumar, S. P. (1988). Anxiety, depression, and hostility in mothers of preterm infants. *Nursing Research, 37*, 213–216.

Brown, J. V., & Bakeman, R. (1978). Relationships of human mothers with their infants during the first year of life: Effect of prematurity. In R. W. Bell & W. P. Smotherman (Eds.), *Maternal influences and early behavior* (pp. 353–373). New York: Spectrum.

Brown, J., & Ritchie, J. A. (1990). Nurses' perceptions of parent and nurse roles in caring for hospitalized children. *Children's Health Care, 19*, 28–36.

Davis, D. H., & Thoman, E. B. (1988). The early social environment of premature and full term infants. *Early Human Development, 17*, 221–232.

Easterbrooks, M. A. (1988). Effects of infant risk status on the transition to parenthood. In G. Y. Michaels & W. A. Goldberg (Eds.), *The transition to parenthood: Current theory and research* (pp. 176–208). New York: Cambridge University Press.

Goldberg, S. (1978). Prematurity: Effects on parent-infant interaction. *Journal of Pediatric Psychology, 3*, 137–144.

Goldberg, S., Brachfeld, S., & DiVitto, B. (1980). Feeding, fussing, and play: Parent-infant interaction in the first year as a function of prematurity and perinatal medical problems. In T. M. Field, S. Goldberg, D. Stern, & A. M. Sostek (Eds.), *High-risk infants and children: Adult and peer interactions* (pp. 133–153). New York: Academic Press.

Goldberg, S., Morris, P., Simmons, R. J., Fowler, R. S., & Levison, H. (1990). Chronic illness in infancy and parenting stress: A comparison of three groups of parents. *Journal of Pediatric Psychology, 15*, 347–358.

Hayes, V. E., & Knox, J. E. (1984). The experience of stress in parents of children hospitalized with long-term disabilities. *Journal of Advanced Nursing, 9*, 333–341.

Holaday, B. (1987). Patterns of interaction between mothers and their chronically ill infants. *Maternal Child Nursing Journal, 16*, 29–45.

Jeffcoate, J. A., Humphrey, M. E., & Lloyd, J. K. (1979). Disturbance in parent-child relationships following preterm delivery. *Developmental Medicine and Child Neurology, 21*, 344–352.

Jones, C. L. (1982). Environmental analysis of neonatal intensive care. *The Journal of Nervous and Mental Disease, 170*, 130–142.

Marino, B. L. (1980). When nurses compete with parents. *Journal of the Association for Care of Children in Hospitals, 8*, 94–98.

Miles, M. S. (1989). Parents of critically ill premature infants: Sources of stress. *Critical Care Quarterly, 12*, 69–74.

Miles, M. S., & Funk, S. G. (1987). *Parental stressors in neonatal intensive care units.* Final grant report submitted to the Division of Nursing, DHHS, Grant Number NU01284.

Miles, M. S., Funk, S. G., & Kasper, M. A. (1991). The neonatal intensive care unit environment: Sources of stress for parents. *AACN Clinical Issues in Critical Care Nursing, 2*, 346–354.

Minde, K., Whitelaw, A., Brown, J., & Fitzhardinge, P. (1983). Effect of neonatal

complications in premature infants on early parent-infant interactions. *Developmental Medicine and Child Neurology, 25*, 763–777.
Office of Technology Assessment. (1987). *Technology-dependent children: Hospital vs. home care* (OTA-TM-H-38). Washington, DC: U.S. Government Printing Office.
Pederson, D. R., Bento, S., Chance, G. W., Evans, B., & Fox, A. M. (1987). Maternal emotional responses to preterm birth. *American Journal of Orthopsychiatry, 57*, 15–21.
Schraeder, B. S. (1980). Attachment and parenting despite lengthy intensive care. *American Journal of Maternal Child Nursing, 5*, 37–43.
Stainton, M. C. (1992). Mismatched caring in high-risk perinatal situations. *Clinical Nursing Research, 1*, 35–49.
Strauss, A., & Corbin, J. (1990). *Basics of qualitative research: Grounded theory procedures and techniques.* Newbury Park, CA: Sage.
Thorne, S. E., & Robinson, C. A. (1989). Guarded alliance: Health care relationships in chronic illness. *Image: Journal of Nursing Scholarship, 21*, 153–157.
Trause, M. A., & Kramer, L. I. (1983). The effects of premature birth on parents and their relationships. *Developmental Medicine and Child Neurology, 25*, 459–465.

[23]

The Behaviors and Nursing Care of Preterm Infants with Chronic Lung Disease

Diane Holditch-Davis and Deborah Assad Lee

Recent advances in the medical and nursing care of critically ill preterm infants have significantly reduced their mortality (Grogaard, Lindstrom, Parker, Culley, & Stahlman, 1990; Hoffman & Bennett, 1990). Survival of infants weighing less than 1500 grams and requiring intensive care now exceeds 80% (Horbar et al., 1988; Kraybill, Bose, & D'Ercole, 1987). However, morbidity remains a significant problem. Approximately 35%–50% of these infants develop chronic lung disease, and the risk of this complication increases as birthweight decreases (Horbar et al., 1988; Kraybill et al., 1987). Although these infants generally show improvement in respiratory status as they grow older (Bozynski et al., 1987), they present major management problems for nurses because of their need for long-term hospital care and their risk for other health and developmental problems.

Even after the initial hospitalization, chronic lung disease is associated with increased morbidity and mortality. Sauve and Singhal (1985), for example, found that lower respiratory tract infections and rehospitalizations were more common in the first year among infants with chronic lung disease than other premature infants (Sauve & Singhal, 1985), and some studies indicate that pulmonary function abnormalities may be still present in these children at 10 years of age (Andreasson, Lindroth, Mortensson, Svenningsen, & Jonson, 1989; Bader et al., 1987, Vohr et al., 1991). Several studies have concluded that infants with chronic lung disease are at risk for growth failure because of their high metabolic demands (Bozynski et al., 1990; Kurzner et al., 1988; Markestad & Fitzhardinge, 1981; Meisels, Plunkett, Roloff, Pasick, & Stiefel, 1986; Sauve & Singhal, 1985; Vohr, Bell, & Oh, 1982). In addition, infants with chronic lung disease have more hearing and visual problems than other premature infants (Sauve & Singhal, 1985).

Infants with chronic lung disease have also been found to have lower cognitive abilities, poorer sensory-motor and language development, and more neurologic abnormalities than other prematurely born children (Bozynski et al., 1987; Goldson, 1984; Meisels, Plunkett, Pasick, Stiefel, & Roloff, 1987; Meisels et al., 1986; Sauve & Singhal, 1985; Skidmore, Rivers, & Hack, 1990; Vohr, Bell, et al., 1982, Vohr, Garcia, et al., 1991). In fact, Landry and others (Landry, Chapieski, Fletcher, & Denson, 1988) found that the development of 3-year-old children who had experienced chronic lung disease in infancy was significantly behind that of normal premature infants and comparable to that of children with Grade III and IV intraventricular hemorrhage. Yet it is not clear that these developmental problems are directly attributable to chronic lung disease. Several investigators have suggested that the problems are more directly related to the growth failure resulting from chronic lung disease and to the neurologic complications, especially intraventricular hemorrhage and periventricular leukomalacia, associated with the low birthweights of these infants (Davidson et al., 1990; Luchi, Bennett, & Jackson, 1991; Markestad & Fitzhardinge, 1981).

Clinically, infants with chronic lung disease have been described as having more difficult temperaments and being more vulnerable to stress during handling for routine nursing and medical procedures. However, there is little empirical data to support these clinical impressions. Only three studies have been conducted on the behaviors of infants with chronic lung disease during their initial hospitalization. Als and others (1986) found that individualized nursing care that minimized infant stress reduced the number of days on the ventilator and the number of days of supplemental oxygen. However, the behaviors of infants who did and did not develop chronic lung disease were not compared in this study. Myers and colleagues (1992) found that at term, infants with chronic lung disease performed more poorly on the interactive and motor clusters of the Neonatal Behavior Assessment Scale than premature infants without this complication. Medoff-Cooper (1988) examined the responses of infants with chronic lung disease to the stress of a neurobehavioral examination. Although these infants exhibited more negative physiological responses than other preterm infants, only three of five behavioral indicators of stress differed significantly between the groups, and then only at one or two of the eight ages studied. Thus, additional study is needed to determine the extent to which the behaviors of infants with chronic lung disease differ from those of other preterm infants during their initial hospitalization, in order to provide an empirical basis for selection of interventions for these infants.

The study reported here examined the sleeping and waking states and other behaviors displayed by infants with chronic lung disease during hospitalization, and compared these behaviors to those of preterm infants without this complication. The demographic characteristics and health status of the infants were also compared to determine if these affected their behaviors. In addition, to determine whether differences in behaviors could be explained by differences in nursing care, the nursing care received by infants in the two groups was compared.

METHOD

Subjects

The research was part of a larger study of behavioral development during the preterm period. All subjects in the larger study were patients in a neonatal intensive care unit (NICU) of a regional tertiary care center in the Southeast. They had high-risk medical conditions as indicated by either a birthweight less than 1500 grams or a requirement for mechanical ventilation; most had both problems. All infants were well enough to be in intermediate care by 36 weeks gestational age.

Infants were classified as having chronic lung disease on the basis of medical diagnosis (clinical and x-ray findings) and oxygen dependence at 36 weeks conceptional age (CA). The criterion of oxygen dependence at 36 weeks was used instead of 28 days of oxygen dependence (an earlier definition of chronic lung disease) (Northway, 1979), because most of the subjects were born prior to 30 weeks gestational age and, as a result, may have required small amounts of oxygen for longer than 28 days for problems unrelated to chronic lung disease, such as apnea. Further, studies have indicated that at 40 weeks CA, the pulmonary status of chronic lung disease infants who are off oxygen by 36 weeks CA does not differ from that of other very low birthweight infants (Greenspan, Abbasi, & Bhutani, 1988; Shennen, Dunn, Ohlsson, Lennox, & Hoskins, 1988).

Infants in the larger study who did not have a medical diagnosis of chronic lung disease, who required mechanical ventilation for less than 20 days, and who were not oxygen dependent at 36 weeks CA were considered to be non-chronic lung disease infants. A maximum length of mechanical ventilation was set to eliminate non-chronic lung disease infants who had prolonged oxygen dependence.

Infants who did not clearly meet the definition of chronic lung disease or non-chronic lung disease (because they had a diagnosis of chronic lung disease without prolonged oxygen dependence or had prolonged oxygen dependence without a diagnosis of chronic lung disease) were not included in the sample.

Procedures

Infants were enrolled in the study as soon as their medical conditions were no longer critical (not receiving mechanical ventilation or in an immediate life-threatening situation) if an additional hospital stay of at least 1 week was anticipated and consent was obtained from the parents. Infants left the study when they were transferred to a community hospital, discharged home, or reached term age. Because the NICU transferred infants to their community hospitals as soon as possible, and the few local infants were discharged home as soon as they were feeding orally and had a stable temperature outside the incubator (usually by 2000 g), infants in the study typically had ongoing problems, such as oxygen dependence or apnea, at the time of the observations.

Weekly naturalistic observations were conducted on each infant from 7:00 pm to 11:00 pm. During the observations the occurrences of infant and nurse behaviors were recorded every 10 seconds using the behavioral scoring system developed by Thoman (Davis & Thoman, 1987, 1988; Thoman, Acebo, Dreyer, Becker, & Freese, 1979) and modified for use with preterm infants (Holditch-Davis, 1990a, 1990b, 1990c). The end of each 10-second epoch was signaled audibly through an ear phone from a small electronic timer on a Tandy 100 portable computer used as an event recorder. At this signal, the observer recorded the behaviors that occurred during the epoch into the event recorder. Multiple occurrences of the same behavior in the same epoch were not recorded. Each observation was conducted by one of two observers; interrater reliabilities (percentage of exact agreement) for the study variables ranged from 66% to 99%.

In addition, to determine the regularity of respiration, the infant's respiration was recorded on a Gulton chart recorder with a piezoelectric sensor pad whenever the infant was asleep. The sensor was placed under the infant's crib pad. Thus, nothing was attached to the infant, and the infant continued on normal heart and apnea monitors.

Variables and their Measurement

Demographic variables The chronic lung and non-chronic lung groups were compared on ten demographic and medical complication variables. There was a single value for six of these variables—gestational age at birth, birthweight, race, sex, overall illness severity, and number of days on mechanical ventilation. The other four variables—current weight, current illness severity, methylxanthines (theophylline or caffeine), and supplemental oxygen—had a different value at each observation. All of these variables were determined from the medical record.

The gestational age at birth of each infant was calculated from the obstetric estimated date of confinement, determined either by the date of the mother's last menstrual period or by an ultrasound examination, assuming that this gestational age agreed within 2 weeks with the results of a simplified version of the Dubowitz examination (Ballard, Novak, & Driver, 1979; Dubowitz, Dubowitz, & Goldberg, 1970) conducted by a pediatrician on admission to the intensive care unit. If the obstetrical dates were considered unreliable, the gestational age from the Dubowitz was used.

Methylxanthines have a long half life in the preterm period (up to 30 hours) (Aranda & Turmen, 1979). Thus, infants were scored as receiving theophylline or caffeine if they had received a therapeutic dose (more than 2 mg per kg) of the drug in the 24 hours before the observation.

The severity of the infant's illness was determined from the Neonatal Morbidity Scale (Minde, Whitelaw, Brown, & Fitzhardinge, 1983). This scale uses objective criteria to rate the severity of 20 common neonatal conditions, such as asphyxia, bleeding tendency, and apnea, at each day of hospitalization. Scores were summed to obtain a daily score. Interrater reliability, the correlation between two independent raters' daily scores, exceeded .92. Overall severity of illness was determined by adding the daily scores from admission to 40 weeks CA. Since this variable was highly skewed, it was normalized for analysis by using the natural log of each subject's score.

The current illness severity at each observation was determined by adding the daily scores for the 5 days surrounding the observation (2 days before, the day of, and 2 days after). This procedure was used because daily scores were heavily weighted with medical treatments. Since medical treatments occur after an illness has been present for some time, a daily score does not always accurately reflect the severity of illness on a particular day, especially during the intermediate care period when treatments occur less frequently.

Nurse contexts The observation period was divided into six mutually exclusive nursing contexts. The infant was considered to be *alone* if the infant was not being touched, held, fed, changed, bathed, or receiving nursing care. Brief interruptions in caregiving, less than 2 minutes in length, were considered to be *pauses in caregiving* and different from alone time. The time when the baby was with the nurse was divided into four contexts: *contact*—nurse is touching, holding, or carrying the infant, but is not involved in caregiving; *routine care*—nurse is feeding the infant by bottle or gavage, or changing and bathing the infant; *low-level nursing care*—nurse is involved in non–invasive examination of the infant such as taking vital signs; *high-level nursing care*—nurse is providing respiratory care, needle stick, or procedures that involve more manipulation of the infant than a simple examination. Contact was scored only if no routine care, low-level nursing care, or high-level nursing care occurred during the 10-second period. If more than one of the other three nurse contexts occurred in the same 10-second period, the one with the highest level of stimulation was scored. The rare instances when babies were touched by caregivers other than nurses were scored in the relevant nurse context.

Nurse behaviors Four nurse behaviors, each representing a different type of interactive stimulation, were examined: *move*—changing the position of the infant's body in space, including rocking the infant; *hold*—holding the infant; *positive touch*—touching the infant in a manner that is positive or affectionate, such as stroking, kissing, or giving pacifier; and *talk*—talking directly to the infant. These behaviors were not mutually exclusive and more than one could be scored in a single 10-second period.

Infant sleep–wake states Sleep–wake states were selected for examination because they are global behaviors that influence the infant's response to care and are thus important to nurses (Colombo & Horowitz, 1987; Korner, 1972). Sleeping and waking reflect the status and maturation of the nervous system (Holditch-Davis, 1990b; Korner et al., 1988; Roffwarg, Muzio, & Dement, 1966), and deviant sleep–wake patterns are predictive of later developmental problems (Anders, Keener, & Kraemer, 1985; Cohen, Parmelee, Beckwith, & Sigman, 1986; Lombroso & Matsumiya, 1985; Thoman, Denenberg, Sieval, Zeidner, & Becker, 1981; Tynan, 1986). Thus, it is possible that chronic lung disease infants, because they are at high risk for developmental problems, might exhibit alterations in sleeping and waking in the preterm period. Also, chronic lung disease is known to alter sleeping patterns in adults (Johnson & Remmers, 1984) and might be expected to affect sleep–wake states in infants as well.

Sleeping and waking states were judged on the basis of muscle tone, motor activity, respiration, and eye movements (Davis & Thoman, 1987; Holditch-Davis, 1990b; Thoman, 1990). These states are mutually exclusive, and if more than one occurred in a single 10-second period, the one that occupied the greatest proportion of the period was scored.

Alert—the infant's eyes are open and scanning. Motor activity is typically low, but the infant may be active.

Non-alert waking activity—The infant's eyes are usually open, dull, and unfocussed. Motor activity varies but is typically high. During periods of high-level activity, the eyes may close.

Fuss—The infant is fussing and emits at least three brief fuss sounds during a 10–second epoch and is usually active, with the eyes open.

Cry—The infant is crying wholeheartedly and is usually active. The eyes are usually closed but may open.

Drowsiness—the infant's eyes are either open but dazed, or opening and closing slowly. Motor activity is typically low, and respiration even.

Sleep–wake transition—the infant is in transition between waking and sleeping. There is generalized motor activity, and eyes are either closed or opening and closing rapidly.

Active sleep—the infant's eyes are closed, and REMs occur intermittently. Sporadic motor movements occur, but muscle tone is low between these movements. Respiration is uneven and primarily costal in nature.

Quiet sleep—the infant's eyes are closed. A tonic level of motor tone is maintained and activity is limited to occasional startles and brief discharges. Respiration is relatively slow, even, and abdominal.

REM variables The intensity of rapid eye movements was scored every 10 seconds during active sleep using criteria developed by Thoman and shown to be reliable for full term and premature infants (Becker & Thoman, 1981, 1982; Booth, Morin, Waite, & Thoman, 1983; Holditch-Davis, 1990b). Since the presence of REMs is a critical criterion of active sleep, these variables provided a measure of the degree of organization of active sleep.

No REM—No rapid eye movements during an entire 10-second epoch of active sleep.

Light REM—Sporadic rapid eye movements or REM with small excursions lasting less than half an epoch of active sleep.

Moderate REM—Small REMs lasting 5–8 seconds or REMs with large excursions lasting less than half an epoch of active sleep.

REM storm—Continuous small REMs for the entire epoch or large REMs for more than half an epoch of active sleep.

Respiratory regularity The respiration tape was scored visually for respiration regularity during quiet sleep using criteria described by Thoman (1975). Reliability was determined by rescoring five respiration tapes more than 6 months after they were originally scored. The percentage of exact agreements ranged from 80.4% to 93.6% for the four variables listed below and averaged 88.5% overall. Since regular respiration is a critical criterion of quiet sleep, these variables provided a measure of the degree of organization of quiet sleep.

Very regular respiration—The smallest breath during the 10-second epoch is at least 80% of the height of the largest breath, and the narrowest peak-to-peak interval is at least 67% of the widest peak-to-peak interval.

Regular respiration—The respiration does not meet the criteria for very regular respiration, but no more than one breath is between 20–50% of the height of the largest breath, and the narrowest peak-to-peak interval is at least 50% of the widest peak-to-peak interval.

Irregular respiration—The respiration is too irregular to be scored as regular respiration, but the epoch does not include apnea, periodic respiration, or continuous movement.

Very irregular respiration—The 10-second epoch includes apnea, periodic respiration, or continuous movement.

Infant behaviors Nine behaviors—large movement, small movement, jitter, startle, hiccup, spit-up or gag, sigh, yawn, and negative facial expressions—were analyzed because they have been suggested to be signs of infant stress or over-stimulation (Als et al., 1986; Als, Lester, Tronick, & Brazelton, 1982; Gorski, Hole, Leonard, & Martin, 1983). A tenth behavior, mouthing, was analyzed because it is used by some infants for self-comforting. Two other behaviors—infant looks at caregiver, and infant smiles—were analyzed because they are early infant social skills. These behaviors were not mutually exclusive, and more than one could be scored in a single 10-second period.

Measures

The nurse contexts, nurse behaviors, infant sleep–wake states, and infant behaviors were measured as percentages of the total observation. These percentages were calculated by dividing the number of 10-second periods in which each behavior occurred by the number of 10-second periods in the observation. The REM variables were measured as percentages of active sleep, and the respiration regularity variables were measured as percentages of quiet sleep.

RESULTS

There were a total of 71 subjects in the larger study, with 289 observations conducted between 27 and 39 weeks CA. Five of these subjects were eliminated from the current study because their medical conditions did not meet the criteria for either group. Only weeks 32 to 36 had adequate numbers of subjects in both groups for statistical analyses. Prior to 32 weeks, fewer than 5 chronic lung disease infants were available each week, and after 36 weeks fewer than 4 non-chronic lung disease infants were available. The final sample consisted of 20 chronic lung disease (CLD) infants with 67 observations and 31 non-chronic lung disease (nonCLD) infants with 79 observations. Table 23.1 shows the number of subjects studied at each age.

Demographic Characteristics

The chronic lung disease (CLD) group had more male infants than the non-CLD group (60% vs 51.6%) although this difference was not statistically

TABLE 23.1 Number of Subjects and Medical Condition of the Chronic Lung Disease (CLD) and Non-Chronic Lung Disease (NonCLD) Infants at the Time of Each Observation

	Postconceptional Age in Weeks				
	32	33	34	35	36
Number of subjects					
CLD	9	10	12	18	18
NonCLD	19	20	18	15	7
% Oxygen Dependent[a]					
CLD	100%	90%	100%	100%	83%
NonCLD	21%	16%	11%	0%	0%
p Level	< .001	< .001	< .001	< .001	< .001
% with Methlzanthines[a]					
CLD	45%	50%	60%	90%	90%
NonCLD	61%	65%	58%	48%	23%
p Level	NS	NS	NS	NS	NS
Mean weight (*SD*)[b]					
CLD	1232 (197)	1402 (227)	1540 (252)	1695 (280)	1823 (289)
NonCLD	1388 (204)	1544 (255)	1590 (391)	1742 (379)	1733 (456)
p Level	< .10	NS	NS	NS	NS
Mean illness severity (*SD*)[b]					
CLD	11.2 (4.8)	10.9 (3.9)	9.7 (4.1)	9.4 (4.6)	8.9 (4.3)
NonCLD	5.7 (4.6)	4.3 (3.6)	2.3 (2.5)	1.8 (0.6)	0.7 (1.9)
p Level	< .01	< .01	< .001	< .001	< .001

aGroups compared using Fisher's exact test at each week.
[b]Groups compared using a *t*-test at each week.

significant. The CLD group was also significantly more likely to be non-white (65% vs 35.5%). They had significantly more medical complications lower birthweights (887.8 g vs 1246.0 g) and younger gestational ages (26.8 weeks vs 29.5 weeks) at birth. They spent more days on mechanical ventilation (24.6 vs 4.7) and had higher overall illness severity(5.5 vs 3.9 on the natural log of the Neonatal Mortality Scale [Minde et al., 1983]). These differences in the medical conditions of infants with and without chronic lung disease are well-known and widely reported (e.g., Davidson et al., 1990; Kraybill et al., 1987; Medoff-Cooper, 1988).

The medical conditions of the chronic lung disease and non-chronic lung disease infants at the time of each observation are given in Table 23.1. These variables were compared at each postconceptional age using *t*-tests for continuous variables and Fisher's exact tests for categorical variables. The mean weights of the two groups and the percentage of subjects receiving methylxanthines did not differ. However, the chronic lung disease infants were far more likely than the other infants to be receiving supplemental oxygen at each week. The mean illness severity score was also significantly higher for the chronic lung disease infants at each observation.

Nursing Activities

Nursing contexts Table 23.2 presents the percentage of the total observation spent in each nursing context by the chronic lung disease and other pre-

TABLE 23.2 The Mean Percentage (and Range[a]) of the Total Observation that the Chronic Lung Disease (CLD) and Non-chronic Lung Disease (NonCLD) Infants Spent in Each Nursing Context and the Nurse Behaviors Experienced.[b]

	CLD		NonCLD	
	Mean	Range	Mean	Range
Nurse context				
Baby alone	85.1	(83.5–97.1)	83.0	(82.3–85.3)
Pauses in caregiving	1.1	(0.8–1.5)	0.8	(0.7–0.9)
Contact	4.3	(3.6–6.6)	5.3	(3.4–7.3)
Routine care	6.6	(4.9–7.8)	9.0	(7.3–10.9)
Low-level nursing care	1.7	(1.1–2.4)	1.2	(0.7–1.6)
High-level nursing care	1.2	(0.8–1.6)	0.6	(0.3–3.3)
Nurse behaviors				
Move	4.6	(3.4–5.3)	6.3	(4.6–9.1)
Hold	4.2	(3.8–10.5)	7.1	(6.0–10.0)
Positive touch	1.2	(1.6–2.9)	1.1	(1.1–3.6)
Talk	1.8	(1.9–4.9)	2.3	(2.0–4.6)

[a]Range is the range of weekly means.
[b]There were no significant differences at any age.

term infants. The nursing contexts were compared using two-factor (group by pattern) repeated measures analyses of variance at each postconceptional age. The time spent in the nursing contexts did not differ for the chronic lung disease infants and other infants at any age.

Differences in the amounts of nurse behaviors for the two groups were compared using a MANOVA at each postconceptional age. There were no significant differences between the groups in the amounts of any nurse behavior. The similarity in the amounts of nurse contexts and behaviors for the two groups indicates that nurses provided similar care to infants with and without chronic lung disease. This means that any behavioral differences found between the two groups probably were true differences, rather than merely responses to differing nursing care.

Infant Activities

Sleep–wake states Table 23.3 presents the percentage of the observation that the infants from the two groups spent in sleeping and waking states at each age. Active sleep was the most common state for both the chronic lung disease and non-chronic lung disease infants. The next most common states were quiet sleep, drowse, and sleep–wake transition. Waking states occurred infrequently in both groups at all ages.

The state patterns of the two groups were compared using two-factor (group by pattern) repeated measures analysis of variance at each postconceptional age. There were no significant differences between the groups in any of these analyses.

Sleep organization Table 23.4 shows the sleep organization variables for the two groups of infants. The groups were compared using two-factor (group by pattern) repeated measures analyses of variance at each postconceptional age. Active sleep and quiet sleep organization were analyzed separately. There were no significant differences between the groups in active sleep organization. Quiet sleep organization, measured by the respiration regularity variables, differed significantly at 32 and 36 weeks CA ,with chronic lung disease infants exhibiting more irregular respiration. Otherwise, however, the sleep–wake patterns and sleep organization of chronic lung disease infants appeared to be very similar to those of other high risk preterm infants between 32 and 36 weeks CA.

Infant behaviors Differences in the percentages of infant behaviors in the two groups were calculated using a t-test at each postconceptional age. The majority of infant behaviors did not differ significantly between the two groups (see Table 23.5). However, the amount of jitter was greater for chronic lung disease infants at all ages. These infants also exhibited less smiling in all weeks except week 32. For other behaviors, there were iso-

TABLE 23.3 The Mean Percentage (and Standard Deviation) of the Total Observation that the Chronic Lung Disease (CLD) and Non-chronic Lung Disease (NonCLD) Infants Spent in the Sleeping and Waking States at Each Postconceptional Age[a]

	Postconceptional age in weeks				
	32	33	34	35	36
Alert					
CLD	0.8 (1.0)	1.6 (2.6)	1.0 (1.4)	1.3 (1.4)	1.3 (2.0)
NonCLD	0.9 (1.6)	1.3 (1.8)	0.8 (0.9)	2.3 (3.7)	2.0 (1.2)
Non-alert waking activity					
CLD	1.6 (1.9)	1.0 (1.3)	1.3 (2.1)	1.1 (1.8)	1.6 (2.0)
NonCLD	0.7 (1.2)	0.7 (0.8)	0.8 (1.1)	1.6 (2.0)	2.3 (2.2)
Fuss					
CLD	0.5 (1.0)	0.7 (1.6)	0.5 (0.7)	0.6 (1.2)	1.4 (2.0)
NonCLD	0.1 (0.2)	1.2 (3.3)	0.5 (1.0)	0.8 (1.0)	2.0 (1.7)
Cry					
CLD	0.0 (0.0)	0.0 (0.1)	0.2 (0.7)	0.3 (0.8)	1.1 (1.7)
NonCLD	0.0 (0.1)	0.2 (0.6)	0.2 (0.4)	0.4 (1.0)	2.4 (4.5)
Drowse					
CLD	4.0 (4.0)	5.0 (4.4)	4.1 (4.0)	5.6 (4.9)	5.5 (5.7)
NonCLD	4.0 (3.2)	5.4 (4.9)	4.5 (4.3)	6.2 (5.2)	6.8 (4.4)
Sleep–wake transition					
CLD	3.7 (1.3)	3.5 (1.9)	3.8 (2.8)	4.8 (3.0)	4.7 (2.3)
NonCLD	3.3 (2.8)	4.5 (3.7)	3.9 (2.3)	4.9 (2.9)	1.9 (1.5)
Active sleep					
CLD	74.1 (9.7)	70.1 (10.8)	69.6 (9.1)	61.1 (10.8)	64.2 (9.9)
NonCLD	74.2 (10.5)	70.9 (9.1)	69.8 (9.6)	62.4 (11.7)	59.4 (8.0)
Quiet sleep					
CLD	15.3 (6.5)	18.1 (6.7)	19.5 (7.8)	25.1(10.9)	20.2 (6.9)
NonCLD	16.7 (9.6)	15.9 (9.0)	19.5 (6.9)	21.3 (7.0)	23.2 (10.1)

[a]There were no significant differences at any age.

lated significant differences: chronic lung disease infants showed more small moves in week 32, more startles in week 36, more sighing in weeks 33 and 35, more spitting-up in week 36, more yawning in week 33, and more mouthing in week 36. However, only two of these behaviors—small movements and sighing—exhibited consistency in the direction of the group differences over all 5 weeks (see Table 23.5). To summarize, although most behaviors of infants with and without chronic lung disease appear very similar from 32 to 36 weeks CA, there is evidence that infants with chronic lung disease exhibit more jitters and fewer smiles and possibly differ in the amounts of small movements and sighing.

TABLE 23.4 The Mean Percentage (and Standard Deviation) of the Total Observation that the Chronic Lung Disease (CLD) and Non-chronic Lung Disease (NonCLD) Infants Spent in Different Sleep Organization States at Each Postconceptional Age

	Postconceptional age in weeks				
	32	33	34	35	36
Active Sleep Organization					
No REM					
CLD	50.6 (11.1)	48.4 (10.3)	43.2 (9.0)	43.5 (11.6)	41.5 (7.9)
NonCLD	50.9 (7.7)	51.1 (8.8)	46.3 (8.3)	46.8 (7.9)	44.2 (9.9)
Light REM					
CLD	39.2 (9.7)	41.1 (7.0)	44.5 (6.5)	42.5 (7.1)	43.7 (5.5)
NonCLD	37.6 (8.2)	37.2 (8.1)	41.9 (8.7)	40.6 (9.2)	39.8 (8.6)
Moderate REM					
CLD	7.9 (3.8)	8.4 (4.5)	10.5 (5.6)	11.6 (5.1)	11.9 (3.6)
NonCLD	8.4 (2.9)	8.7 (4.8)	9.0 (4.3)	9.3 (4.4)	11.2 (4.0)
REM Storm					
CLD	2.4 (1.4)	2.1 (2.1)	1.7 (0.8)	2.5 (1.6)	2.9 (1.7)
NonCLD	3.1 (2.4)	3.1 (2.9)	2.8 (3.1)	3.3 (2.9)	4.7 (3.5)
p Level	NS	NS	NS	NS	NS
Quiet Sleep Organization					
Very regular respiration					
CLD	14.5 (11.3)	22.6 (17.9)	20.0 (16.6)	27.3 (12.8)	24.4 (13.7)
NonCLD	27.5 (11.3)	23.2 (8.9)	22.3 (9.2)	32.8 (15.2)	42.6 (12.0)
Regular respiration					
CLD	45.0 (11.0)	43.1 (8.7)	51.7 (11.1)	46.3 (11.8)	50.5 (9.9)
NonCLD	41.2 (9.0)	48.1 (6.3)	47.5 (12.2)	44.3 (11.7)	38.8 (6.2)
Irregular respiration					
CLD	34.4 (12.1)	28.9 (13.9)	24.9 (8.6)	21.1 (8.0)	21.4 (11.7)
NonCLD	25.0 (8.0)	22.7 (8.4)	21.7 (10.6)	17.3 (7.3)	11.4 (4.9)
Very irregular respiration					
CLD	6.1 (4.8)	5.3 (3.2)	3.4 (2.7)	5.3 (5.4)	3.7 (3.2)
NonCLD	6.4 (5.2)	6.0 (4.4)	8.5 (15.2)	5.7 (5.3)	7.3 (7.7)
p Level	< .01	NS	NS	NS	< .01

DISCUSSION

It is clear that between 32 and 36 weeks CA, the sleep–wake states and behaviors of infants with chronic lung disease are very similar to those of high-risk preterm infants without this complication. The similarities occur despite dramatic differences in gestational age at birth, birthweight, sever-

TABLE 23.5 The Mean Percentage (and Standard Deviation) of the Total Observation that the Chronic Lung Disease (CLD) and Non-chronic Lung Disease (NonCLD) Infants Exhibited Specific Infant Behaviors at Each Postconceptional Age

	Postconceptional age in weeks				
	32	33	34	35	36
Large movement					
CLD	23.8 (7.1)	24.8 (4.9)	24.7 (4.5)	23.2 (5.3)	25.6 (6.0)
NonCLD	22.4 (6.6)	24.1 (8.9)	22.8 (6.1)	24.6 (5.9)	22.0 (3.4)
Small movement					
CLD	24.6 (6.9)[c]	22.6 (9.2)	19.8 (4.7)	19.6 (7.9)	18.2 (5.6)
NonCLD	17.1 (4.7)	18.9 (6.2)	17.0 (5.9)	17.4 (5.0)	16.3 (7.1)
Jitter					
CLD	15.0 (9.4)[b]	13.3 (5.8)[c]	10.7 (4.8)[c]	9.6 (5.3)[b]	7.8 (3.9)[b]
NonCLD	7.6 (4.3)	7.7 (3.6)	6.0 (2.8)	5.7 (2.8)	3.9 (2.6)
Startle					
CLD	2.1 (0.8)	2.3 (0.9)	2.0 (0.9)	1.5 (0.8)	1.5 (0.6)[b]
NonCLD	2.2 (1.0)	2.3 (1.2)	2.1 (1.0)	1.8 (0.9)	1.1 (0.2)
Hiccup					
CLD	2.6 (2.3)	3.2 (2.3)[a]	1.9 (2.6)	1.5 (2.4)	1.7 (2.7)
NonCLD	2.3 (2.0)	1.5 (2.2)	1.7 (1.8)	2.0 (2.1)	1.3 (1.7)
Sigh					
CLD	4.5 (2.0)	4.7 (1.9)[c]	3.7 (1.9)	4.0 (1.7)[b]	3.0 (1.6)
NonCLD	3.9 (1.9)	3.0 (1.4)	3.6 (1.7)	2.8 (1.4)	2.3 (2.4)
Spit up or gag					
CLD	0.4 (0.5)	0.4 (0.5)	1.2 (2.1)	0.7 (1.4)	0.7 (0.8)[b]
NonCLD	0.3 (0.3)	0.4 (0.4)	0.4 (0.5)	0.5 (0.6)	0.2 (0.2)
Yawn					
CLD	0.6 (0.5)	0.4 (0.4)[b]	0.5 (0.3)[a]	0.5 (0.4)[a]	0.8 (0.6)
NonCLD	0.7 (0.6)	0.9 (0.7)	0.8 (0.6)	0.9 (0.7)	0.7 (0.6)
Negative facial expression					
CLD	5.2 (3.2)	5.2 (3.3)	5.7 (3.6)	6.7 (4.5)	8.7 (5.6)
NonCLD	4.2 (2.6)	6.7 (7.6)	5.2 (2.9)	6.4 (4.1)	9.5 (6.6)
Mouthe					
CLD	22.3(11.6)	21.0 (9.2)	25.3(10.3)	22.5 (8.1)	27.2 (7.4)[b]
NonCLD	22.4 (6.9)	22.5 (8.5)	24.3 (7.1)	23.1 (6.4)	19.4 (7.7)
Look at caregiver					
CLD	0.0 (0.0)	0.0 (0.0)[a]	0.0 (0.1)	0.1 (0.1)	0.0 (0.1)
NonCLD	0.0 (0.0)	0.1 (0.1)	0.0 (0.1)	0.1 (0.1)	0.1 (0.1)
Smile					
CLD	0.6 (0.5)	0.2 (0.2)[d]	0.4 (0.5)[b]	0.3 (0.3)[c]	0.3 (0.2)[a]
NonCLD	0.9 (1.0)	0.9 (0.8)	1.0 (0.7)	0.7 (0.5)	0.5 (0.3)

[a] Groups differ, $p < .10$.
[b] Groups differ, $p < .05$.
[c] Groups differ, $p < .01$.
[d] Groups differ, $p < .001$.

ity of illness, days of mechanical ventilation, and need for supplemental oxygen. Thus, nurses and parents can expect that chronic lung disease infants will behave generally like other intermediate-care preterm infants.

It cannot be known from our data whether these similarities would be seen at other points in the infants' hospitalizations. The behaviors of chronic lung disease infants might differ from those of other high-risk preterm infants during critical illness or after discharge. Myers et al. (1992), for example, found that the interactive and motor behaviors of chronic lung disease infants at term age were poorer than those of other premature infants. Also, Medoff-Cooper (1988), studying preterms over a wider age range than we used in this study, found isolated differences (5 of 24 tests) in the stress behaviors that infants with and without chronic lung disease showed in response to handling. Some of these differences, however, may have come from comparing the infants at different points in their hospitalizations. Infants without chronic lung disease are not a homogeneous group. For example, 14 subjects from our larger study recovered from their illnesses so quickly that they were transferred back to their community hospitals before 32 weeks CA. The behaviors of these healthier non-chronic lung disease infants might differ from those of intermediate care infants both with and without chronic lung disease. Additional research is needed to determine the relative impact of chronic lung disease on preterm infant behaviors at different points in the illness trajectory.

The behavioral differences that we found, though subtle, may have implications for the development of infants with chronic lung disease and for their relationships with nurses and parents. Infants with chronic lung disease exhibited approximately twice as many jitters and half the number of smiles as other infants. They also exhibited slightly more small movements. Thus, they may appear to parents and nurses to be more immature and to react less positively to handling than other preterm infants.

In addition, the chronic lung disease infants had significantly less regular respiration in quiet sleep during 2 of the 5 weeks. At all points, chronic lung disease infants exhibited more irregular respiration and less very regular respiration than other preterm infants. These differences in quiet sleep organization might reflect underlying changes in the central nervous systems of the chronic lung disease infants that may foreshadow later developmental problems. However, the findings may be due to the direct effect of chronic lung disease on respiration, with no implications for later outcome. Since the two groups also differed on another respiratory variable—that is, the chronic lung disease infants sighed more often each week, and this difference was significant for 2 weeks—the second explanation appears the more likely.

One of the surprising findings of this study was that other than quiet sleep organization, no behaviors theoretically related to neurological status or developmental outcome differed between infants with and without chronic lung disease. There are a number of possible explanations for this. First, it is possible that chronic lung disease is not directly responsible for the increased morbidity in these infants. Other medical complications, such as intraventricular hemorrhage, that occur more commonly in infants with chronic lung disease than in other preterm infants, might cause the developmental problems (Markestad & Fitzhardinge, 1981). It is also possible that studies finding poorer developmental outcomes for infants with chronic lung disease had healthier infants in their comparison group than we did. Thus, the apparent greater risk of developmental problems in infants with chronic lung disease might be an artifact of poorly matched samples. In preliminary analyses of the first 24 infants in our larger study to reach age 3 years, we found that over 40% had IQs in the borderline or retarded range and 70% exhibited suspect performance in two or more areas of development (Holditch-Davis, Miles, & Huber, 1991), indicating that our whole sample is at risk for developmental problems. Finally, it is possible that the increased risk for poor development in chronic lung disease infants is entirely due to the very poor outcomes of the small proportion of chronic lung disease infants who remain dependent on mechanical ventilation after term. These infants were not healthy enough to be included in this study.

Nurses working with infants with chronic lung disease need to be aware of the importance of individualizing their care based on the behaviors of the infants. Generalizations about behavior or outcome may not apply to specific individuals. Research has shown that nursing interventions that are individualized based on the behaviors of specific infants are most likely to reduce length of mechanical ventilation and, thus, the severity of chronic lung disease (Als et al., 1986; Becker, Grunwald, Moorman, & Stuhr, 1991). In addition, our findings indicate that the behaviors of the majority of chronic lung disease infants do not differ from those of other high-risk preterm infants. Thus, this study did not support the most common clinical generalization about chronic lung disease infants—that they are more irritable and react more negatively to care than other preterm infants.

The danger of this type of generalization is that it might become a self-fulfilling prophecy. Expecting more negative behaviors, nurse and parents might provide different handling and stimulation for chronic lung disease infants while they are in the hospital. As a result, these infants might have fewer opportunities to develop appropriate skills, might be less successful social partners after hospital discharge, and might even experience developmental problems because of lack of social stimulation in the home. A possible example of the consequences of this type of stereotyping comes from a study by Jarvis and colleagues (Jarvis, Myers, & Creasey, 1989). At 4 and 8 months after term, they found that mothers of infants who had chronic lung disease were less sensitive to infant cues, were less responsive to infant distress, and provided less social-emotional growth fostering in a teaching situation than did mothers of high-risk preterm infants without this complication—despite the fact that the behaviors of the two groups of infants did not differ.

It is important that clinicians model for parents appropriate ways to interpret infant behaviors. Instead of dismissing irritability as typical of chronic lung disease infants, nurses can help parents find explanations. In young preterm infants, hypoxia, sepsis, pain, and over-stimulation are likely causes. Generally, it will be necessary to intervene and observe infant responses to changes in order to differentiate these possibilities. Infants older than 1 month after term also become irritable because they want attention. These infants are content while being held but then cry as soon as they are put down. Although this behavior may be difficult for nurses in a busy NICU to handle, it is actually a sign that the infant is developing appropriately and an opportunity to get parents more directly involved in the infant's care. When nurses assess behaviors of infants with chronic lung disease and modify their care based on these behaviors, they will be better able to meet the needs of both the infants and their families.

NOTE

The nurse contexts, sleep–wake states, REM variables, and respiration regularity variables each summed to 100%. Therefore, group differences in these variables were determined using a two-factor (group by pattern) repeated measures analysis of variance for each of these four clusters of variables. These analyses had one non-repeated factor—group (chronic lung disease versus non-chronic lung disease infants)—and one repeated factor—pattern (the various variables within each cluster). Thus, there were six levels of pattern in the nurse context analyses, eight levels in the sleep–wake state analyses, four levels in the REM analyses, and four levels in the respiration regularity analyses. Since these clusters of variables sum to 100%, the F value for pattern in each of the analyses was expected to equal 0. Therefore, it was the group by pattern interaction that indicated whether there was a significant difference between the two groups.

ACKNOWLEDGMENTS

We wish to thank Debra B. Miller, Diane C. Hudson, Paul Bernthal, Charlene Garrett, and John Carlson for technical assistance.

The preparation of this chapter was supported by Grant No. 1 R29 NR01894 from the National Center for Nursing Research, National Institutes of Health.

REFERENCES

Als, H., Lawhon, G., Brown, E., Gibes, R., Duffy, F. H., McAnulty, G., & Blickman, J. G. (1986). Individualized behavioral and environmental care for the very low birth weight preterm infant at high risk for bronchopulmonary dysplasia: Neonatal intensive care unit and developmental outcome. *Pediatrics, 78,* 1123–1132.

Als, H., Lester, B. M., Tronick, E. C., & Brazelton, T. B. (1982). Manual for the assessment of preterm infants' behavior (APIB). In H. E. Fitzgerald, B. M. Lester, & M. W. Yogman (Eds.), *Theory and research in behavioral pediatrics* (Vol. 1, pp. 65–132). New York: Plenum.

Anders, T. F., Keener, M. A., & Kraemer, H. (1985). Sleep–wake organization, neonatal assessment and development in premature infants during the first year of life. II. *Sleep, 8,* 193–206.

Andreasson, B., Lindroth, M., Mortensson, W., Svenningsen, N. W., & Jonson, B. (1989). Lung function eight years after neonatal ventilation. *Archives of Disease in Childhood, 64,* 108–113.

Aranda, J. V., & Turmen, T. (1979). Methylxanthines in apnea of prematurity. *Clinics in Perinatology, 6,* 87–107.

Bader, D., Ramos, A. D., Lew, C. D., Platzker, A. C. G., Stabile, M. W., & Keens, T. G. (1987). Childhood sequelae of infant lung disease: Exercise and pulmonary function abnormalities after bronchopulmonary dysplasia. *The Journal of Pediatrics, 110,* 693–699.

Ballard, J. L., Novak, K. K., & Driver, M. (1979). A simplified score for assessment of fetal maturation of newly born infants. *The Journal of Pediatrics, 95,* 769–774.

Becker, P. T., Grunwald, P. C., Moorman, J., & Stuhr, S. (1991). Outcomes of developmentally supportive nursing care for very low birth weight infants. *Nursing Research, 40,* 150–155.

Becker, P. T., & Thoman, E. B. (1981). Rapid eye movement storms in infants: Rate of occurrence at 6 months predicts mental development at one year. *Science, 212,* 1415–1416.

Becker, P. T., & Thoman, E. B. (1982). Intense rapid eye movements during active sleep in infants: An index of neurobehavioral instability. *Developmental Psychobiology, 15,* 203–210.

Booth, C. L., Morin, V. N., Waite, S. P., & Thoman, E. B. (1983). Periodic and nonperiodic sleep apnea in premature and fullterm infants. *Developmental Medicine and Child Neurology, 25,* 283–296.

Bozynski, M. E. A., Albert, J. M., Vasan, U., Nelson, M. N., Zak, L. K., & Naughton, P. M. (1990). Bronchopulmonary dysplasia and postnatal growth in extremely premature black infants. *Early Human Development, 21,* 83–92.

Bozynski, M. E. A., Nelson, M. N., Matalon, T. A. S., O'Donnell, K. J., Naughton, P. M., Vasan, U., Meier, W. A., & Ploughman, L. (1987). Prolonged mechanical ventilation and intracranial hemorrhage: Impact on developmental progress through 18 months in infants weighing 1,200 grams or less at birth. *Pediatrics, 79,* 670–676.

Cohen S. E., Parmelee, A. H., Beckwith, L., & Sigman, M. (1986). Cognitive development in preterm infants: Birth to 8 years. *Journal of Developmental and Behavioral Pediatrics, 7,* 102–110.

Colombo, J., & Horowitz, F. D. (1987). Behavioral state as a lead variable in neonatal research. *Merrill-Palmer Quarterly, 33,* 423–437.

Davidson, S., Schrayer, A., Wielunsky, E., Krikler, R., Lilos, P., & Reisner, S. H. (1990). Energy intake, growth, and development in ventilated very-low-birth-weight infants with and without bronchopulmonary dysplasia. *American Journal of Diseases of Children, 144,* 553–559.

Davis, D. H., & Thoman, E. B. (1987). Behavioral states of premature infants: Implications for neural and behavioral development. *Developmental Psychobiology, 20,* 25–38.

Davis, D. H., & Thoman, E. B. (1988). The early social environment of premature and fullterm infants. *Early Human Development, 17,* 221–232.

Dubowitz, L. M. S., Dubowitz, V., & Goldberg, C. (1970). Clinical assessment of gestational age in the newborn infant. *The Journal of Pediatrics, 77,* 1–10.

Goldson, E. (1984). Severe bronchopulmonary dysplasia in the very low birth weight infant: Its relationship to developmental outcome. *Journal of Developmental and Behavioral Pediatrics, 5,* 165–168.

Gorski, P. A., Hole, W. T., Leonard, C. H., & Martin, J. A. (1983). Direct computer recording of premature infants and nursery care: Distress following two interventions. *Pediatrics, 72,* 198–202.

Greenspan, J. S., Abbasi, S., & Bhutani, V. K. (1988). Sequential changes in pulmonary mechanics in the very low birth weight (≤1000 grams) infant. *The Journal of Pediatrics, 113,* 732–737.

Grogaard, J. B., Lindstrom, D. P., Parker, R. A., Culley, B., & Stahlman, M. T. (1990). Increased survival rate in very low birth weight infants (1500 grams or less): No association with increased incidence of handicaps. *The Journal of Pediatrics, 117,* 139–146.

Hoffman, E. L., & Bennett, F. C. (1990). Birthweight less than 800 grams: Changing outcomes and influences of gender and gestation number. *Pediatrics, 86,* 27–34.

Holditch-Davis, D. (1990a, April). *Development of activity and behaviors in preterm infants: Relation to sleep–wake states.* Poster presented at the biennial International Conference on Infant Studies, Montreal. (Abstract published in *Infant Behavior and Development, 13* [Special ICIS Edition], 421.)

Holditch-Davis, D. (1990b). The development of sleeping and waking states in high-risk preterm infants. *Infant Behavior and Development, 13,* 513–531.

Holditch-Davis, D. (1990c). The effect of hospital caregiving on preterm infants' sleeping and waking states. In S. G. Funk, E. M. Tornquist, M. T. Champagne, L. A. Copp, & R. A. Wiese (Eds.), *Key Aspects of Recovery: Improving Nutrition, Rest, and Mobility* (pp. 110–122). New York: Springer Publishing Co.

Holditch-Davis, D., Miles, M. S., & Huber, C. (1991, April). Parenting experiences of mothers of 3-year-old prematurely born children: Impact on utilization of intervention services. Presented as part of a symposium, *The Changing Face of Neonatology—Impact on Parents,* J. Oehler, chair. Biennial Conference of the Society for Research in Child Development, Seattle. (Abstract published in *SRCD Abstracts, 9,* 102.)

Horbar, J. D., McAuliffe, T. L., Adler, S. M., Albersheim, S., Cassady, G., Edwards, W., Jones, R., Kattwinkel, J., Kraybill, E. N., Krishnan, V., Raschko, P., & Wilkinson, A. R. (1988). Variability in 28-day outcomes for very low birth weight infants: An analysis of 11 neonatal intensive care units. *Pediatrics, 82,* 554–559.

Jarvis, P. A., Myers, B. L., & Creasey, G. L. (1989). The effects of infant illness on mothers' interactions with prematures at 4 and 8 months. *Infant Behavior and Development, 12,* 25–35.

Johnson, M. W., & Remmers, J. E. (1984) Accessory muscle activity during sleep in chronic obstructive pulmonary disease. *Journal of Applied Physiology: Respiratory, Environmental, and Exercise Physiology, 57,* 1011–1017.

Korner, A. F. (1972). State as variable, obstacle, and as mediator of stimulation in infant research. *Merrill-Palmer Quarterly, 18,* 77–94.

Korner, A. F., Brown, B. W., Jr., Reade, R. P., Stevenson, D. K., Fernback, S. A., & Thom, V. A. (1988). State behavior of preterm infants as a function of development, individual, and sex differences. *Infant Behavior and Development, 11,* 111–124.

Kraybill, E. N., Bose, C. L., & D'Ercole, A. J. (1987). Chronic lung disease in infants with very low birth weight. *American Journal of Diseases of Children, 141,* 784–788.

Kurzner, S. I., Garg, M., Bautisa, D. B., Bader, D., Merritt, R. J., Warburton, D., & Keens, T. G. (1988). Growth failure in infants with bronchopulmonary dysplasia: Nutrition and elevated resting metabolic expenditure. *Pediatrics, 81,* 379–384.

Landry, S. H., Chapieski, L., Fletcher, J. M., & Denson, S. (1988). Three year outcomes for low birth weight infants: Differential effects of early medical complications. *Journal of Pediatric Psychology, 13,* 317–327.

Lombroso, C. T., & Matsumiya, Y. (1985). Stability in waking-sleep states in neonates as a predictor of long-term neurologic outcome. *Pediatrics, 76,* 52–63.

Luchi, J. M., Bennett, F. C., & Jackson, J. C. (1991). Predictors of neurodevelopmental outcome following bronchopulmonary dysplasia. *American Journal of Diseases in Children, 145,* 813–817.

Markestad, T., & Fitzhardinge, P. M. (1981). Growth and development in children recovering from bronchopulmonary dysplasia. *The Journal of Pediatrics, 98,* 597–602.

Medoff-Cooper, B. (1988). The effects of handling on preterm infants with bronchopulmonary dysplasia. *Image: Journal of Nursing Scholarship, 20,* 132–134.

Meisels, S. J., Plunkett, J. W., Pasick, P. L., Stiefel, G. S., & Roloff, D. W. (1987). Effects of severity and chronicity of respiratory illness on cognitive development of preterm infants. *Journal of Pediatric Psychology, 12,* 117–132.

Meisels, S. J., Plunkett, J. W., Roloff, D. W., Pasick, P. L., & Stiefel, G. S. (1986). Growth and development of preterm infants with respiratory distress syndrome and bronchopulmonary dysplasia. *Pediatrics, 77,* 345–352.

Minde, K., Whitelaw, A., Brown, J., & Fitzhardinge, P. (1983). Effect of neonatal complications in premature infants on early parent-infant interactions. *Developmental Medicine and Child Neurology, 25,* 763–777.

Myers, B. J., Jarvis, P. A., Creasey, G. L., Kerkering, K. W., Markowitz, P. I., & Best, A. M., III. (1992). Prematurity and respiratory illness: Brazelton Scale (NBAS) performance of preterm infants with bronchopulmonary displasia (BPD), respiratory distress syndrome (RDS), or no respiratory illness. *Infant Behavior and Development, 15,* 27–42.

Northway, W. H. (1979). Observations on bronchopulmonary dysplasia. *Journal of Pediatrics, 95,* 815–818.

Roffwarg, H. P., Muzio, J. N., & Dement, W. C. (1966). Ontogenetic development of the human sleep–dream cycle. *Science, 152*, 604–619.

Sauve, R. S., & Singhal, N. (1985). Long-term morbidity of infants with bronchopulmonary dysplasia. *Pediatrics, 76*, 725–733.

Shennen, A. T., Dunn, M. S., Ohlsson, A., Lennox, K., & Hoskins, E. M. (1988). Abnormal pulmonary outcomes in premature infants: Prediction from oxygen requirement in the neonatal period. *Pediatrics, 82*, 527–532.

Skidmore, M. D., Rivers, A., & Hack, M. (1990). Increased risk of cerebral palsy among very low-birthweight infants with chronic lung disease. *Developmental Medicine and Child Neurology, 32*, 325–332.

Thoman, E. B. (1975). Early development of sleeping behaviors in infants. In N. R. Ellis (Ed.), *Aberrant development in infancy: Human and animal studies* (pp. 122–138). New York: John Wiley & Sons.

Thoman, E. B. (1990). Sleeping and waking states in infancy: A functional perspective. *Neuroscience and Biobehavioral Reviews, 14*, 93–107.

Thoman, E. B., Acebo, C., Dreyer, C. A., Becker, P. T., & Freese, M. P. (1979). Individuality in the interactive process. In E. B. Thoman (Ed.), *Origins of the infant's social responsiveness* (pp. 305–338). Hillsdale, New Jersey: Lawrence Erlbaum.

Thoman, E. B., Denenberg, V. H., Sieval, J., Zeidner, L., & Becker, P. (1981). State organization in neonates: Developmental inconsistency indicates risk for developmental dysfunction. *Neuropediatrics, 12*, 45–54.

Tynan, W. D. (1986). Behavioral stability predicts morbidity and mortality in infants from a neonatal intensive care unit. *Infant Behavior and Development, 9*, 71–79.

Vohr, B. R., Bell, E. F., & Oh, W. (1982). Infants with bronchopulmonary dysplasia: Growth pattern and neurologic and developmental outcome. *American Journal of Diseases of Children, 136*, 443–447.

Vohr, B. R., Garcia Coll, C., Lobato, D., Yunis, K. A., O'Dea, C., & Oh, W. (1991). Neurodevelopmental and medical status of low-birthweight survivors of bronchopulmonary dysplasia at 10 to 12 years of age. *Developmental Medicine and Child Neurology, 33*, 690–697.

[24]

Cost Burden of Low Birthweight

Susan Gennaro, Dorothy Brooten, Audrey Klein, Marilyn Stringer, Ruth York, and Linda Brown

Around the world, low birthweight (LBW ≤ 2500 g) is a major determinant of infant mortality. The lower the birthweight, the less likely the infant is to survive. Low birthweight survivors have a greater incidence of handicaps, poorer general health in the first year of life, and lower projected life-time earnings; the financial and human costs of their care are staggering. The high cost of providing care to LBW infants is of concern to those making public policy decisions as well as health care providers, insurers, and families. Costs include charges for hospitalization, related medical costs, and nonmedical costs.

In 1984, average charges for the initial hospitalization of LBW infants in the United States ranged from $39,420 to $111,670 (Office of Technology Assessment, 1987). In 1986 the additional cost over the cost of caring for a healthy term newborn was $5,236 (Institute of Medicine, 1990). In 1992, a Florida study found the average daily hospital charge per admission for a LBW infant was $5,111 (Imershein, Turner, Wells, & Pearman, 1992). In addition to initial hospitalization, rehospitalization is reported to occur in between 25%–50% of very low birthweight (VLBW) (≤ 1500 g) and LBW infants, compared with 8% of normal weight infants (McCormick, 1985; McCormick, Shapiro, & Starfield, 1980; Mutch, Newdick, Lodwick, & Chalmers, 1986; Termini, Brooten, Brown, Gennaro, & York, 1990). During rehospitalizations the length of stay for both LBW and VLBW infants is also longer than for normal birthweight infants (> 2500 g) (McCormick et al., 1980). The average number of physician visits in the first year of life is 14 to 16 for VLBW infants, compared to 10 for normal weight infants (McCormick, 1985). And many infants are discharged to their homes dependent upon technology, including apnea monitors, ventilators, etc., with their associated costs. The outpatient health care costs for neonatal intensive care unit graduates have been estimated at $31 a month for children without handicaps, $86 a month for children with mild handicaps, and $109 a month for children with moderate to severe handicaps (Shankaran, Cohen, Linver, & Zonia, 1988). While some of these outpatient costs are paid by third party payors, many are not. McCormick and colleagues (McCormick, Stemmler, Bernbaum, & Farran, 1986) reported higher out-of-pocket expenses for hospitalization, ambulatory care, and medical equipment for VLBW infants than for full-term normal weight newborns.

Although many of the hospital and related medical costs are well documented, few data are available on the nonmedical costs associated with LBW, including costs of visiting the infant during lengthy hospitalizations, extra transportation costs, parking costs, child care for siblings, additional food costs, and lost family wages. Median weekly out-of-pocket nonmedical expenses of $39.70 have been reported for families of children with cancer. This figure did not include lost wages, though about half of the families experienced a loss in wages. When the lost wages were included, weekly out-of-pocket cost was $88.20. In over half of the families, the combined out-of-pocket expenses and loss of wages came to more than 25% of the annual family budget (Lansky et al., 1979).

In families of VLBW infants who require surgery, transportation and babysitting costs have been documented as a substantial financial burden (McCormick, Bernbaum, Eisenberg, Kustra, & Finnegan, 1991). Another potential nonmedical cost of LBW is its effect on family functioning. Studies of children with chronic or catastrophic illness suggest that family functioning may be disrupted substantially; major problems include marital instability, decreased social contacts and vacations, problems with other children in the family, and increased workload for mothers (Institute of Medicine, 1985).

This longitudinal study examined the costs to families of having a VLBW (≤ 1500 grams) infant for the first 6 months after the infant was discharged home. The specific costs examined included out-of-pocket expenses directly attributable to having a VLBW infant as well as changes in family functioning (an indirect cost) and changes in family economic status (monthly income, employment status, and public assistance status). Costs were compared for families at varying income levels.

METHOD

Sample

A convenience sample of 44 mothers of VLBW infants born in a university hospital in the Northeastern United States from August 1988 through

March 1990 provided data for the study. Mothers were eligible for the study if their infant was born weighing 1500 grams or less and without congenital anomalies.

The mean age of study mothers was 26 years (*SD* = 7). Most were African-American (75%), unmarried (73%), multiparas (75%) who delivered vaginally (53%). Thirty-seven percent had graduated from high school, 31% had less than a high school education, and 32% had more. Mean birthweight of the infants was 1061 grams (*SD* = 436), and mean gestational age at birth was 28 weeks (*SD* = 2.8). The mean length of infant hospital stay was 57 days (*SD* = 21.2); 41% of the infants were discharged home on an apnea monitor.

Half of the mothers were insured by Medicaid; 38% had private insurance and 12% were uninsured. Yearly reported income was as follows: ≤ $5,000, 31%; $5,001–$7,000, 22%; $7,001–$24,000, 26%; over $24,000, 21%. In national multicenter studies in the United States, a higher incidence of prematurity has been found in lower socioeconomic groups (Lieberman, Ryan, Monson, & Schoenbaum, 1987; McCormick et al., 1980) and the sample in this study was consistent with these national statistics.

Procedure

Mothers were interviewed regarding family economic status (income and out-of-pocket expenses), changes in employment, and family functioning at infant discharge and at 1, 3, and 6 months post infant hospitalization. Data were collected through face-to-face interviews at infant discharge and telephone interviews thereafter. All mothers either had telephones in their own homes or had ready access to a telephone at a neighbor's or a relative's home.

Family Economic Status Data on out-of-pocket costs attributable to the home care of the very low birthweight infant were collected for the first 6 months after infant discharge using a diary of expenses. Out-of-pocket expenses were considered to be those that would not normally be incurred after giving birth to a full-term low-risk infant. Out-of-pocket costs included medications, special equipment or supplies for the infant's care at home (e.g., apnea monitoring), travel to specialty clinics or specialists, and unreimbursed expenses for infant rehospitalizations or infant medical and nursing care (unreimbursed cost for specialists, private nursing, health aid workers, etc.). To enhance reliability, mothers kept logs and were also interviewed about out-of-pocket expenses.

Data on changes in parental employment and changes in family income were also collected for the first 6 months following infant discharge, using a standardized form listing job titles, hours worked per week, and monthly income. Monthly income was defined as all income obtained by people residing in the same household who were related through birth, marriage, or adoption, and money received from members of other households. In this sample, monthly income was probably underestimated because if mothers said they could not give information about a family member's income (such as a sister's or mother's income), no further attempt was made to obtain this information. Yet these family members, when living in the same household, often provided some economic resources such as help with rent and groceries. At discharge, both employment and income data were validated whenever possible using hospital records; after discharge, reported income was validated against known standards (as in the case of public assistance) to assure that reported incomes fell within standard guidelines (55 Pennsylvania Code, 1986).

Impact on Family Scale The Impact on Family Scale was administered to mothers in interviews at discharge and at 1, 3, and 6 months post discharge. This instrument yields a total score reflecting the impact of having a preterm infant on various components of family life: the financial situation, social interaction within and outside the home, subjective distress felt by the parent, and the sense of mastery which may emerge from coping with stress (Stein & Riessman, 1980). Although the Impact on Family Scale was originally designed to be used with families of ill children, it has been used previously with families of preterm infants (McCormick et al., 1986). Content validity of the scale was supported by deriving items from the literature, from interviews with mothers, and from interviews with care providers of ill children.

Scores on the Impact on Family Scale range from 24 to 96, with higher scores indicating greater impact on the family. In the current study, internal consistency reliability was examined using Cronbach's alpha at discharge and 1, 3, and 6 months post discharge. The reliability coefficient for the total scale was .69 at infant discharge, .75 at 1 month post discharge, .76 at 3 months post discharge, and .78 at 6 months post discharge.

RESULTS

For the families in this study, the cost burden of very low birthweight infants included out-of-pocket expenses and changes in family employment; however, there were no significant changes in monthly income or in family functioning over the 6 month study period.

Out-of-Pocket Expenses

All families reported out-of-pocket expenses associated with the care of a VLBW infant. The greatest expenses were for transportation during the infant's hospitalization and for health-related costs incurred from 3 to 6 months post discharge that were not covered by third party insurers. These included physician bills and bills for appliances such as breast pumps and apnea monitors. The mean amount of money spent by families for each category of expense is reported in Table 24.1.

When the differences in expenses of the four income groups were examined, significant differences between the groups were found [F (3,27) = 3.96, p = .02] (see Table 24.2). Families with the highest income had significantly higher out-of-pocket expenditures at every time period. There was no difference from one time period to another in the amount of money that families spent [F (3,27) = 2.7, p = .07], and no interaction between income group and time period [F (9,81) = 1.3, p = .24].

The percentage of family income used for out-of-pocket expenses was calculated based upon mean yearly income. A considerable percentage of economic resources was devoted to caring for the VLBW infant—resources that would not have been spent if the infant had been born healthy and at term. Families in the lowest income group spent 2% of their annual income on out-of-pocket expenses, and families in other income categories spent 1% of their income on out-of-pocket expenses for the care of their VLBW infant.

Family Employment

Only unexpected changes in employment that were a direct result of having had a VLBW infant were considered as employment changes. At infant discharge, 35% of mothers were employed, but 15% of those had decreased the number of hours they worked. At 6 months post infant discharge, only 30% of mothers were still employed and 7% of these mothers had de-

TABLE 24.1 Out-of-Pocket Expenses in Dollars by Categories

	Months post discharge							
	Discharge		Month 1		Month 3		Month 6	
Category	*M*[a]	*SD*[b]	*M*	*SD*	*M*	*SD*	*M*	*SD*
Transportation	188.48	471	13.78	19	11.48	18	9.19	20
Medication	1.00	2	6.23	19	2.45	8	2.40	8
Food	23.43	85	.21	1	1.00	3	1.90	7
Health	0.00	0	14.42	69	11.45	30	53.87	156
Appliances	0.00	0	11.63	45	5.35	28	35.16	109
Babysitting	6.89	31	18.00	56	0.00	0	0.00	0

[a] *M* = Mean
[b] *SD* = Standard Deviation

TABLE 25.2 Out-of-Pocket Expenses in Dollars by Income Group (N = 44)

	Post Discharge							
	Discharge		Month 1		Month 3		Month 6	
	M[a]	*SD*[b]	*M*	*SD*	*M*	*SD*	*M*	*SD*
All	221.38	517	64.61	135	40.63	76	117.81	247
Group 1: ≤ $5,000 (*n* = 15)	114.81	116	25.50	23	17.60	25	24.66	11
Group 2: $5,001 – $7,000 (*n* = 10)	83.33	115	4.00	4	16.57	11	13.25	18
Group 3: $7,001 – $24,000 (*n* = 10)	113.55	97	37.00	47	59.62	100	66.00	95
Group 4: > $24,000 (*n* = 9)	617.44	1018	185.77	230	81.71	119	407.33	416

[a] *M* = Mean
[b] *SD* = Standard Deviation

creased the number of hours of their employment. Those mothers who were employed at infant discharge but unemployed 6 months later had not planned on leaving the work force but were forced to do so because of caretaking needs of the VLBW infant. Thirty-eight percent of fathers who lived in the same household as the mother and infant were employed at infant discharge, but only 34% were employed 6 months later. Two fathers reported losing their jobs because of the need for additional leave time resulting from having a VLBW infant. At the same time, three fathers and five mothers reported increasing their employment hours.

Monthly Income

Most families (58%) had no changes in monthly income over the course of the study. The mean monthly family income at discharge was reported as \$1352 (SD = \$1581) and the median monthly family income was \$716. The mean monthly family income 6 months later was \$1550 (an increase of \$198, SD = \$1763). The median family income at 6 months was \$847, an increase of \$131.

Because economic changes might have different effects on families depending on their economic resources, changes in monthly income were examined within each of the four income groupings. All families had a higher mean income at 6 months post infant discharge than they did at discharge, except for families with incomes of \$5,001 to \$7,000; their monthly income decreased by \$139. Twenty-seven mothers reported receiving public assistance at infant discharge; 6 months later an additional four mothers were receiving public assistance. Overall the majority of families in each group did not experience changes in monthly income though they did have increased out-of-pocket expenses.

Family Functioning

In studying children with a variety of chronic illnesses, Stein and Jessop (1984) found that the mean score on the Impact on the Family Scale was 48, with a standard deviation of 8.2. McCormick et al. (1986), working with families of VLBW infants, reported a mean impact score of 37.1 (SD = 9.0). The mean impact score for the families in this study was 41 (SD =8.0) at the infant's discharge. At 1, 3, and 6 months post infant discharge, the scores were 42, 38, and 38, respectively (with a standard deviation of 9.0 at each of these time points). Using a repeated measures analysis of variance, no differences in family functioning were seen between the four income groups [F (3, 27) = .01, p = .99]. There was also no difference in the pattern of family functioning over time [F (3,27) = 1.8, p = .16] and no difference in functioning over time in families at different income levels [F (9,81) = .28, p = .97].

DISCUSSION

Having a VLBW infant necessitated changes in employment for almost half of the mothers who worked. However, the economic impact of low birthweight on the labor force is underestimated by this figure, because only 35% of study mothers worked at infant hospital discharge. This is a lower percentage than that found in a previous study, in which 43% of mothers worked at infant hospital discharge (Gennaro, Hornberger, & Brooten, 1990), and it is lower than the national figures: 57% of married and 70% of divorced women with children under the age of 6 work outside the home (Bureau of the Census, 1989). In future studies the economic impact of lost wages needs to be examined to see more fully the cost of having a VLBW infant both to families and to society.

The fathers (7%) who increased their working hours did so to increase income. However, the mothers (12%) who increased working hours over the 6 months of the study were returning to prepregnancy patterns of employment. Many working mothers had decreased hours because of problems with their pregnancy or because they needed to care for their infant. As time went on, these mothers were returning to their normal patterns of employment.

Most families (58%) did not have any change in their income. However, some families had an increase in family income (20%), perhaps because fathers were working longer hours, or because public assistance increased. Yet 22% of families had a decrease in income at the same time that the amount of money they needed for the care of the VLBW infant was increasing. Families with limited economic resources spend a higher percentage of total income on necessities such as food and rent and therefore have less expendable income. Families with more limited economic resources thus have less choice about where spending can be changed to cover increased health costs.

The greatest out-of-pocket costs were transportation at discharge, and health care costs and appliances from 3 to 6 months. Transportation has also been found to be one of the greatest out-of-pocket expenses for families of VLBW infants requiring surgery (McCormick et al., 1991) and families of children with cancer (Lansky et al., 1979).

The impact of having a VLBW infant on family functioning appears to have been minimal for the families in this study. Initial impact scores were very similar to those reported by McCormick et al. (1986) for a group of families with infants of similar birthweight. However, the lack of change seen in family functioning scores over time conflicts with the findings of other studies (Leventhal, 1981; Sabbeth & Leventhal, 1981) that having a premature infant or a child with chronic health problems caused disruptions in family functioning.

The findings of this study regarding employment changes are important for public policy. All changes in employment were unplanned—made not because families had a new baby but because that baby was born early and at very low birthweight. Although the recently enacted Family Leave Bill would have helped many mothers (and the two fathers who were fired) to remain in the work force, uncompensated leave is only a beginning. The out-of-pocket expense of 1%–2% of family income resulting directly from the infant being born VLBW may be extremely burdensome for families with limited expendable income. For those families whose employment was disrupted, the percentage of income spent on the VLBW infant would actually be higher if lost wages were factored in.

The high transportation costs during the infant's hospitalization need to be examined in relation to visiting patterns of families. In other studies, poorer mothers have been found to visit their VLBW infants less frequently than mothers with more economic resources, perhaps in part because in the United States, no social service programs exist to cover the cost of transportation to the hospital (Brown, Brooten, York, Jacobsen, & Gennaro, 1989). Although occasional attempts are made to provide help for mothers who have economic barriers to frequent visiting, there is no overall commitment to ensuring that economic barriers do not needlessly separate a mother from her child. Other forms of contact, such as telephone calls and notes from nurses, take on particular importance when barriers to visiting exist.

In this study, between 3 and 6 months, unreimbursed health care costs were being paid by families. The impact of these costs on the family's use of preventive health care services needs to be further examined. In the United States, routine follow-up is poorly reimbursed by many insurance carriers, and utilization of well child care may be more difficult for families who have limited economic resources and high health care bills. Therefore, in future research the impact of the out-of-pocket costs to families having a VLBW infant needs to be examined in relation to whether or not the family is able to continue to access health care.

REFERENCES

55 Pennsylvania Code } 171.22. Family allowance provisions (1986).

Brown, L., Brooten, D., York, R., Jacobsen, B., & Gennaro, S. (1989). Very low birthweight infants: Parental visiting and telephoning during initial infant hospitalization. *Nursing Research, 38,* 233–266.

Bureau of the Census. (1989). *Statistical abstracts of the United States, 1989* (109th ed.). Washington, D.C.: U. S. Department of Commerce.

Gennaro, S., Hornberger, K., & Brooten, D. (1990). Family costs associated with having a low birthweight infant. *Proceedings of NAACOG Third National Re-*

search Conference: Making a difference in women's and infant's health (p. 84). Denver, CO.

Imershein, A., Turner, C., Wells, J., & Pearman, A. (1992). Covering the costs of care in neonatal intensive care units. *Pediatrics, 89*, 56–61.

Institute of Medicine. (1985). *Preventing low birthweight*. Washington, DC: National Academy Press.

Institute of Medicine. (1990). *Science and babies: Private decisions, public dilemmas*. Washington, DC: National Academy Press.

Lansky, S., Cairns, N., Clark, G., Lowman, J., Miller, L., & Trueworthy, R. (1979). Childhood cancer: nonmedical costs of the illness. *Cancer, 43*, 403–408.

Leventhal, J. (1981). Risk factors for child abuse: Methodologic standards in case-control studies. *Pediatrics, 68*, 684–690.

Lieberman, E., Ryan, K, Monson, R., & Schoenbaum, S. (1987). Risk factors accounting for racial differences in the rate of premature birth. *New England Journal of Medicine, 317*, 743–748.

McCormick, M. (1985). The contribution of low birthweight to infant mortality and childhood morbidity. *New England Journal of Medicine, 312*, 82–90.

McCormick, M., Bernbaum, J., Eisenberg, J., Kustra, S., & Finnegan, E. (1991). Costs incurred by parents of very low birthweight infants after the initial hospitalization. *Pediatrics, 88*, 533–541.

McCormick, M., Shapiro, S. & Starfield, B. (1980). Rehospitalization in the first year of life for high risk survivors. *Pediatrics, 66*, 991–999.

McCormick, M., Stemmler, M., Bernbaum, J., & Farran, A. (1986). The very low birthweight transport goes home: Impact on the family. *Developmental and Behavioral Pediatrics, 7*, 217–223.

Mutch, L., Newdick, N., Lodwick, A., & Chalmers, I. (1986). Secular changes in rehospitalization of very low birthweight infants. *Pediatrics, 78*, 164–171.

Office of Technology Assessment. (1987). *Neonatal intensive care for low birthweight infants: Cost and effectiveness*. (OTA-HCS38). Washington, DC: U.S. Government Printing Office.

Sabbeth, B., & Leventhal, J. (1981). Marital adjustment to chronic childhood illness: A critique of the literature. *Pediatrics, 68*, 684–690.

Shankaran, S., Cohen, S., Linver, M., & Zonia, S. (1988). Medical care costs of high-risk infants after neonatal intensive care: A controlled study. *Pediatrics, 81*, 372–378.

Stein, R., & Jessop, D. (1984). *Evaluation of a home care unit as an ambulatory ICU*. (Final report grant No. MC-R360402). Springfield, VA: National Technical Information Services.

Stein, R., & Riessman, C. (1980). The development of an impact-on-family scale: Preliminary findings. *Medical Care, XVIII*, 465–472.

Termini, L., Brooten, D., Brown, L., Gennaro, S., & York, R. (1990). Reasons for acute care visits and rehospitalizations in very low-birthweight infants. *Neonatal Network, 8*, 23–26.

[25]

Parental Role Alterations Experienced by Mothers of Children with a Life-Threatening Chronic Illness

Margaret Shandor Miles, Jennifer Piersma D'Auria, Ellen M. Hart, Debra A. Sedlack, and Melody Ann Watral

Parenting, as defined by Leal (1983), is the state in which a single adult (or a pair of adults) undertakes by conscious choice or biological demand the care and keeping of a child. The success of parenting can be observed in the optimal functioning of the child in accordance with his or her stage and phase of psychosocial, emotional, adaptive, and temperamental development, and in keeping with the child's capacities and potential. In her theoretical essays on mothering, Ruddick (1989) says that children demand that their lives be preserved and their growth fostered. Ruddick contends that to be a mother, one must be committed to meeting the demands of preservation and growth, while also training the child for social acceptability. Thus, the parental role encompasses many responsibilities, including the provision of basic necessities such as food, protection from harm, emotional nurturing, and teaching. The responsibility of being a parent is challenging and continues through the young adult years.

Much of the literature on parental roles and responsibilities focuses on parenting a healthy child. However, a growing body of literature is examining the experience of parents whose children have a chronic illness. During the 1960s and 1970s this work focused on negative or dysfunctional parenting behaviors used in response to a child with chronic illness (Binger, Albin, & Feuerstein, 1969; Fife, 1978; Glaser, Harrison, & Lynn, 1964). Anxiety, guilt, fear of death, and chronic sorrow experienced by parents, especially mothers, were thought to lead to distorted child-rearing practices such as overprotectiveness, overindulgence, and overinvolvment with the child (Shapiro, 1983).

More recently, "normalization" has been identified as a salient aspect of family management of the chronically ill child. Normalization is defined as the strategies parents use to convey to others the normality of their child (Anderson, 1981; Krulik, 1980). Normalization involves defining family life and the social consequences of the child's illness as normal, while at the same time acknowledging the existence of the illness (Anderson, 1981; Deatrick, Knafl, & Walsh, 1988; Knafl & Deatrick, 1986). Thus, normalization refers to strategies used to normalize family life despite having a child with a serious illness, as well as strategies used to normalize the child. Closer examination of the concept suggests that even with normalization, some aspects of the parental role are changed as a result of the child's illness. Anderson (1981), for example, found that even though parents of chronically ill children defined their child as normal, their behaviors with the child reflected a restrictive parenting style. Few studies, however, have looked at how the overall parental role is altered when a child has a serious chronic illness.

Parents of chronically ill children are challenged to adequately nurture, teach, and protect their children. Depending on the illness and related treatments, the child's response to the illness, and the parental response to the situation, some aspects of the parental role may be difficult to achieve. In addition, new roles may need to be assumed, particularly by mothers, who handle most of the care of their chronically ill children (Anderson, 1981; Anderson & Elfert, 1989).

The nursing diagnosis "altered parenting" identifies parents who are unable to provide an environment that nurtures the growth and development of a child because of personal, social, or environmental problems (Carpenito, 1989). This diagnosis is extremely broad, however, and does not adequately address many of the issues faced by parents of children who are ill. A more recent diagnosis, "parental role conflict," refers to "the state in which a parent or primary caregiver experiences or perceives a change in role in response to external factors" (Carpenito, 1989, p. 566). This diagnosis is more directly focused on parenting the child who is ill, but the defining characteristics of the diagnosis are vague and the contributing or etiological factors are not clearly identified; furthermore, the title of the diagnosis does not match the defining characteristics. Although these diagnoses are commonly used in nursing practice, little research has been done to clarify or validate them, especially with parents of chronically ill children.

It is important to understand changes in the parental role experienced by parents of children who have a chronic condition—especially one that can be considered life-threatening. Life-threatening conditions include diseases that hold the potential for death from the progression or complications of the disease, sequelae of treatment regimes, and other complications that could occur because of vulnerabilities related to the disease. Life-threatening chronic conditions are characterized by intense treatment regimens that necessitate frequent visits to outpatient clinics and frequent and sometimes long-term hospitalizations for treatments, relapses, or secondary problems. The study reported here was designed to explore changes in the parental role experienced by mothers of children with two life-threatening chronic conditions—cancer and immunodeficiency diagnoses. The study also identified aspects of the parental role perceived as stressful.

METHOD

Thirty-one mothers of children with a chronic, life-threatening illness constituted the parent sample. The mothers were primarily Caucasian and came from a wide variety of socioeconomic levels. The majority had a high school education and some had a college or professional education; however, several had not graduated from high school. Most were married and many worked outside the home. Mothers rated their perceptions of the severity of their child's health problem at the time of the interview using a 5-point scale, with "1" indicating not serious and "5" indicating the most serious condition possible. Their mean rating indicated that these mothers viewed the severity of their child's illness as moderate ($M = 2.3$).

Their children were being treated at two different Southeastern university medical centers. Sixteen of the children had a diagnosis of primary immunodeficiency, and 15 had cancer diagnoses, including leukemia, osteogenic sarcoma, Ewing's sarcoma, lymphoma, retinoblastoma, rhabdomyoscarcoma, sacroccygeneal teratoma, medulloblastoma, and neuroectodermal tumor. The ages of the children ranged from 3 to 18 years. Mothers of children with cancer diagnoses participated in the study during the hospitalization of their child, while mothers of children with a diagnosis of primary immunodeficiency participated during an outpatient clinic visit.

Both qualitative and quantitative data were collected. A semi-structured interview guide was used to identify mothers' perceptions of their parental role with their chronically ill child. The interview guide focused broadly on overall parental role changes, including role changes during hospitalization, and aspects of parenting viewed as most stressful. Probes were used to explore salient topics. The interviews lasted 30 to 60 minutes and were tape-recorded and transcribed.

Interview data were analyzed using a constant comparative method. First, broad themes were identified for each interview. These themes were then evaluated across all interviews. Next the themes were clustered and relevant sub-categories were identified. Finally, interviews were reviewed again to verify themes and clarify their breadth and content.

Mothers also completed the Parental Role Alteration Stress Scale (PRASS) (Miles, Nelson, Poprawa, & Cooper, 1991), which is designed to assess the amount of stress parents experience in parenting the chronically ill child. The tool was adapted from the parental role alteration subscales of the Parental Stressor Scale: Pediatric Intensive Care Unit (Carter & Miles, 1989) and the Parental Stressor Scale: Neonatal Intensive Care Unit (Miles, Funk, & Carlson, in press). Items were expanded based on a review of the literature on parenting the chronically ill child; the PRASS focus is on illness-related caregiving, meeting the child's special needs, and changes in normal aspects of parenting. Mothers in this study rated the level of stress they experienced using a 5-point scale with "1" indicating not at all stressful and "5" indicating extremely stressful. The internal consistency alpha for the PRASS using a sample of 31 parents of children with cancer was .73 (Miles et al., 1991).

RESULTS

The mothers' accounts of their experience emphasized the significance of the role changes required in parenting the child with a chronic, life-threatening illness. Mothers indicated that two parenting styles were used: normalizing and compensating. The mothers also noted that four aspects of the parental role were altered as a result of their child's illness: advocating, protecting, caregiving, and supporting. Sequelae of these altered parental roles included the erosion of the mother's time for self and other family members, including the siblings and spouse. Also, several mothers experienced a "never-ending feeling of responsibility." This relentless feeling was especially prominent in mothers whose children had more severe problems or complications accompanying the disease.

Parenting Styles: Normalizing and Compensating

The normalizing parenting style involved keeping the child's life as normal as possible, given the limitations of the illness. Normalization was done to ensure that the child had every opportunity to be like other children and to develop appropriately despite the illness. Normalization involved socialization of the child into the family, peer group, school, and community. It also involved trying to have routines for daily living and attempting to treat the child as siblings were treated.

The compensatory parenting style involved doing things for the child that one would not ordinarily do for or with a healthy child. Compensation was made because of guilt related to the child's diagnosis and feelings of helplessness related to the child's pain and suffering, or to make sure that the child had every opportunity to overcome problems imposed or caused by the illness. Compensation included spending extra time or giving extra attention to the child, doing special things to ensure that the child's educational and developmental progress was adequate, and providing extra experiences such as trips to special places. In addition, compensating often involved reducing demands on the child, especially those related to discipline.

Parental Role Changes

Advocating Mothers continually communicated with other people to inform them about the child's needs. This was done to ensure that the child's normal developmental needs were met, while making sure special needs related to the illness were considered. Advocating was done with spouses, siblings, other family members, teachers, peers, and others in the community, and involved informing them about the child's illness, especially the prognosis of the illness and related health care needs.

Protecting Protecting was the enhanced vigilance mothers used to foster the child's well-being. The mothers had to be careful about their child's exposure to infections and to the possibility of injury at home, at school, and at play. They also watched their children for signs and symptoms of complications of the illness; several referred to this as "constant watching." This vigilant protectiveness continued when the child was in the care of health professionals. Many mothers reported watching and checking on nursing and medical staff to make sure the treatments provided for the child were necessary and were done correctly and expeditiously.

Nurturing Nurturing involved providing special support to help the child cope with the illness and related treatments. It included helping the child to see himself as normal, informing the child about the illness and treatments, preparing the child for hospitalizations and clinic visits, and being understanding of the child's emotional responses. It also involved parental presence—being with the child during stressful times such as painful or frightening health care encounters. In being supportive of their children, the mothers had to cope with the child's mood swings, demanding behavior, and resistance to repeated and painful treatments and diagnostic procedures.

Caregiving Caregiving required expanding parental activities to manage the child's complex medical regimen, including taking the child to clinic visits, monitoring symptoms, giving medications, and providing treatments such as catheter care, tracheotomy care, and administration of hyperalimentation fluids. In managing the medical regimen, mothers had to be concerned about normalizing the child's life while imposing very unusual activities and treatments on the child. Caregiving also encompassed communicating with the child's health care team.

Parental Role Alteration Stress

Data from the PRASS provided information on the specific aspects of the parental role viewed as stressful by these mothers. The two most stressful aspects were "being separated from the child during hospitalizations" (mean [*M*] = 3.8) and "not being able to protect the child from pain and painful procedures" (*M* = 3.7). Also stressful were "coping with the child's mood changes and upset feelings" (*M* = 3.3) and "not knowing how to comfort the child" (*M* = 3.2).

DISCUSSION

This study indicates that mothers employ two different parenting styles with their chronically ill children—normalizing and compensating. Normalizing has been identified as a strategy used by families of chronically ill children to maintain a normal family life (Deatrick et al., 1988; Knafl & Deatrick, 1986) or to emphasize the normality of the child (Anderson, 1981). In this study the normalizing strategy most frequently reported involved normalizing the child's life in spite of a chronic life-threatening condition that necessitated changes in the usual childhood activities and regimens. This is similar to the findings of Krulik (1980), who noted that mothers attempted to reduce the child's sense of being different by normalizing the child's life to the extent possible.

The compensating parenting style might be considered similar to "overprotection" (Fife, 1978) or the parental approach called "restrictiveness" (Anderson, 1981). However, the concepts of overprotection and restrictiveness imply a negative process and outcome, whereas the findings of this study suggest that compensating may have positive benefits for the child. It might present problems, however, for siblings in the family if the chronically ill child is treated more favorably.

These mothers of children with life-threatening chronic illnesses experienced a number of alterations in their usual parental role. Advocating, supporting, protecting, and caregiving were greatly expanded among the mothers. They emphasized the relentless and daily need to assess their children while realigning other roles. Stressful problems in parenting these chronically ill children included coping with mood swings and helping the child deal with repeated painful tests and procedures. Parents were also stressed by the separation imposed by hospitalizations.

Parental vigilance was a dominant theme in carrying out the parental role of protecting. Similarly, Miles and Carter (1985) found that vigilance was important for coping with the experience of having a critically ill child in the pediatric intensive care unit. Burke, Kauffmann, Costello, and Dillon (1991) view parental vigilance as a "way of taking charge" or coping with the stress of repeated hospitalizations of chronically ill children. Ray (1988) found this constant vigilance to be a caregiving burden for parents providing home care for technologically dependent children. Another theme that emerged was parental presence. Mothers reported using this to help their children cope with particularly stressful events.

Mothers of chronically ill children generally spend more time in care and medical management of the ill child and less time with other family members (Seligman & Darling, 1989). As expected, the mothers in this study reported that the requirements for parenting the chronically ill child were time consuming and added to their already busy schedule. The illness also created a financial drain on the family, especially if the mother stopped working outside the home to meet the child's needs, and led to changes in the parental role with the other children. Many mothers indicated at the end of the interviews that the erosion of their time and the separation from other family members during hospitalizations were very stressful.

Nursing Diagnosis and Parental Role

Although this study was not designed to validate a specific nursing diagnosis, "parental role conflict" (PRC) appears to be the most appropriate label for the parental role changes these mothers experienced (Carpenito, 1989). The mothers met the major defining characteristics for PRC in that they expressed concern about changes in their parental role and discussed disruptions in care and routines related to parenting and family life. A number of the minor defining characteristics of PRC also were expressed, particularly concerns about the effects of the child's illness on the family and the care of siblings. The mothers described a "never-ending feeling of responsibility" in parenting these children that conflicted with other responsibilities. Several potential aspects of parental role conflict, which are not presently identified in this nursing diagnosis, were uncovered in this study: feeling the need to protect the child in a wide variety of settings including the hospital; advocating for the child with spouses, teachers, and others; supporting the child (especially when the child is demanding, moody, and resistant); and following complex medical care regimens. These parental role changes appear to be an adaptive response to parenting the chronically ill child; it is not clear, however, whether or how they might be problematic for the parent, child, or family.

The major and minor characteristics of the diagnosis "parental role conflict" were developed primarily using samples of mothers. These criteria need to be validated with fathers because fathers are assuming more parenting tasks with their children. The findings from this study also suggest that additional nursing diagnoses related to parenting need to be developed. The parental vigilance and parental presence observed among these mothers suggest the possibility of additional diagnoses and related interventions for mothers with chronically ill children.

Clinical Implications

The findings from this study indicate that the day-to-day management of a child with a life-threatening chronic illness is much more complicated than the snapshot of management we see during an acute crisis or a brief outpatient encounter. Mothers experience many challenges in parenting their children and make many adaptations to the parental role. Nurses working with these mothers must be aware of the parents' experiences in parenting their child, the parenting styles assumed by these mothers, and the parental role changes the mothers have undergone. Furthermore, it is important to identify the impact of the expanded parental responsibilities on the entire family.

One approach is to use a nursing interview focused on parenting issues; this interview should allow the mother to "tell her story" about her experiences in parenting the child, to identify her unique approaches to parenting, and to tell the nurse about her needs. Periodic additional nursing assessments may be done using clinical logs, genograms, and computer-designed databases to track patterns of parental role changes in mothers of chronically ill children. This information can form the foundation for timely intervention at critical points during the trajectory of the child's illness. Our diagnoses and interventions with parents must reflect their own priorities, particularly as they seek to conserve their time and energy so they can meet all their family obligations and reduce role conflicts. Thus, planning for the child's care should be done in full partnership with parents.

Finally, nurses working with parents of seriously ill children need to be prepared for the challenging role they assume. Working with parents who are coping with difficult issues around the care and needs of a child with a life-threatening illness is complicated. Orientation programs, inservices, and nursing rounds should focus on both the responses and needs of parents and on approaches to helping them. These activities should be based on the latest literature on parenting—especially research and theoretical papers that advance knowledge. Research findings such as these must be disseminated and debated among nursing colleagues to advance knowledge in the area of parenting the chronically ill child.

REFERENCES

Anderson, J. M. (1981). The social construction of illness experience: Families with a chronically ill child. *Journal of Advanced Nursing, 6,* 427–434.

Anderson, J. M., & Elfert, H. (1989). Managing chronic illness in the family: Women as caretakers. *Journal of Advanced Nursing, 14,* 735–743.

Binger, C., Albin, A., & Feuerstein, R. (1969). Childhood leukemia: Emotional impact on patient and family. *New England Journal of Medicine, 280,* 414–418.

Burke, S. O., Kauffmann, E., Costello, E. A., & Dillon, M. C. (1991). Hazardous secrets and reluctantly taking charge: Parenting a child with repeated hospitalizations. *Image: Journal of Nursing Scholarship, 23,* 39–45.

Carpenito, L. J. (1989). *Nursing diagnosis: Application to clinical practice.* Philadelphia: J. B. Lippincott Co.

Carter, M., & Miles, M. S. (1989). The Parental Stressor Scale: Pediatric intensive care unit. *Maternal-Child Nursing Journal, 18,* 187–198.

Deatrick, J., Knafl, K., & Walsh, M. (1988). The process of parenting a child with a disability: Normalization through accommodations. *Journal of Advanced Nursing, 13,* 15–21.

Fife, B. L. (1978). Reducing parental overprotection of the leukemic child. *Social Science & Medicine, 12,* 117–122.

Glaser, H. H., Harrison, G. S., & Lynn D. B. (1964). Emotional implications of congenital heart disease in children. *Pediatrics, 31,* 367–379.

Knafl, K., & Deatrick, J. (1986). How families manage chronic conditions: An analysis of the concept of normalization. *Research in Nursing and Health, 9,* 215–222.

Krulik, T. (1980). Successful 'normalizing' tactics of parents of chronically ill children. *Journal of Advanced Nursing, 5,* 573–578.

Leal, C. A. (1983). Successful parenting in the black community. In V. J. Sasserath (Ed.), *Minimizing high-risk parenting* (pp. 11–16). Skillman, NJ: Johnson & Johnson.

Miles, M. S., & Carter, M. C. (1985). Coping strategies used by parents during their child's hospitalization in an intensive care unit. *Children's Health Care, 14,* 14–21.

Miles, M. S., Funk, S., & Carlson, J. (in press). The Parental Stressor Scale: Neonatal Intensive Care Unit. *Nursing Research.*

Miles, M. S., Nelson, A., Poprawa, C., & Cooper, H. (1991). *Stress and health in parents of children recently diagnosed with cancer.* Unpublished proposal.

Ray, L. (1988). *Parents' perceptions of coping with the burdensome home care of their chronically ill child.* Unpublished master's thesis, Dalhouse University, Halifax, Nova Scotia.

Ruddick, S. (1989). *Maternal thinking: Toward a politics of peace.* Boston: Beacon Press.

Seligman, M., & Darling, R. B. (1989). *Ordinary families, special children*. New York: Guilford Press.
Shapiro, J. (1983). Family reactions and coping strategies in response to the physically ill or handicapped child: A review. *Social Science & Medicine, 17*, 913–931.

[26]

Family Response to a Child's Chronic Illness: A Description of Major Defining Themes

Kathleen A. Knafl, Agatha M. Gallo, Bonnie J. Breitmayer, Linda H. Zoeller, and Lioness Ayres

> We're on a schedule. It's just like if you had to take a teaspoon of medicine or something. It's no big deal. Now that it's in control, it's like brushing your teeth or changing your shoes.
>
> Diabetes is a very big change. The average American family doesn't understand what diabetes is and that's why we're not the average American family. It's overwhelming. It affects everything even though you don't want it to. It controls your life.

Estimates of the prevalence of chronic illness in children vary depending on how chronic illness is defined and the methods used to collect prevalence data. Recent estimates based on data from the National Health Interview Survey (NHIS) suggest that 31% of children in the United States are affected by chronic illness (Newacheck & Taylor, 1992): 20% experience mild chronic conditions which do not limit their activities; 9% experience conditions of moderate severity, and 2% of children experience severe chronic conditions. The NHIS sample included 17,110 children and adolescents under the age of 18. A condition was considered to be chronic if it had an expected duration of over 3 months.

Most children with chronic illness are cared for at home by family members. However, few studies have examined how the family responds to a member's chronic illness. As the above quotations illustrate, this response can vary tremendously even among families experiencing the same illness. This chapter reports data from a study that used a grounded theory approach to characterize how families define and manage a child's chronic illness (Knafl, Breitmayer, Gallo, & Zoeller, 1987). Our interest in studying the family's subjective experience of chronic illness was spurred by Schwenk and Hughes's (1983) extensive review of the literature. They found that:

> The way in which the family perceived the illness or accident . . . was directly related to the eventual level of family stability and coping. Specific diseases appeared to cause no consistently predictable outcomes, and the actual level of prior family stability also seemed to have little predictive value. (p. 9)

The design of the study was guided by a conceptualization of the family's response to illness as a configuration formed by individual family members' definitions of their situation, their management behaviors, and the sociocultural context in which these occurred (Knafl & Deatrick, 1990). This chapter presents data on how parents viewed the child with a chronic illness, the illness, and the treatment regimen, as well as their parenting philosophy. We also provide case presentations to illustrate typical configurations of these themes in the families we studied.

METHOD

Sample

The study sample was composed of 63 families with a school-age child who had a chronic illness, defined as an illness with (1) a duration greater than 3 months, (2) a stable or progressive course, (3) a relatively normal life span despite impairment, and (4) a requirement of active management by family members to minimize serious consequences. In order to participate in the study, family members had to be English-speaking. The child with the chronic illness had to be between 7–14 years old and have no other major physical or mental impairments. Both parents (when available), the child with the chronic illness, and a well, school-age sibling were invited to participate in the research. Participation by at least one parent and the child with chronic illness was required for inclusion in the sample.

The 63 participating families were recruited from one central Illinois and two Chicago medical centers. The sample included 65 children (two families had two children with a chronic illness), 62 mothers, 55 fathers, and 28 well siblings. Twenty children from 19 families had been diagnosed for less than a year; the remainder had been diagnosed for more than 2 years. There were 35 children who had diabetes, 9 who had juvenile rheumatoid arthritis or ankylosing spondylitis, and 7 who had asthma; the remaining 14 had a variety of other illnesses cared for in specialty clinics. The families were diverse in demographic characteristics. Of the 55 families reporting annual household income, 6 reported a total income of less than $15,000 and 13 reported an income exceeding $50,000; 37% of the mothers and 34% of the fathers had a high school degree, and 19% of the mothers and 39% of the fathers had a college or postgraduate degree.

Procedure

Family members (parents, the child with chronic illness, and the well sibling) participated in two tape-recorded interviews conducted 12 months apart in the family's home. Family members were interviewed individually by research assistants who were graduate students in nursing. Interviews included a series of open-ended questions on how family members defined and managed their situation. Separate guides were developed for first- and second-year interviews with parents, the children with chronic illness, and siblings. The second-year interview guides focused on changes in the family's situation over the past year and themes which had been identified during preliminary analysis of the first interviews. In addition, family members completed several structured measures, including the Feetham Family Functioning Survey (FFFS) (Feetham, 1988)—completed by parents—and the Harter Self-Perception Profile (Harter, 1985)—completed by the child with chronic illness and the sibling.

The FFFS asks about the respondent's satisfaction with three aspects of family functioning: the relationship between the family and broader social units, the relationship between the family and its subsystems, and the relationship between the family and its individual members. It yields a discrepant score which is the difference between the actual amount of activity and the desired amount of activity. A higher discrepant score is indicative of greater dissatisfaction with family life. Each parent completed the FFFS. The Harter Self-Perception Profile (Harter, 1985) assesses children's self-perception across six areas of functioning: scholastic competence, social acceptance, athletic competence, physical appearance, behavioral conduct, and global self-worth. It was completed both by the child with chronic illness and by the well sibling.

All interviews were transcribed and coded using descriptive categories developed from a subset of interviews. In addition, detailed case summaries were completed for the family to gain a more integrated view of the family. Both coded data and case summaries were reviewed in order to identify themes characterizing families and family members' responses to illness.

RESULTS

Many families experience chronic illness as a manageable, taken-for-granted part of their everyday existence. However, for some families it is an enduring burden or tragedy that separates them from the mainstream of American family life. This section describes the different ways the parents in our sample defined their ill child and the illness, their parenting philosophy, and their view of the treatment regimen. Differences are outlined in Table 26.1.

Defining Themes

Parents were asked a number of questions about their image of the child. As shown in Table 26.1, parents were divided on how they viewed their

TABLE 26.1 Comparison of Mothers and Fathers across Defining Themes

	Percentage[a]	
Defining themes	Mothers	Fathers
View of child		
Normal	66	82
Not normal	34	18
View of illness		
Manageable condition	55	59
Ominous situation	38	32
Hateful restriction	5	5
Uninformed	2	5
Parenting philosophy		
Accommodative	72	75
Restrictive	13	14
Minimizing	2	9
Shifting	13	2
Treatment regimen management		
Confidence	60	66
Burden	36	9
"Not My Job"	4	25

[a]Percentages may not sum to 100 due to rounding.

child. Most continued to see the child as *normal* in spite of the illness; however, some parents who no longer viewed the child as normal described how in their mind the child had become either a tragic figure or a problem child. Parents who viewed their child as a *tragic figure* emphasized how his or her life chances had been irreparably compromised as a result of the illness. Parents who described a *problem child* noted how the illness had combined with other academic or behavioral problems to create a difficult parenting situation. Mothers were less likely than fathers to continue to define the child as normal. In only 6 of the 42 families (14%) in which both parents participated did the parents *disagree* in their view of the child.

Parents' beliefs about their child's illness included not only their technical understanding of the chronic illness but also their perceptions of the subjective experience of living with illness. Most parents described the illness as a *manageable condition* which could be accommodated without becoming the focus of family life. For these parents, life went on in spite of the illness, which typically was viewed as less serious than other chronic conditions. The possibility of future complications was downplayed in favor of emphasizing successful adaptation in the present. However, about one-third of both mothers and fathers saw the illness as an *ominous situation*. They emphasized the seriousness of the illness and the possibility of future complications. Many of these parents described themselves as successfully managing the illness, while still being fearful of the future. A few parents viewed the illness as a *hateful restriction*, something that significantly decreased the quality of their own life or the life of their child. These parents also stressed the serious nature of the illness, but their comments had an intensity not reflected in other illness views. They saw the illness as an enemy intruder who had invaded their home and diminished their chance for happiness. A small number of parents also indicated that they had a very *limited understanding* of the illness. There were no striking differences between the views of mothers as a group and fathers as a group. On the other hand, in 11 of the 42 couples (26%), parents had discrepant views of the illness.

Parents' ideas about parenting a child with a chronic illness reflected several distinct parenting philosophies. These philosophies included both parenting goals as well as strategies and behaviors parents used to implement the goals. Parents with an *accommodative* philosophy emphasized the importance of assuring a normal childhood for their offspring. This typically entailed encouraging the child to take part in usual school and extracurricular activities and making whatever arrangements might be needed to make such participation a reality. Other parents expressed a *restrictive* philosophy, which emphasized sheltering the child from possible harm rather than assuring participation in usual childhood activities. These parents described the importance of placing appropriate restrictions on their child and teaching the child to recognize the limitations imposed by the illness. In sharp contrast to the restrictive group, other parents *minimized* the seriousness of the illness and downplayed the necessity of making *any* accommodations to the treatment regimen. Finally, some parents could best be described as having a *shifting* or missing philosophy. Their comments about parenting the ill child contained conflicting, ambiguous descriptions of their goals and strategies. At one point in the interview they would espouse a restrictive philosophy; at another point they would express their commitment to an accommodative stance. Mothers were more likely to have a shifting philosophy than fathers, but there were no other major differences between mothers and fathers. Fourteen couples (32%) had discrepant parenting philosophies.

When discussing the child's treatment regimen and the ease or difficulty of managing the illness, most parents said illness management had become a routine part of family life and expressed *confidence* in their ability to carry out the treatment regimen and deal with unexpected situations or emergencies. Some parents, however, emphasized the difficulties they were experiencing in managing the illness. Their descriptions focused on their own sense of inadequacy as well as conflicts with the ill child over adherence to the treatment regimen. These parents viewed the treatment regimen as a *burden* which had not been integrated into the family's usual routine. Another group of parents, primarily fathers, viewed illness management as "*not my job.*" While they typically expressed confidence in their wife's management abilities, these fathers did not view themselves as sharing responsibility for illness management. As a group, mothers were considerably more likely to view the treatment regimen as a burden; fathers were more likely to see it as "not my job." Seventeen couples (42%) had discrepant views about the ease of managing the treatment regimen.

Case Illustrations of Defining Clusters

Through matrix display and analysis of our thematically coded data, we found that parents' views of the illness and treatment regimen and their parenting philosophy varied with their view of the ill child (Knafl, Gallo, Zoeller, Breitmayer, & Ayres, in press; Miles & Huberman, 1984). When both parents viewed their child as normal, they both also tended to view the illness as a manageable condition, to maintain an accommodative parenting philosophy, and to view the treatment regimen as a routinized component of family life which they were competent to manage. In contrast, when neither parent defined the child as normal, the parents tended to have a more negative view of other aspects of their situation. Such parents were more likely to view the illness as ominous or hateful, hold a restrictive or shifting parenting philosophy, and view the treatment regimen as a burden. Finally, parents who disagreed on their view of the child tended to disagree on the other defining themes. In these couples it was the mother who usually held the more negative view of the situation. These defining clusters are illustrated below by case presentations of three families in which the child had diabetes. We selected these families in order to highlight how the same disease can be experienced in very different ways by different families. (The names are all fictitious to preserve the families' anonymity.)

The Jordan Family: Both Parents View the Child as Normal Both Mr. and Mrs. Jordan defined their 12-year-old daughter Sarah, who had had diabetes for 4 years, as a normal adolescent. Mrs. Jordan said:

> I think a lot of how I feel about this has to do with who she is. If I were to come in and describe Sarah, I certainly would mention something about her having diabetes. But I don't know if that would be any more important than the fact that she is short and that she likes to read and dance and play baseball. It's just part of who she is; that's how she is.

Mr. Jordan's comments mirrored those of his wife. He, too, stressed how he saw diabetes as a relatively unimportant component of his daughter's identity:

> If somebody were to say, "Tell me about Sarah," I would never say that she has diabetes. I would say that she talks on the phone for thousands of hours, and she is a certain age, and she has brown hair, and she does certain kinds of things. I think that the diabetes would almost be an afterthought to me.

Consistent with their view of their child, these parents espoused an accommodative management philosophy in which they emphasized that diabetes had not altered their expectations of Sarah and there was no need to restrict her activities because of the illness. Mrs. Jordan said, "When I think about Sarah and how we are with her, the word determination comes to mind—determination that her life won't be different from her brother's and sister's lives." Mr. Jordan agreed with this view, saying, "Maybe her diabetes has become so normal to us that I just don't see how we could treat her differently. We don't think that she should be treated any differently." Both parents also viewed the illness as a manageable condition and felt confident of their ability to manage it. Both pointed out that over the years they had learned when they were capable of managing the illness on their own and when it was necessary to confer with a physician. Mrs. Jordan reported:

> On a day-to-day type of thing, it's just something that we have to do. I don't even think about it or spend a lot of time worrying about it. In the beginning I

> relied on the doctor for everything, but now I rely much more on what I know. I don't call the doctor unless she starts vomiting, and that makes me freaky.

While Mr. Jordan expressed some concern about future complications, he also viewed the illness as essentially manageable. He said:

> My wife and I don't really talk about it that much. My biggest worry is that with her getting it so young, it may affect her eyes. But that's not something we talk about a lot. We pretty much manage things on our own. If she's sick enough that it's affecting her diabetes, we consult with the doctor—like if she is 30 or 40 points out of whack.

As reflected in these quotations, this family took a stable, adaptive approach to the situation, which supported the integration of the illness into the parents' view of a normal life. The demands of the illness were accommodated without becoming the focus of the family.

The Williams Family: Neither Parent Views the Child as Normal Mr. and Mrs. Williams presented a very different view of family life with a child with diabetes. Their 11-year-old son James had had diabetes for most of his life, and both parents' descriptions of him were colored by a sense of tragedy. For example, Mrs. Williams said:

> He can do things the other kids can, but it's really hard for him. It's rough having to take a blood test twice a day and shots twice a day. That really hurts. It bothers him, too, when someone brings treats to school and he can't eat them, and that bothers me even more.

Mr. Williams' comments also stressed how difficult he believed it must be for his son to have diabetes: "It starts the day off. He has to do the blood test and the insulin, first thing. That's probably when I feel the most sorry for him. I shouldn't, but I do." Both these parents admitted to feeling sorry for their son, and their parenting philosophy reflected a restrictive stance. However, while they emphasized the need to protect James from further harm, they described efforts to indulge him as a way to compensate for the tragedy of his diabetes. For example, Mrs. Williams said:

> I guess I am over-protective of him. He probably should assume more responsibility for his care, but I just feel better about it if I do it. I think that I give him more attention than the others. You don't always realize it, but you do.

Mr. Williams pointed out that his son's illness had been an impetus for becoming more involved in his activities, such as Little League, as a way to assure his son's safety. Like his wife, he felt that he was more indulgent with James than his other children:

> I can say "no" to the other kids a lot easier than I can to him. It's just I feel guilt. I feel sorry for him. You know there are things that he can't have, so I just want him to have the things that he wants and he can have.

Not surprisingly, both these parents expressed an intense hatred of the illness. When asked what the word acceptance meant to her, Mrs. Williams said, "I accept it. I mean, I know that I have to deal with it, but I hate it. I really do. I envy other people who have kids that are happy. I really do." Mr. Williams said that he and his wife avoided talking about the long-term complications of diabetes because such discussions usually ended with both of them in tears. When asked if he thought he had accepted the illness, he said, "It's a forced acceptance. I don't think that I have totally accepted it. I'm pretty mad that he has it—mad at the world in general." Both these parents also described the treatment regimen as a burden. Mrs. Williams described treatment as a "constant worry." Mr. Williams questioned his ability to manage the illness and described the agonizing self-doubts he experienced:

> The other night he said that he was going to have a big dinner but ended up having a small one. You always worry then about the dosage. I was awake that night worrying if he was going to be all right. That happens about once a week. I ended up having a terrible night's sleep over it.

Unlike the previous family, diabetes was very much in the foreground of family life for these parents. It colored their view of their child and their approach to parenting. For both of them it was a constant source of worry, sadness, and burdensome responsibility. Moreover, they appeared less confident of their views and their approach to managing the illness than the previous family. This self-doubt was reflected in comments such as, "I really shouldn't feel this way," scattered throughout the interviews. Such comments suggest that these parents were critical of both their views and their behaviors.

The Armstrong Family: Parents Have a Discrepant View of the Child Bill Armstrong was 8 years old at the time of the first interview and had been diagnosed with diabetes for 3 years. Mr. Armstrong stressed how normal his son was, saying, "I'm not going to put any kind of self-pity on him. I don't baby him or anything. There's no reason to." On the other hand, Mrs. Armstrong pointed out many things in her son's life that were "not like a normal kid." Her view of Bill was further reflected in her descriptions of her restrictive parenting philosophy. She was quite protective of Bill. For example, she went on most class field trips and to birthday parties with Bill because she would be "worried sick" if she didn't. In contrast, Mr. Armstrong said that Bill's diabetes had not changed his ideas about being a parent. On the other hand, he did concede that:

> You've got to keep after him. But I don't take anything from him. Sometimes he complains about how I give the shot, but I tell him, "Look, if I'm going to give the shot, I'm just going to do it." I don't worry about asking his preferences any more.

In contrast to his wife, Mr. Armstrong was very matter-of-fact about his parenting philosophy. He saw himself as doing what needed to be done to manage this illness but did not see the diabetes as influencing his overall view of parenting. At one point in the interview he summed up his position, saying, "You know what you have to do to arrest this disease and you do it." These parents also held rather discrepant views of the illness. It was difficult for Mrs. Armstrong not to dwell on negative aspects of the illness and her fears of future complications. She said:

> I pray, and I ask God just to get me through this day. I try to keep myself busy so I don't sit there and think about it. If I did, I would crack up. I think that my biggest fear is that he will be blind. I would crack up over that.

Her very conscious efforts not to be overwhelmed by her fears of what might lie ahead stood in sharp contrast to her husband's view of the illness. After saying that he had accepted his son's diabetes, he spent a great deal of time discussing how difficult the situation had been for his wife. "My wife can tell you what she wants, but I don't think she ever really accepted this. She's not the same since this happened. I don't think that the total initial shock has ever left her." The implication of many of his remarks was that in contrast to his wife, he dealt with the illness situation very well. Mr. Armstrong was confident of his ability to manage the illness. For example, at one point in the interview he provided four pages of detailed examples of all the "tricks of the trade" he had learned over the years to manage his son's illness. In contrast, Mrs. Armstrong emphasized the uncertainty of managing her son's diabetes and her lack of confidence in her management abilities. She said:

> It's like you don't know what to do. It's like you are always thinking about it when you are grocery shopping—worrying about what to buy and what's he going to eat. It's like when we go out to eat, what are all the equivalents? What's he going to be able to eat?

Their son's illness was a very different experience for Mr. and Mrs. Armstrong. Their differing views of their child were reflected in differing parenting philosophies and different views of the illness and treatment regimen. Although they recognized their differing views, each also acknowledged that the spouse's view was neither entirely understood nor supported.

Comparison of Defining Clusters

These three defining clusters were seen in a variety of chronic illnesses. While our case examples compared three families in which a child had diabetes, in the overall sample, children whose parents viewed them as normal had very different chronic illnesses, including diabetes, lupus, asthma, juvenile rheumatoid arthritis, and renal disease. Children whose parents viewed them as a tragic figure or a problem also had different illnesses—diabetes, juvenile rheumatoid arthritis, renal disease, scleroderma, and asthma. The number of children in the sample with each illness was small (except diabetes), so making comparisons is difficult, but there appeared to be *no* clear relationship between the child's diagnosis and the parent's view of the child. It is interesting to note, however, that five of the six couples with a discrepant view of the child had a child with diabetes.

It is also of interest that parents in different defining clusters differed in their perception of the impact of the illness on their family life and their satisfaction with family life, as measured by the Feetham Family Functioning Survey (FFFS). Couples who defined their child as normal minimized the impact of the illness on their family life. For example, Mrs. Jordan described the impact of her daughter's diabetes:

> We have adjusted very well. We were determined that things were going to fit in and that this wasn't going to be a problem. I think we just have a philosophy that it's not going to change anything. We just incorporated it and I think we do well.

Mr. Jordan also minimized the impact of his daughter's illness. He said, "I don't see it as having any effect. We are a really close family. I don't see any big change in our lives because of this." In contrast, the Williams family, who did not view their child as normal, believed their child's illness had had a major impact on their family life. Mrs. Williams described this impact as something that had brought her and her husband closer as a couple:

> I think we're closer as a couple because we discuss this so much. It's not that we argue about it or blame each other for this, we try to handle it together. Every day after the kids go to bed, we spend half an hour or so talking about it and trying to figure out what to do.

Mr. Williams described a different kind of impact on his family. He thought the illness had introduced a level of tension into family relationships that would not have been there otherwise. He said, "I think there is a tension that comes with an illness. There is a tendency for things to be blown out of proportion." For these parents there was a clear sense of being a different family as a result of the illness.

The Armstrongs, who had different views of their child, also had different views of the impact of the illness. Although Mrs. Armstrong described the impact thus: "We always have to be around and be available, about three-fourths of my life revolves around it," her husband maintained, "We do what we are supposed to do. I don't classify it as a burden or anything." At the same time, both Mr. and Mrs. Armstrong described how their differing views had imposed an added stress on their marital relationship.

Considering the sample as a whole, parents in the three defining clusters differed on the FFFS. On this scale a lower score reflects greater satisfaction with family life. When both mothers and fathers viewed the child as normal, mothers had an average discrepant score of 19.1. In contrast, the average score was 33.3 for mothers when both they and the fathers viewed the child as not normal, and 31.6 for mothers whose view of the child differed from that of the father. Analysis of variance (ANOVA) revealed significant differences among these three groups [$F(2,35) = 3.75, p < .05$]. Post hoc analysis of these differences using Fisher's Least Significant Differences method indicated that mothers who viewed their child as not normal, or who held a different view of the child from the husband, differed significantly on their satisfaction with family life from those who viewed the child as normal. For fathers, those who, along with the mother, viewed their child as normal had an average score of 21.7, while those who viewed the child as not normal (along with the mother) had an average score of 34.7. Those fathers whose view of the child differed from the mother had an average score of 30.0 [$F(2,37) = 3.05, p < .06$]. Post hoc analysis of the results of the ANOVA indicated significant differences between those fathers who viewed the child as normal and those who viewed the child as not normal. Those fathers whose view of the child differed from that of the mother did not differ significantly from either fathers who viewed the child as normal or fathers who viewed the child as not normal.

Children's self-perception also varied across the three groups. Based on a rating scale of 1–4, children whose parents viewed them as normal had an average Global Self Worth score of 3.5; those whose parents viewed them as not normal had a average score of 2.9. Children whose parents held discrepant views had average Global Self Worth scores of 3.7. Interestingly, all the children in this latter group had one parent who continued to see the child as normal. Analysis of variance indicated significant differences between these groups [$F(2,37) = 6.54, p < .01$], and further analysis indicated that children whose mothers *and* fathers viewed them as *not* normal had significantly *lower* scores on the Global Self Worth scale of the Self-Perception Profile than either children whose parents viewed them as normal or whose parents had discrepant views.

DISCUSSION

Parents' views of the illness situation as reflected in the defining themes and clusters we have described provide a perspective for examining the illness experience from a family's point of view. These themes may be considered "windows of opportunity" for developing productive working relationships with families and for helping to shape definitions of the situation that simultaneously support appropriate illness care, family members' well-being, and family functioning.

These data support the importance of understanding parents' definitions of the illness situation, for these definitions provide insights into the functioning of the family unit and family members. The data also suggest the various ways in which illness control, treatment regimen, and disease course are interpreted and the different meanings they have for parents. The parents' view of the child seems an especially useful way to understand their experience of the child's illness because it is linked to how the parents view the illness, their parenting philosophy, and their view of the treatment regimen. It is also a fairly easy dimension to assess. We directly engaged parents in a discussion of whether they thought it was desirable and possible to treat their ill child normally. In the clinical setting such an approach would suggest openness and acceptance of the parents' viewpoint without cutting off the possibility of working to reshape that view in a more positive direction.

In addition to questioning mothers and fathers about their individual views of the situation, there are numerous standardized instruments available for measuring various aspects of family functioning and coping. Speer and Sachs (1985) summarized a number of such instruments they judged to be of particular relevance to nursing, and Grotevant and Carlson (1989) compiled a broad array of family assessment tools. Readers interested in considering a more formalized assessment of the families with whom they work are referred to these sources.

In general, an understanding of the parents' stance provides an important foundation for individualizing interactions and interventions, *not* just to the disease/illness but to the family's experience of the illness. These data highlight the hazards of assuming one parent is representing the *family* viewpoint and the importance of assessing each parent's view of the situation. Spouses' rate of disagreement ranged from 14% on their view of the child to 42% on their view of the treatment regimen. Moreover, the nature of these differences suggests that mothers are more likely to have a negative view of the situation. Today in nursing there is tremendous interest in viewing the family as the primary unit of care. Although we wholeheartedly support this family focus, we believe that it should not overshadow the importance of individual family members. We agree with Ransom, Fisher, Phillips, Kokes, and Weiss (1990): "It seems that to gaze at the [family] 'system' makes it easy to forget a most interesting and inescapable feature of a family: the individuals who make it up" (p. 63).

REFERENCES

Feetham, S. (1988). *Feetham Family Functioning Survey.* (Available from Suzanne Feetham, National Center for Nursing Research, Washington, DC.)

Grotevant. H., & Carlson, C. (1989). *Family assessment: A guide to methods and measures.* New York: Guilford.

Harter, S. (1985). *Manual for Self-Perception Profile for Children.* Denver: University of Denver.

Knafl, K., Breitmayer, B., Gallo, A., & Zoeller, L. (1987). *How families define and manage a child's chronic illness.* Unpublished grant proposal (NCNR, Public Health Service Grant #NR01594).

Knafl, K. A., & Deatrick, J. A. (1990). Family management style: Concept analyses and development. *Journal of Pediatric Nursing, 5,* 4–14.

Knafl, K., Gallo, G., Zoeller, L., Breitmayer, B., & Ayres, L. (1993). One approach to conceptualize family response to chronic illness. In S. Feetham, J. Bell, S. Meister, & C. Gilliss (Eds.), *Advances in nursing of families* (Vol. 2) (pp. 70–78). Newbury Park, CA: Sage.

Miles, M., & Huberman, M. (1984). *Qualitative data analysis: A sourcebook of new methods.* Newbury Park, CA: Sage.

Newacheck, P., & Taylor, W. (1992). Childhood chronic illness: Prevalence, severity, and impact. *American Journal of Public Health, 82,* 364–371.

Ransom, D., Fisher, L., Phillips, S., Kokes, R., & Weiss, R. (1990). The logic of measurement in family research. In T. W. Draper & A. C. Marcos (Eds.), *Family variables: Conceptualization, measurement, and use* (pp. 48–63). Newbury Park, CA: Sage.

Schwenk, T., & Hughes, C. (1983). The family as patient in family medicine: Rhetoric or reality. *Social Science & Medicine, 17,* 1–16.

Speer, J., & Sachs, B. (1985). Selecting the appropriate family assessment tool. *Pediatric Nursing, 11,* 349–355.

[27]

Quality of Life and Family Relationships in Families Coping with Their Child's Chronic Illness

Becky J. Christian

Chronic illness was once lethal during childhood, but technological advances in health care have increased the child's life span. As a result, children and their families are confronted with managing, coping, and adjusting to the chronic illness over an extended period (Thompson, 1985). Home care for the chronically ill child is generally more cost-effective than institutional care, since the family provides the majority of care services (Texas Senate Committee on Health & Human Services, 1989). Moreover, continuity of services and stabilization of the chronic illness trajectory result when the home becomes the center of care (Strauss & Corbin, 1988). Therefore, with appropriate assistance, home care may be as effective as a hospital in promoting the child's health and quality of life over the long-term chronic illness trajectory (Congress of the United States, Office of Technology Assessment, 1987).

However, chronic illness in a child makes heavy demands on the family system and requires family members to make permanent sacrifices (Griffin, 1980). Regardless of the particular diagnosis, the family must adapt to the child's illness. First, family members are challenged to learn about the nature of the illness and home management. Second, they must provide a network of support, readjust role functions, promote coping strategies, and develop resources, while maintaining relationships among family members. Finally, the family must establish an environment that facilitates growth and change within the family system. Managing both illness and home can overwhelm family caregivers, causing them to feel stretched to the limits of energy and tolerance (Strauss et al., 1984). Thus, realistic appraisal of the challenges and care needs of vulnerable families faced with home management of their child's care is needed.

Clearly the most important issue for the family of a chronically ill child is how to achieve a satisfactory quality of life, or overall sense of life satisfaction and well-being (Lubkin, 1986). The purpose of this study, therefore, was to explore parents' perceptions of the impact of the child's chronic illness on family relationships, family coping, and satisfaction with quality of life.

METHOD

Sample

This was part of a larger descriptive correlational study of 55 families with chronically ill children between the ages of 4 and 12 years diagnosed with insulin-dependent diabetes mellitus, juvenile rheumatoid arthritis, or spina bifida. The sample was obtained from the list of chronically ill children followed by the outpatient care services programs at a Children's Hospital in a Southwestern city. Families were given a questionnaire to be completed independently by both parents or other caregivers. Semi-structured interviews were conducted with a subset of 11 families (n = 5 insulin-dependent diabetes mellitus, n = 3 juvenile rheumatoid arthritis, n = 3 spina bifida), using open-ended questions to clarify perceptions about the impact of the child's chronic illness on the family and how the family managed the child's care at home. The mean age of the chronically ill children was 8.3 years, while the mean age of both mothers and fathers was 35 years. All of the parents were married, and both parents were employed. Ten of the families were Caucasian and one was Hispanic. Only the findings from the 11 families interviewed are reported here.

Instruments

The Family Concerns Interview is a semi-structured interview composed of open-ended questions designed to clarify parent perceptions of the impact of a child's chronic illness on the family and the quality of life. Seventeen open-ended questions were developed by the investigator to examine five areas of interest: 1) family life and chronic illness; 2) management of the child's care; 3) social support and resources; 4) coping strategies; and 5) health care services. The parent interviews lasted approximately 1 to 2 hours and were conducted in the family's home and tape recorded for verbatim transcription.

RESULTS

The constant comparative method was used to analyze data from the interviews. Efforts to reframe the impact of the child's chronic illness on the family's quality of life, and attempts to control the family environment were the predominant themes.

Controlling the Child's Chronic Illness

Families who participated in this study described the impact of the child's chronic illness on the family as a process of "shifting gears" that required changing perceptions, changing priorities and, ultimately, changing family life-style. When their child had a chronic illness, families were overwhelmed with managing and learning to care for the child. Moreover, the child's chronic illness threatened family functioning. In order to survive this transition, families reframed their perceptions of life. Their quality of life reflected these efforts to reframe the environment to create a sense of health and well-being. Moreover, the family had to reframe perspectives across three levels or contexts: individual, family, and environment.

The families' reframing task involved moving beyond parenting to learn how to provide care for their child with a chronic illness. To this end, the families' energy became focused on maintaining family health by controlling the individual members, the family system, and the environment. Not only did families describe events in terms of controlling the child's illness and preventing complications, but they also were concerned about normalizing attitudes and perceptions, controlling time and managing schedules, as well as coordinating care and gaining access to systems. Their feelings of loss of control (Dimond & Jones, 1983; Lubkin, 1986) and powerlessness (Miller, 1983) were typical of the responses of individuals with a chronic illness. Specific aspects of controlling were minimizing, normalizing, balancing, managing, and advocating.

Minimizing Families sought to control the situation by minimizing the severity of the child's chronic illness or ignoring problems. In fact, some families were convinced that although their child had been diagnosed with a chronic illness, the child was "essentially well." For example, the mother of a diabetic noted:

> It just doesn't seem like a big deal to us, especially because she does everything herself. It is just something that has to be done and she is not ill. So, it really does not affect us negatively in any way because it is not like I have to deal with anything.

When describing the impact of the child's juvenile rheumatoid arthritis on the family, one mother explained:

> I think at times there is a lot of stress, but you kind of get used to it and work through it. You've got to take things and make it work.

Thus, families minimized the changes they had undertaken to cope with the impact of the chronic illness (Hymovich & Hagopian, 1992). Essentially, these families reframed the situation to gain control over their lives.

Normalizing Even individual and family attitudes and perceptions were controlled. Contact was limited with extended family if they did not accept the child as "just like any other child." Deliberate attempts were made to prevent the child's disease from becoming the central focus of family life. Many families described the chronic illness as just a "normal part of life." Explaining how their family maintained a sense of normalcy, the mother of a child with juvenile rheumatoid arthritis summarized it thus:

> I guess we decided a long time ago to let some things go. Conventional things, like neatness. You just can't do it all. You can't, so we decided that raising our children and spending time with them was really important to us. . . . So, weekends are sort of mini relief valves, in that we just decide to let a lot of the other things go.

Parents were upset about the school system treating the child "differently." The mother of a diabetic explained:

> They can be just like any other children. They can do anything that anybody else does and they have feelings just like everybody else. Don't make them feel different.

Normalization has been widely reported as a method families use to accommodate a child's chronic illness and promote the child's development (Deatrick, Knafl, & Walsh, 1988; Holaday, 1984; Knafl & Deatrick, 1986; Strauss et al., 1984). These families controlled the child's chronic illness by making it a part of their lives and recognizing that they could manage even if they were overwhelmed.

Balancing All families were overwhelmed by the demands of caring for a child with a chronic illness. The central question was how to balance the care needs of the child with the needs of the family and the other individuals within the family. Prime concerns were managing time, establishing a routine, and juggling activities. In an effort to control the overload, families described numerous attempts to establish a routine schedule. For example, the mother of a child with spina bifida explained it this way:

> I think we just try to balance everything out so that . . . if financially things are tough, you try to not do without everything, you know, or try to just take advantage of different things and that sort of thing. Keep a routine.

Although these routines helped families manage time better, they provided organization at the expense of personal time. The balancc between rigidity and flexibility was a constant interplay and affected family functioning. The importance of flexibility in coping with family stress has been documented (McCubbin, 1989). These families identified the importance of "always being prepared" and "being flexible." The father of one diabetic child said:

> Time management is probably the most difficult thing to deal with. Managing your time and your schedule, having to make sacrifices of individual time and family time. Having to deal with it.

Several family members even carried beepers so they could be instantly in control of any situation and were "continuously on call." Many families explained that they were "postponing" their lives and described the personal "sacrifices" they had made. All families identified how they had changed their priorities in their lives.

Managing In order to maintain a satisfactory level of care, families must learn to coordinate services with the health care system, school system, and insurance industry. Families select a management style based on how they define significant events and manage their daily lives, and depending on how the sociocultural context influences the situation (Knafl & Deatrick, 1990). Moreover, the time demands of trying to interface with each of these systems can be overwhelming. Many families in this study felt that they could not trust the school, day care, or respite care to provide appropriate care for their child. Thus, they would periodically "check in" to find out about the condition of their child.

Not only must the family control the child's care, but they must also control family life, the work environment, community and financial resources, and access to the school system, health care system, and the insurance industry. One family of a child with spina bifida described the most important thing that was helpful to them:

> Just mainly to have a routine and try to periodically sit back and evaluate and look and see what should you be doing that would be an improvement. Of course, that is restricted by the resources that you have to use. But, just try to make it through the day the best you can.

For these families, lack of time and learning how to prioritize needs and work together were the central issues facing them. Interestingly, parent perceptions of spouse concerns about the child's chronic illness were more important to the family's adaptation than perceptions of health professionals about family adaptation (Christian, 1989).

Advocating Conflict occurs when families confront systems in attempting to gain access to them or to control the services that the child needs. Learning to access the health care system was one of the major themes in this study. This was important not only to maintain the child's health, but also to obtain appropriate services. In order for the school to manage a diabetic child's diet, several parents either prepared all the child's meals themselves or they taught the dietician how to prepare the child's diet. One mother of a child with juvenile rheumatoid arthritis, frustrated by the family's difficulty in convincing the school system of her daughter's care needs, described the situation in this way:

> At school, she cannot get around very well at all. So, I have to go up there for a lot of things. I have to drag both boys with me because we can't afford a sitter at this point in time. Take them both up there with me and do whatever she needs done because it is not provided. I still have to make sure that she is getting what she needs.

Many families believed that the insurance industry created unnecessary barriers to care. Whether the barriers involved increased financial demands or continuing coverage, the struggle was constant. In fact, those who were health conscious or who participated in health-promoting activities were penalized for behaviors that would provide long-term cost savings. The mother of a child with spina bifida expressed her dissatisfaction with the health care system and insurance industry in this way:

> We have paid out tens of thousands of our own money, as well as what the insurance has paid. But, I think that the focus is not enough on preventive measures that you take. To me, we have been penalized because we take care of our equipment and we take care of our jobs. . . . I think that the health care industry needs restructuring.

Clearly, families of children with chronic illness are concerned about controlling the quality of their lives. Minimizing the demands of the child's illness serves to decrease the impact of the chronic illness. Normalizing allows families to control the changes in their lives. Balancing provides families a way to maintain stability in family functioning. Managing care activities allows families to coordinate their lives and schedules. Advocating provides families a way to confront the system. In these ways, families maintain the quality of their lives by reframing the family's health.

DISCUSSION

Analysis of these family interviews indicates that when a child is diagnosed with a chronic illness, the family is confronted with a crisis. This crisis challenges the family to adapt to the situation. The family has lost control of every aspect of their lives. In order to function effectively, the family must regain control. Moreover, the family of a chronically ill child must reframe the situation to survive. Reframing family health captures the process of change and adaptation that the family undergoes.

Implications for Practice

Identifying the process of reframing family health is central to understanding the effect of the child's chronic illness on the family. It explains why some families adapt to the illness better than others. The more families are able to control their lives, the better their response to the child's chronic illness. It is critical for nurses who care for families and children with chronic illness to understand how families reframe their lives to accommodate the new demands of the illness. With this knowledge, nurses can play a vital role in the family's successful adaptation. Just as families must reframe the quality of their lives, so must nurses reframe their approach to families of children with chronic illness. We must learn why some families are not adapting successfully to the child's chronic illness, and take steps to help them.

Strategies to Enhance Family Health

All families have the capacity to achieve a positive outcome in adapting to the child's chronic illness, even when the barriers appear insurmountable. Nurses must accept some of the blame for the inability of families to manage the child's chronic illness. We must ask ourselves what barriers we impose on families. We must consider how we control families to meet the needs of the health care system.

Nursing strategies to enhance family health require that nurses change their priorities and reframe their own nursing practice. We must consider whether we act as advocates for the family's health. We must teach families not only how to care for their child, but also how to teach their families, friends, and schools about the child's care. We must give families control over the management of their child's health. This means that health care providers must trust the family to really direct the child's care: We must trust the family's intuition and vigilance; we must trust the family's cry for our help; we must care enough to listen. It is our responsibility to link families with other families, not only for the support they can provide, but also for the management techniques they can share. It is only with this shared commitment that families can learn to balance the demands of the illness and manage time.

We must challenge families to become their own advocates for family health. In order to be successful advocates, families need to know what they need. It is our responsibility to teach families what their rights are. We all teach families about available resources, but we also need to teach them how to ask for what they want and need. We need to teach them how to access community services; and how to confront the school system, the health care system, and the insurance industry. We must also be willing to assist them to interface with these systems and intervene if necessary.

It is imperative that nurses intervene with families. Nurses can enhance family health by teaching families how to live with the child's chronic illness and maintain a satisfying quality of life. Sustaining a family environment that is supportive of individual family members, family relationships, and the family unit is vital to the family and their adaptation to the child's chronic illness.

ACKNOWLEDGMENT

The author gratefully acknowledges the assistance of the following graduate research assistants in this study: Deborah Bechtel, MSN, RN; Deborah Northrup, MSN, RN; Maureen O'Brien, MSN, RN; Deborah Wymer, BSN, RN; and Eva Nystrom, BSN, RN. This study was supported in part by grants from The University Research Institute at The University of Texas at Austin and by the Ed and Molly Smith Fellowship in Nursing.

REFERENCES

Christian, B. J. (1989). *Family adaptation to childhood chronic illness: Family coping style, family relationships, and family coping status—implications for nursing*. Unpublished doctoral dissertation, The University of Texas at Austin.

Congress of the United States, Office of Technology Assessment. (1987). *Technology-dependent children: Hospital vs. home care* (#87–13362). Washington, DC: Office of Technology Assessment.

Deatrick, J., Knafl, K., & Walsh, M. (1988). The process of parenting a child with a disability: Normalization through accommodations. *Journal of Advanced Nursing, 13*, 15–21.

Dimond M., & Jones, S. (1983). *Chronic illness across the life span*. Norwalk, CT: Appleton-Century-Crofts.

Griffin, J. (1980). Physical illness in the family. In J. R. Miller & E. Janosik (Eds.), *Family-focused care* (pp. 245–268). New York: McGraw-Hill.

Holaday, B. (1984). Challenges of rearing a chronically ill child. *Nursing Clinics of North America, 19*(2), 361–368.

Hymovich, D. P., & Hagopian, G. A. (1992). *Chronic illness in children and adults: A psychosocial approach*. Philadelphia: Saunders.

Knafl, K. A., & Deatrick, J. A. (1986). How families manage chronic conditions: An analysis of the concept of normalization. *Research in Nursing and Health, 9*, 215–222.

Knafl, K. A., & Deatrick, J. A. (1990). Family management style: Concept analysis and development. *Journal of Pediatric Nursing, 5*, 4–14.

Lubkin, I. (1986). *Chronic illness: Impact and interventions*. Boston: Jones & Bartlett.

McCubbin, M. (1989). Family stress and family strengths: A comparison of single- and two-parent families with handicapped children. *Research in Nursing and Health, 12*, 101–110.
Miller, J. (1983). Epilogue. In J. F. Miller (Ed.), *Coping with chronic illness: Overcoming powerlessness* (pp. 301–304). Philadelphia: Davis.
Strauss, A., Corbin, J., Fagerhaugh, S., Glaser, B., Maines, D., Suczek, B., & Wiener, C. (1984). *Chronic illness and the quality of life*. St. Louis: Mosby.
Strauss, A., & Corbin, J. (1988). *Shaping a new health care system: The explosion of chronic illness as a catalyst for change*. San Francisco: Jossey-Bass.
Texas Senate Committee on Health & Human Services. (1989). *The needs of medically fragile and chronically ill children and their families* (Staff Report). Austin, TX: Author.
Thompson, R. (1985). Coping with the stress of chronic childhood illness. In A. O'Quinn (Ed.), *Management of chronic disorders of childhood* (pp. 11–41). Boston: G. K. Hall Medical Publishers.

[28]

Impact of Childhood Cancer on Families at Home

Ida M. Martinson

In the United States approximately 6,550 children under 15 years of age are newly diagnosed each year as having cancer (Miller, 1989). Although science cannot yet prevent childhood cancers, in recent years it has changed the trajectory of the illness dramatically. The diagnosis of cancer is no longer a death sentence; indeed, the life expectancy of children with cancer has increased 50%–90% (Foley & Whittam, 1990). However, although the mortality rate has decreased, lengthy treatment regimens, often accompanied by multiple complications, make childhood cancer a chronic disease requiring assessment and treatment over many years. Most of the time the child's treatment is at home, with limited time being spent in the hospital.

The magnitude of the illness experienced by children with cancer and the effects of this illness on the child's parents and siblings warrant serious concern. The purpose of the investigation reported here was to extend our knowledge about the impact of cancer on the child, the parents, and the healthy siblings through an examination of longitudinal data on 40 families. The specific aims were to:

1. describe the impact of childhood cancer on the child at diagnosis;
2. describe the impact of childhood cancer on the family at the time of diagnosis and afterward (up to 5 years);
3. describe the impact of childhood cancer on healthy siblings.

METHOD

Forty families entered the study consecutively over a 12-month period. Though the sample was not random, all but five families who were asked to participate in the study did so. Therefore, the sample approximated all cases of childhood cancer diagnosed at a major cancer center during a 1-year period. All families were invited to participate during the child's initial hospitalization at the center.

After giving written consent, one or both parents were interviewed about their experiences during the diagnostic phase of the child's illness. When the ill child was older than 4 years, he or she also was interviewed. All interviews were semi-structured. At the first interview, parents were also asked to complete the Symptom Checklist 90 Revised (SCL-90-R) (Derogatis, 1983), and ill children were asked to complete the Thematic Apperception Test (TAT) (Murray, 1943).

The SCL-90-R has been used to measure current psychological symptom status in a broad array of clinical and medical contexts (Derogatis, 1983). It is considered a particularly good indicator of responses to the kind of distress expected when a child is diagnosed with cancer. The SCL-90-R is a self-administered paper-and-pencil inventory that can be scored and interpreted on nine primary symptom dimensions and three global indices of distress. Each of the 90 symptom-associated items is rated on a 5-point scale of distress, ranging from "not at all" to "extremely." The current revised version of the SCL-90 has good internal consistency (.77–.90) and good 1-week test-retest reliability (.78–.90) (Derogatis, 1983). Published evidence supports its criterion validity, and concurrent validity has been established through comparisons with other similar instruments, including the Minnesota Multiphasic Inventory (Derogatis, 1983).

The TAT is a projective test developed by Murray (1943) that involves presentation of a series of pictures with ambiguous content; subjects' responses reveal information about their emotions and needs, conscious or unconscious. Interpretation of the TAT is subjective, and validity is always open to question. The same is true of interviews. However, objectivity is maintained by eliciting standard material, by limiting the field of observation, by recording all responses, and by using a quantitative scoring system.

In this study data collection was repeated annually, in the home, until the child's death or the end of the 5 years of the study. Healthy siblings were interviewed at these annual contacts. If a child died, the family was visited within 1 month of the death and participated in a semi-structured interview on their postdeath experiences; parents again completed the SCL-90-R at that time. Data collection was repeated for these families at 6 months after the death of the child and then annually up to the end of the 5-year study. All interviews were audio taped.

RESULTS

For preliminary analysis of the family data, 10 families were selected from the larger cohort, 5 with living children and 5 with deceased children, in order to identify similarities and differences in the families' experiences and responses. For analyses of children's responses, 13 children with cancer were selected from the larger sample, and 22 siblings were selected from 18 families of children with cancer.

In the family subsample, mothers were 21 to 45 years old and fathers were 25 to 47 years old. All but one mother had completed high school and two were college graduates. All fathers had some college education, and 6 were college graduates. Initial analysis focused on identifying the ways in which these 10 families perceived, interpreted, and responded to childhood cancer, beliefs that guided or evolved from their experience, and the meaning the families attached to the long-term survival or death of the child. The themes that emerged from their interviews and family histories were unpreparedness, information needs, dependence on the medical center, growing dissatisfaction with the quality and quantity of information, home, normalization, taking one day at a time, fear of coming home, ambiguity, fear of recurrence, relief through death, relinquishing and reclaiming control, self-determination, social stigma, anniversaries of stressful times, vulnerability, new understandings and changing values, and symbols and rituals as coping strategies (Martinson & Cohen, 1988). Characteristics of these themes are summarized in Table 28.1.

We had predeath and postdeath scores on the SCL-90 for six families.[1] In five of the six families, the predeath total SCL-90 scores were higher than

[1]A pre-death SCL-90 was available for a sixth family and thus was included in the analysis.

TABLE 28.1 Family Themes and Their Characteristics

Theme	Characteristic
Unpreparedness	While parents had realized that something was wrong, they were unprepared for the seriousness of the cancer diagnosis.
Initial relinquishing of control	The parents, in attempting to cope, relinquished all control over the medical situation and wanted to provide comfort, food, and social experiences for their child.
Initial need for information was satisfied	Basically the parents were pleased with the honesty at the time of diagnosis as well as the manner in which the information was given.
Strategies for managing probabilistic information	The likelihood of their child's survival was expressed in terms of probability, which was interpreted by different families as either reassuring or threatening, independently of the actual risk quoted.
Fears about bringing the child home	The experience of bringing the patient home from the hospital for the first time after diagnosis was frightening for many of the families.
The need to normalize family life	The parents were eager to restore prediagnosis routines and relationships as soon as possible. Many families followed the health care professionals' recommendation to adopt the attitude of one-day-at-a-time. This allowed them to function during the most stressful times.
Dependence on the medical center	As time evolved, the families relied more and more on the expertise of the medical treatment center rather than relying on the competence of their local physician.
Reclaiming of control	Parents later in the course of treatment reclaimed control and became assertive advocates for their child.
Fear of a recurrence	Stress continued for the families whose child had survived. The fear increased at routine follow-up appointments or when symptoms of any illness appeared, no matter how minor.
Dissatisfaction with information as death approached	As the child's condition deteriorated, parents became more dissatisfied with the information provided to them by health care professionals.
Relief through death	The parental grief over the loss of their child was mixed with a sense of relief from the daily stresses of the illness.
Use of symbols and rituals to cope with illness and death	Sunsets were noted at the time of death, and the release of balloons at the funeral was noted as especially meaningful for family members.
Anniversaries of stressful time	If the child had died, the date of the death and the child's birthday were times of increased sense of loss. If these dates were around a holiday, the feelings of loss and depression occurred in spite of the happiness of the holiday. If the child had survived, the date of diagnosis was remembered and became a milestone in stacking odds in the child's favor.
Fear that a sibling would develop cancer	With any symptom of illness in another sibling, cancer was immediately feared.
Difficulty managing the responses of siblings	Not all parents were sensitive to the needs and responses of siblings related to the patient's illness and treatment.

TABLE 28.2 Means of Predeath and Postdeath Total SCL-90 Scores by Family

	Total score[a]	
Family	Predeath	Postdeath
01	61.0	59.0
02	30.0	12.0
03	15.0	12.0
04	23.3	32.0
05	16.6	4.3
06	40.0	34.2

[a]Scores ranged from 4.3 to 61.0. Lower scores indicate less distress, higher scores indicate greater distress.

the postdeath scores (see Table 28.2). A matched pair Wilcoxin Signed Rank Test was used to compare the mean of the total SCL-90 taken before the death with the mean of the postdeath scores. Although the difference was not statistically significant, the decrease in the total SCL-90 score suggests that families tend to experience greater distress during the predeath period than after the death of their child. In an earlier study, parents whose child had died told of even greater distress at the time of diagnosis, which underscores the importance of being alert not only to parents' current expressions of distress but to changes over time (Martinson, 1976).

The 13 children with cancer included 8 females and 5 males. They ranged in age from 4½ to 17 years with a mean of 10.6 years. The diagnoses included 3 leukemia, 2 acute myelocytic leukemia, 1 Burkett's lymphoma, 1 Ewing's sarcoma, 1 Hodgkins, 1 malignant glioma, 2 rhabdomyosarcoma, and 2 Wilm's tumor.

The interview transcriptions were reviewed, and a list of child concerns was developed and categorized as psychological, social, or physical concerns. The stories from the TAT were analyzed by a psychologist experienced in interpreting this test; the psychologist listed the themes and affect arising out of the ideational content. The interview and TAT lists then were examined to assure that all concerns from both sources were included in the larger categories. Responses to the TAT indicated concern about body vulnerability, but the TAT did not provide the specific data that the interviews did. Children expressed their concerns according to the developmental stage they had achieved. Children under 6 years of age showed separation anxiety, fear of abandonment, and loneliness. Those 6–10 years old focused on body integrity and showed greater fear of needles and operations. After age 10, the concept of irreversibility was grasped and fear of permanent body functioning loss was internalized (Rudin, Martinson, & Gilliss, 1988).

To examine the impact of childhood cancer on healthy siblings, 22 siblings were selected from 18 families in the larger sample. Among these 18 families, 6 had a child who had died from cancer and in the remaining 12 families the child with cancer was living. The healthy siblings' ages ranged from 4 to 19 years with the majority being between 7 and 11 years of age. Siblings who were preschool age did not remember being told specific information about the cancer diagnosis. Their emotional experience was one of fearing for their sibling's physical safety and wishing for warm secure objects or another sibling. School-age children retained the information given them and understood that their sibling could die from the illness but that a healthy life was also possible. They experienced loneliness and reported missing siblings and parents. They thought cancer was the "scariest" disease but did not think they would catch it. Adolescent siblings felt they were informed about the diagnosis and knew the outcome could be death or a healthy life. They missed their sibling and found it most difficult to answer friends' and relatives' questions about the sick child when they did not feel that they had adequate or up-to-date information themselves (Martinson, Gilliss, Coughlin, Freeman, & Bossert, 1990).

DISCUSSION

The findings of this study point to the need for increased support and services at the following times: immediately after discharge and for the first week at home; during times of illness of either the affected child or of otherwise healthy siblings; when routine follow-up appointments are scheduled; and at times of significant anniversaries. Interventions might include:

1. helping parents develop the skills to recount and re-explain death or illness to children as they develop, especially children who are too young at the time of diagnosis to use abstract thought;
2. providing continuous access to services to families whose children have survived and apparently are doing well;
3. sensitively sharing control of decisions about the child's care as the parents' ability to do so fluctuates;
4. preparing parents to adjust constructively to stigmatizing experiences.

Most parents in the study reported that the things that helped most were concrete services such as babysitting, financial assistance, food preparation, and a few hours to spend on themselves. Therefore, attention should be directed to offering these services along with psychological support and counseling.

Nurses can address both the physical and social concerns of children with cancer, thereby facilitating adjustment. Nurse clinicians may act as liaisons between school and hospital, providing education about the children's concerns to teachers and students. Peer relationships are a major concern for any child, and they are especially difficult for those experiencing an illness. Support groups during hospitalization and outpatient clinic visits may be invaluable, and parent education about age-appropriate concerns may facilitate parental support for the child. The nurse clinician can act as an emotional and psychological advocate for the child through frequent peer meetings and nursing rounds. The nurse should act as the child's confidant as well as meeting his or her physical needs.

We also need a variety of approaches that will help us understand the child's expressions of feelings. From the siblings' interviews we learned that parents generally perceive their children's expressions of feelings correctly; the children, however, experience more feelings than they are able to process verbally and therefore express themselves physically and behaviorally. Children ages 4–11 have difficulty processing their grief and need help from adults to understand and share their feelings and to resolve their feelings consciously. Nurses must help parents be available to healthy siblings, especially if the ill child is expected to die.

We must alert parents to the continuing emotional needs of the siblings at home; encourage attendance at support groups for siblings; and educate the parents on the developmental aspects of the physical and behavioral responses of healthy siblings to an ill child. I strongly urge public health nurses or visiting nurses to get involved with every family who has a child with cancer. If you become involved at the time of diagnosis, you have time to become knowledgeable about the disease and its treatment, and also to get to know the family. They will need you throughout the course of treatment, whether it results in long-term survival or death.

ACKNOWLEDGEMENT

Funding in part from the American Cancer Society, Minnesota and California Divisions, to Ida M. Martinson, the St. Paul Foundation; and the Home Care Research Fund.

REFERENCES

Derogatis, L. (1983). *SCL-90 (revised) manual*. Baltimore, MD: Johns Hopkins University.

Foley, G., & Whittam, E. (1990). Care of the child dying of cancer: Part I. *CA-A Cancer Journal for Clinicians, 40*, 327–354.

Martinson, I. M. (1976). [Home Care for the Child with Cancer Project]. Unpublished data.
Martinson, I. M., & Cohen, M. (1988). Themes from a longitudinal study of family reaction to childhood cancer. *Journal of Psychosocial Oncology, 6*(3/4), 81–98.
Martinson, I. M., Gilliss, C., Coughlin, D., Freeman, M., & Bossert, E. (1990). Impact of childhood cancer on healthy school age siblings. *Cancer Nursing, 13*, 183–190.
Miller, R. (1989). Frequency and environmental epidemiology of childhood cancer. In P. Pizzo & D. Poplack (Eds.), *Principles and practice of pediatric oncology*, (p. 4). Philadelphia: J. B. Lippincott Co.
Murray, H. (1943). *Thematic apperception test: Manual.* Cambridge, MA: Harvard University Press.
Rudin, M., Martinson, I., & Gilliss, C. (1988). Measurement of psychosocial concerns of adolescents with cancer through projective and interview techniques. *Cancer Nursing, 11*, 144–149.

[29]

The Effects of an Asthma Education Program on Selected Health Behaviors of School-Aged Children with Asthma

Laurel R. Talabere

Asthma is the leading cause of school absenteeism and a significant cause of pediatric hospital admissions and emergency health care. It is also increasing in school-aged children in the United States (Clark et al., 1986; Evans et al., 1987; National Heart, Lung, and Blood Institute Data Fact Sheet, 1989). This chronic illness challenges the family to manage a complex regimen and minimize the disruptions of daily living at home and school. Thus, the need for asthma self-management skills is clear. Asthma education programs are the vehicle for learning asthma self-management. They have been shown to reduce health care utilization, school absences, and altered breathing episodes and to increase knowledge and the self-management of asthma by children and their parents (Blessing-Moore, Fritz, & Lewiston, 1985; Clark & Shope, 1986; "Efficacy of asthma education," 1989; Parker & Wolfe, 1987; Wilson, Fish, Page, Stancavage, & Rolnick, 1990).

In most successful asthma education programs, the parent, child, and health professional are co-managers, and the unique knowledge of each is respected. It is recognized that parent and child exercise a high degree of independent decision-making in managing the asthma on a day-to-day basis, and the context for the management of asthma varies, depending on the child's status, the environment, and the knowledge and skills needed. The child is taught to become as competent as possible in asthma self-management, and it is acknowledged that management tasks are most likely to be undertaken when they fit the family's life-style (Clark, 1989, 1990; Wasilewski, 1990).

Unfortunately, only 2 of the 20 asthma education programs reported in the last 2 decades decreased school absences significantly (Fireman, Friday, Gira, Vierthaler, & Michaels, 1981; Hindi-Alexander & Cropp, 1984). Emergency health care visits for asthma also decreased significantly in only 2 programs (Clark, Feldman, Evans, Wasilewski, & Levison, 1984; Lewis, Rachelefsky, Lewis, de la Sota, & Kaplan, 1984). There was a significant increase in asthma self-management in 4 programs (Clark et al., 1986; Evans, Clark, et al., 1987; Hindi-Alexander & Cropp, 1984; Whitman, West, Brough, & Welch, 1985). Asthma episode frequency was reduced significantly in 3 programs (Evans, Clark, et al., 1987; Fireman et al., 1981; Staudenmayer, Harris, & Selner, 1981). The number of hospitalizations decreased significantly in 3 programs (Clark et al., 1986; Lewis et al., 1984; Staudenmayer et al., 1981). A significant knowledge gain was a result in only 2 programs (Whitman et al., 1985).

The low number of asthma education studies producing statistically significant improvements points to a need for studies that pay greater attention to research design and statistical analysis. The purpose of the study reported here (Talabere, 1991) was to determine whether or not an asthma education program for school-aged children and their parents could (1) reduce the number of hospitalizations and emergency health care visits, (2) decrease school absences and episodes of altered breathing, (3) increase the child's knowledge about asthma, and (4) change the child's and parent's perception of the child's asthma.

METHOD

Design

A pretest–posttest control group design was used to test the effectiveness of the Asthma Education Program (AEP). The children and their parents were assigned randomly to an experimental or control group, using a blocking technique to control for gender, race, and age.

Sample

The subjects selected for study were 50 children, 8 through 12 years old, receiving treatment at Columbus Children's Hospital (CCH) for a primary medical diagnosis of asthma. They were selected from children admitted for asthma to inpatient units that offered the Asthma Education Program, which was the study intervention, and children seen in the emergency room (ER) for acute asthma. All subjects had recently experienced an acute episode requiring either an emergency room visit or hospitalization. Children were excluded from the study if they had additional chronic health problems, needed a community health nurse referral for postdischarge follow-up, or were participating in a concurrent asthma education program. No attempt was made to exclude children who had previously participated in asthma camp, an asthma support group, or another asthma education program. As noted above, children were randomly assigned to the experimental or control group. Eleven experimental group subjects were inpatients and 14 were recruited from the ER. Fourteen control group subjects were inpatients and 11 were recruited from the ER.

The Intervention

Developed in collaboration with staff nurses at the hospital, the AEP used for the experimental group met the objectives for the asthma teaching plan at CCH. The AEP consisted of two 1-hour sessions involving both parent and child. Class I focused on normal lung anatomy and physiology, changes occurring in the lungs during an asthma episode, triggers and their avoidance, early warning signs of an asthma episode, and medication actions and side effects. Class II provided a brief review of Class I plus a return demonstration by the child of breathing exercises and inhaler technique, more in-depth information about child-specific triggers and how to manage them, additional discussion of early warning signs, what to do when an asthma episode first begins, when to get medical help, feelings of the parent and child, school concerns, support groups, and camps. Discussion was individualized, questions were encouraged, and printed materials and props reinforced the content for both child and parent. Written and graphic materials for the course included patient teaching sheets, a diagram of asthma-related lung changes, articles on dust and mold-spore allergies, an asthma find-the-word game, a body relaxation guide, information on asthma camps and support groups, and information for school personnel.

The 25 children and parents in the experimental group were taught individually in the child's home ($n = 16$), in the child's hospital room ($n = 8$), or in the hospital cafeteria ($n = 1$). If the child was hospitalized, the AEP was taught by the nursing staff or researcher after the child was medically stable and at a time when the parent could be present. If the child was at home, the AEP was taught at the earliest time mutually convenient for the parent, child, and researcher.

AEP instruction was provided by registered nurses who were (1) regular staff on the unit to which the child was admitted, (2) had had previous experience teaching children with chronic health problems and their parents, (3) had completed a 2½ hour continuing education program conducted by the researcher, and (4) had taught AEP sessions prior to teaching participants in the study.

Instruments

Five instruments, either adapted from existing questionnaires or designed by the researcher, were administered to both the experimental and control groups to measure the program's effectiveness. Data were collected over a 12-week period.

Nursing Assessment of the Child with Asthma and the Family This 31-item questionnaire, designed by the investigator, provided baseline information about the health history and the child's and parent's knowledge, attitudes, and behaviors related to asthma. Sixteen items provided data about previous emergency health care visits, hospitalizations, and school absences as well as patterns of health care and demographic factors. Fifteen items provided the nurse teaching the AEP with data about the learning needs of the parent and child. For example, the parent was asked, "What do you do first when your child has an asthma episode?" The parent and child were also asked to give examples of the ways in which they learned best. This instrument was administered during the initial meeting with the parent and child and helped establish initial rapport with the family.

Asthma Knowledge Questionnaire (AKQ) This 16-item questionnaire, designed by the researcher, was administered to the child at the beginning and end of the 12-week study period to measure the child's knowledge of asthma and its management. The child labeled a line drawing of the respiratory system and answered multiple-choice questions. For example, the child was asked, "What does the word trigger mean when you are talking about asthma?" Choices included: (1) something that makes your asthma better, (2) your asthma medicine, (3) something that starts your asthma episode, and (4) your extra hard breathing. In a pilot study with 13 subjects, the AKQ had a test–retest reliability of .81.

Asthma Attitude Survey (AAS) This 20-item, 5-point Likert scale, adapted by the researcher from the Asthma Attitude Survey developed by Reynolds and Creer (1987), was also completed at the beginning and end of the study period by the child. Based on a test–retest reliability of only .66 in the pilot study, several items were clarified prior to the main study. The AAS assessed the child's attitudes and behaviors related to asthma self-control. For example, the child was given the statement, "There are things I can do to help my asthma" and asked to mark it as false, mostly false, sometimes true and sometimes false, mostly true, or true.

Survey of Asthma Problems and Severity (SAPS) This 12-item multiple-choice questionnaire, adapted by the researcher from the Survey of Asthma Problems and Severity by Reynolds and Creer (1987), was administered as a pretest and posttest. The SAPS gave parents an opportunity to express their perceptions of their child's asthma. For example, the parent was asked: "On the average, how often has asthma interfered with your child's recreational and social activities?" Choices included: (1) less than once a month, (2) more than once a month but less than once a week, (3) more than once a week but less than once a day, (4) once a day, or (e) more than once a day. The SAPS has a reported test-retest reliability of .82 – .88.

Parent Diary This self-report calendar instrument, designed by the researcher, was used by parents during the 12-week study period to record five specific events related to asthma: (1) hospitalizations, (2) emergency health care visits, (3) school absences, (4) altered breathing episodes, and (5) the name, frequency, and route of asthma medications. A cover sheet of instructions, including examples, was provided. Parents received a reminder phone call every 2 weeks, encouraging them to maintain the diary, and they were provided the researcher's phone number should questions arise.

Data Collection

On entry into the study, the Nursing Assessment of the Child with Asthma and the Family, and the AKQ, AAS, and SAPS instruments were administered to both the experimental and control groups. Then the children and parents in the experimental group participated in the AEP. For the next 12 weeks each parent in both the experimental and control groups maintained the Parent Diary. Within 2 weeks of the completion of the 12-week study period, the AKQ, AAS, and SAPS were mailed to the child and parent's home (to be completed by the same parent who completed the SAPS before the study). A cover letter reminded the parent that the tests for the child were to be completed without parental assistance. There were also instructions for returning the questionnaires plus the Parent Diary in an enclosed self-addressed stamped envelope.

When the poststudy questionnaires and Parent Diary were returned, a thank-you note and a specially designed T-shirt were sent to the child. Those in the control group also received a packet of the educational materials prepared for the AEP.

In addition to the data collected during the 12-week study period, data on the number of hospitalizations and emergency health care visits were also collected for three prestudy periods: (1) the 12 months prior to the child's entry into the study, (2) the 12-week period in the previous year that corresponded to the same 12-week calendar segment as the study period, and (3) the 12-week period immediately preceding the study period. The second of these prestudy periods provided a basis for comparison with the study period that had approximately the same school calendar and seasonal variations. Data were not available for these three prestudy periods on the number of school absences and altered breathing episodes.

RESULTS

Major Findings and Tests of Significance

The experimental and control groups were similar in number of emergency visits for each of the three prestudy periods—the preceding 12 months, the same 12-week period one year prior to the study, and the 12-week prestudy period. Analysis of covariance (ANCOVA) showed a significant greater decrease [$F(1,47) = 4.67, p = .036$] in emergency visits among children in the experimental group than those in the control group when controlling for the number of visits during the corresponding period in the previous year, but not when controlling for visits during the 12 weeks immediately prior to the study [$F(1,47) = 2.26, p = .139$] (see Table 29.1). The mean number of ER visits during the 12-week period 1 year prior to the study was 0.36 for the experimental group and 0.24 for the control group. During the 12-week study period the mean was 0.44 for the experimental group and 1.08 for the control group. As noted above, children were randomly assigned to the experimental or control group. Eleven experimental group subjects were inpatients and 14 were recruited from the ER. Fourteen control group subjects were inpatients and 11 were recruited from the ER.

TABLE 29.1 Comparison of Experimental and Control Groups on Emergency Health Care Visits

		Total sample		Study groups: Experimental group		Study groups: Control group	
Time periods	Range	*M*	*SD*	*M*	*SD*	*M*	*SD*
12 Months prior to the study	1–8	2.56	1.69	2.32	1.62	2.80	1.76
12-Week period one year prior to study[a]	0–2	0.30	0.58	0.36	0.64	0.24	0.52
12-Week prestudy period[b]	1–5	1.74	0.94	1.48	0.82	2.00	1.00
12-Week study period	0–4	0.76	1.12	0.44	0.77	1.08	1.32

[a]The 12-week period in the previous year that corresponds to the same 12-week calendar segment as the study period.
[b]The 12-week period immediately before the study period.

An ANCOVA also showed a significant increase in asthma knowledge for children in the experimental group [$F(1,47) = 4.94$, $p = .031$] when the posttest scores were compared with pretest scores. Prior to the study, the two groups were similar in their basic knowledge of asthma [$F(1,48) = .07$, $p = .80$] (see Table 29.2).

Changes in the number of hospitalizations [$F(1,47) = 2.15$, $p = .149$], the number of school absences [$F(1,42) = 1.74$, $p = .194$], and the parent's perception of the child's asthma [$F(1,47) = 1.67$, $p = .203$] were positive for the experimental group but not statistically significant (see Table 29.3).

TABLE 29.2 Comparison of Experimental and Control Groups on Asthma Knowledge Questionnaire (AKQ) Scores

		Total sample		Study groups: Experimental group		Study groups: Control group	
Scores	Range	*M*	*SD*	*M*	*SD*	*M*	*SD*
Pretest	2–14	9.40	3.23	9.28	3.60	9.52	2.89
Posttest	6–14	11.58	2.20	12.20	1.96	10.96	2.30
Change[a]	-4–11	2.18	3.34	2.92	3.56	1.44	3.00

[a]The difference between the pretest and posttest scores.

TABLE 29.3 Descriptive Data for the Experimental and Control Groups for the 12 Week Study Period

	Experimental group			Control group		
Dependent variables	Range	*M*	*SD*	Range	*M*	*SD*
Number of hospitalizations[a]	0–1	0.08	0.28	0–10	0.12	0.33
Number of hospitalizations[b]	0–2	0.60	0.50	0–2	0.76	0.52
Number of school absences[c]	0–8	1.36	2.52	0–14	2.60	3.75
Number of altered breathing episodes[d]	0–93	6.68	18.67	0–76	10.04	17.13
AAS scores[e]						
Pretest	55–96	73.80	8.85	55–96	77.48	9.01
Posttest	55–98	79.94	10.21	55–98	80.00	9.43
Change	– 11–27	6.14	9.67	– 11–27	2.52	6.30
SAPS scores[e]						
Pretest	30–57	47.16	1.11	30–57	44.76	7.21
Posttest	30–58	49.68	6.87	30–58	45.86	7.57
Change	– 16–10	2.52	4.18	– 16–10	1.10	5.53

[a]Adjusted for the 12-week period 1 year prior to the study.
[b]Adjusted for the 12-week prestudy period (immediately before the study period).
[c]Adjusted for absences in previous school year.
[d]Not adjusted; no prestudy data were available.
[e]Posttest and change scores adjusted for pretest scores.

Changes in the attitudes of the child toward assuming responsibility for self health care [$F(1,47) = 1.23$, $p = .273$] and in the frequency of altered breathing episodes [$F(1,48) = .44$, $p = .51$] showed these variables to be least affected by the AEP.

Eight factors that might have contributed to the differential improvements in the groups were analyzed: grade in school, previous participation in asthma camp and previous participation in asthma support groups, age at the onset of asthma, primary care provider, first action taken by the child or parent at the onset of an asthma episode, the presence of smokers, and the presence of pets in the household. Measures of association and nonparametric analysis of categorical data showed no significant differences between the experimental and control groups on these factors prior to the study.

When ANCOVA was used to analyze the effects of instructor and location on experimental group results, there were no significant effects. This suggests that the AEP achieves similar results when conducted in the hospital or at home by different nurses.

DISCUSSION

Major Findings

In this study of school-aged children with asthma and their parents, the AEP significantly reduced the frequency of emergency health care visits in the experimental group during the 12-week study period and significantly increased the child's knowledge about asthma. Although not statistically significant, the improvements in the experimental group in the number of hospitalizations, the number of school absences, and the parents' perceptions of asthma-related problems and their severity suggest that the AEP has the potential to have a positive impact in these areas. The AEP was least effective in improving the attitudes of the child toward assuming responsibility for self-health care and in decreasing the frequency of altered breathing episodes.

These findings provide evidence that a short, targeted asthma education program may significantly reduce the frequency of emergency health care visits and significantly increase the school-aged child's knowledge of asthma. This AEP may be useful in and adaptable to a variety of health care settings. We have a number of suggestions which should help ensure success.

In the AEP, a course outline and reference notebook guided the planning of teaching sessions and assured reasonable consistency among instructors. However, we recognized that these detailed resource materials could lead a novice instructor to overemphasize content and neglect the real learning needs of families. Thus, teacher preparation is an important component of the program.

In our program all instructors had had previous experience in teaching children with chronic health problems and had completed a 2½ hour continuing education program about teaching in the AEP. We recommend using similar criteria in selecting instructors in other settings.

The depth and sequencing of content in the AEP varied with the learning needs of parents and children. The individualized discussion format created a relaxed and nonthreatening context for learning in which child and parent experiences were shared. Thus, children and parents helped shape each session. For example, the importance of taking medications regularly and avoiding allergens was emphasized with all parents and children, but discussions of particular medications and allergy avoidance approaches were child-specific. Also, while the targeted time was 1 hour per session, emphasis was placed on covering the information and answering the child's and parent's questions. Thus, class length ranged from 45 to 75 minutes.

In this study the AEP was limited to two 1-hour individual sessions because the average length of hospitalization for a child with asthma is about 3 days. However, this amount of time is not adequate to help the parent and child assess altered breathing patterns. Inaccuracies in the Parent Diaries as well as many parent questions on when to seek help suggest that these are important areas to emphasize. Also, more time was needed to discuss the child's and parent's feelings associated with asthma episodes. Other areas to expand include problem-solving strategies for actual situations that might arise, the use of prn medications, and the concept of self-management.

Most successful asthma education programs, including ours, are characterized by five educational principles and seven curricular elements. Any adaptation of an asthma education program should retain these core elements.

Five principles:

1. The parent, child, and health professional are co-managers.
2. The context of learning is individualized to the needs of the child and parents.
3. The child is taught competence as well as knowledge in self-management.
4. The family's independent role in decision-making is acknowledged.
5. The asthma management is congruent with the family's life-style.

Seven core curricular elements:

1. The signs and symptoms of an acute asthma episode.
2. How to remain calm when these signs and symptoms occur.
3. How to administer prescribed therapy.
4. When to get emergency care.
5. How to reduce exposure to triggers.
6. How to normalize activities.
7. How to communicate with health and education professionals.

Finally, the participation of staff nurses in the research led directly to the utilization of the findings. Staff nurses were actively involved at every level. The study evolved from nursing audit findings that showed a deficit in parental knowledge about asthma medications. Staff nurses helped develop the asthma education program, collect data, teach children and parents, and critique the program outcomes. It was through their efforts that institutional approval was gained for the Asthma Education Program, and it is staff nurses who are currently implementing the AEP. Staff nurse involvement has fostered a strong sense of commitment to the program.

ACKNOWLEDGMENT

Financial support for this research was received from Columbus Children's Hospital Clincial Studies Center.

REFERENCES

Blessing-Moore, J., Fritz, G., & Lewiston, N. J. (1985). Self-management programs for childhood asthma: A review. *Chest, 87*(6), 107S–110S.

Clark, N. M. (1989). Asthma self-management education research and implications for clinical practice. *Chest, 95*(5), 1110–1113.

Clark, N. M. (1990). *Educating children with chronic disease: Models for asthma: Part 1.* (Cassette Recording No. 98). Boston, MA: American Thoracic Society.

Clark, N. M., Feldman, C. H., Evans, D., Duzey, O., Levison, M. J., Wasilewski, Y., Kaplan, D., Rips, J., & Mellins, R. B. (1986). Managing better: Children, parents and asthma. *Patient Education and Counseling, 8,* 27–38.

Clark, N. M., Feldman, C. H., Evans, D., Wasilewski, Y., & Levison, M. J. (1984). Changes in children's school performance as a result of education for family management of asthma. *Journal of School Health, 54,* 143–145.

Clark, N. M., & Shope, G. T. (1986). The current knowledge base for health education programs for chronically ill children. *Advances in Health Education and Promotion, 2,* 91–105.

Efficacy of asthma education — selected abstracts: Expanding the opportunities in patient care. (1989). NY: American Lung Association.

Evans, D., Clark, N. M., Feldman, C., Rips, J., Kaplan, D., Levison, M., Wasilewski, Y., Levin, B., & Mellins, R. B. (1987). A school health education program for children with asthma aged 8–11 years. *Health Education Quarterly, 14,* 267–279.

Evans, R. E., Mullally, D. I., Wilson, R. W., Gergen, R. J., Rosenberg, H. M., Grauman, J. S., Edmonds, J. C., & Feinleib, M. (1987). National trends in the morbidity and mortality of asthma in the USA: Prevalence, hospitalization, and death from asthma over two decades: 1965–1984. *Chest, 91*(6), 65S–74S.

Fireman, P., Friday, G. A., Gira, C., Vierthaler, W. A., & Michaels, L. (1981). Teaching self-management skills to asthmatic children and their parents in an ambulatory care setting. *Pediatrics, 68,* 341–348.

Hindi-Alexander, M. C., & Cropp, G. J. A. (1984). Evaluation of a family asthma program. *Journal of Allergy and Clinical Immunology, 74,* 505–510.

Lewis, C. E., Rachelefsky, G., Lewis, M. A., de la Sota, A., & Kaplan, M. (1984). A randomized trial of ACT (Asthma Care Training) for kids. *Pediatrics, 74,* 478–486.

National Heart, Lung, and Blood Institute data fact sheet: Asthma statistics. (1989, December). Bethesda, MD: U.S. Department of Health and Human Services.

Parker, S. R., & Wolfe, J. M. (1987). Asthma self-management: A second generation of research programs: Forward. *Health Education Quarterly, 14,* 265–266.

Reynolds, R. V., & Creer, T. L. (1987). *A multisite, statewide evaluation of asthma camp: A research proposal.* Unpublished manuscript, Ohio University, Athens.

Staudenmayer, H., Harris, P. S., & Selner, J. C. (1981). Evaluation of a self-help education-exercise program for asthmatic children and their parents: Six-month follow-up. *Journal of Asthma, 18,* 1–5.

Talabere, L. R. (1991). The effects of an asthma education program on selected health behaviors of school-age children who have recently experienced an acute asthma episode. (Doctoral dissertation, The Ohio State University, Columbus, OH, 1990). *Dissertation Abstracts International*, *51*(12–A), 4030.

Wasilewski, Y. M. (1990). Educating children with chronic disease: Models for asthma: Part 1. (Cassette Recording No. 98). Boston, MA: American Thoracic Society.

Whitman, N., West, D., Brough, F. K., & Welch, M. (1985). A study of a self-care rehabilitation program in pediatric asthma. *Health Education Quarterly, 12*, 333–342.

Wilson, S., Fish, L., Page, A., Stancavage, F., & Rolnick, C. (1990). Evaluation of four pediatric self-management programs. *American Review of Respiratory Disease*, *141*(4, Pt. 2, Abstracts), A495.

Part IV

CARING FOR THE CHRONICALLY ILL: IMPLICATIONS FOR THE FUTURE

[30]

Clinical Implications of Research on Caring for Chronically Ill Adults and Children: Where Can We Go from Here?

Barbara Germino

The research included in this volume, from Angela McBride's call to action through studies of family caregiving in chronic illness, clarifies once again that the essence of nursing care in chronic illness is enhancing and facilitating the best possible quality of life for the chronically ill, their families and their caregivers.

Quality of life for the chronically ill has physical/functional, psychological, social, economic, and spiritual dimensions; and according to the research highlighted in these chapters, there are a variety of interventions which address many of the dimensions of quality of life. The challenge now is to take the results of these studies and to begin applying them to the nursing care of the chronically ill in the hospital, in transitions to home, in long-term care facilities, in home care, and in community settings. This chapter discusses the three major categories of nursing interventions which emerge from analysis of this collection of work and considers some key issues in testing such interventions in nursing practice.

The first major area of intervention comes from an idea which goes back to Florence Nightingale, but which is as relevant to today's rapidly changing health care system as it was to nursing in the last century—creating *environments that fit the needs of the chronically ill or of special groups within that population.* Studies included here indicate that in the hospital, attention to the physical environment and use of carefully planned clinical protocols can prevent loss of function, enhance patient–staff interaction, decrease the need for restraints, reduce costs, and increase staff satisfaction as well as preventing acute confusion. What do we do with this information? For those who practice in hospital and long-term care settings, the work provides data on the effectiveness of tailoring environments to the needs of certain groups of chronically ill. In the acute care hospital this may not be an initially appealing idea, but outcomes like reduced costs, enhanced staff satisfaction, and diminished complications such as further confusion or functional decline will carry weight because they fit the system's goals. They also address the overall objective of enhancing quality of life. The challenge, if a special care unit or environment is needed, is to document that need and to use the results of research presented here and other published research to make the case for such a unit. Armed with such information, it is possible to take a leadership role in getting support for, planning, and implementing such a unit. This information can also be useful in documenting the unit's effectiveness in enhancing patient and family quality of life, reducing costs, shortening stays, lowering readmission and complication rates, and improving patient, family, and staff satisfaction.

Another aspect of fitting the environment to the needs of the chronically ill involves planning for transitions from home to hospital and from hospital to home. The challenge here is to commit appropriate people and adequate time to planning for such transitions, to improve communications among all those involved (not forgetting that chronically ill persons and their families are the central characters of concern), and to remember that professionals and patients and families may have differing perceptions and priorities which need attention.

Creating a home environment in which families can not only care for an ill child but also maintain their quality of life is a challenge raised by Christian in her study of families caring for chronically ill children: "Sustaining a family environment that is supportive of individual family members, family relationships and the family unit is vital to the family and their adaptation to the child's chronic illness" (p. 311). This work reminds us as well that individual family members' perceptions of their own and others' concerns may be more important to adaptation than the way professionals define and interpret family adaptation.

There are several points of importance here: *First*, the findings of studies presented here validate ideas that have been discussed in nursing for some time, including the importance of patient and family perceptions, continuity of care, personalized care, the expertise of advanced practitioners, and communication throughout a fragmented system not designed to meet the needs of the chronically ill. *Second*, we have rarely had or sought the nursing resources and flexibility to do this kind of planning and facilitation well. *Third*, with shortened stays, increases in many chronically ill populations, and availability of nurses with special expertise in many settings, the time has never been better to put these ideas into action. Several chapters in this volume provide examples of how this might be done and evaluated. Angela McBride suggests that this should be the *era of nursing demonstration projects*. The research in these chapters can be used to propose and support such projects. Consultation can be sought with experts in planning, testing, and evaluating these and many other approaches to the many transitions that characterize chronic illness trajectories.

A second major challenge is to *open up our ideas not only about the kinds of interventions which can enhance quality of life, but also about the particular groups who could benefit from them and the settings in which they could be implemented.* For example, we need to test the feasibility and effectiveness of programs of intervention at home and in community and occupational settings. We must focus on realistic and cost-effective ways to move outside institutions to address the nursing care needs of the majority of chronically ill and their families, who are living at home with their illness. In particular, the needs of those in rural areas demand our attention.

This volume certainly offers creative ideas in this regard. The use of a small group and an in-home setting to do exercise training with frail elderly, and the use of a planned and progressive program of exercise for people with some degree of functional loss like hemiparesis or impaired respiratory function, or with significant cardiovascular disease, easily lend themselves to trials with other chronically ill populations in other settings. The clinical challenge is to maximize what chronically ill persons can learn to incorporate in their activities of daily living, at home or in groups, which can enhance their functional abilities, self-esteem, sense of well-being and quality of life—whether one is talking about exercise and activity, improved nutrition, or management of uncertainty. Why not seek out settings where people with chronic illnesses come together in the community—adult day care centers, senior centers, nutrition sites, support groups, and organizations for people with particular illnesses like multiple sclerosis, diabetes, and Alzheimer's disease? Many of these places and groups welcome ideas for projects which are geared to enhancing quality of life, and enthusiastic participation is a plus.

Special populations of chronically ill persons and their families demand particular kinds of intervention. Many of these special interventions are not new in principle but are new in their fit with special needs or characteristics. Holditch-Davis and Lee remind us that role modeling for other nurses and for parents the interpretation and response to infant cues enhances nurse-infant and parent-infant interactions and facilitates more individualized care of infants with such problems as chronic lung disease.

Nurses will also benefit from understanding the difficulties of parenting an acutely ill hospitalized infant and the importance of negotiating roles with parents to facilitate both illness care and parent care. Both of these issues call for expert nurses who can educate nursing staff and parents, and perhaps thus prevent many problems in caring for very young children who are chronically ill.

A third type of intervention challenging nurses is *facilitating a good quality of life for patients and families with chronic illness*. Studies by Martinson and Miles et al. in this volume remind us that such efforts must occur throughout the trajectory of illness, because needs and concerns change over time. Also, there are key points at which efforts need to be intensified in anticipation of increased stress and possible depletion of resources.

The economic impact of chronic illness on quality of life is not always visible in the process of planning and giving care. The research of Gennaro et al. conveys the powerful message that, in addition to the possibility of their being uninsured or underinsured, families with chronically ill children have out-of-pocket costs which peak at various times. While the percentage of family income required for out-of-pocket expenses is small, families with limited economic resources and less expendable income will feel the impact of such expenses more acutely. In addition, unplanned changes in employment may occur for the parents of premature, low birthweight babies, and these may add to the economic burden. Facilitating a positive quality of life for such families must include attention to economic factors so the family can continue functioning effectively in a stressful situation.

Daly, in her chapter, makes the point that chronically ill persons have survived by learning to manage their treatment regimen, balancing illness demands with the rest of their life—learning to juggle a number of aspects of their own care and lives at the same time. We know that chronically ill persons vary in their view of the illness experience, the trajectory of their illness, and the amount of uncertainty involved. There is a well-known teaching/learning principle implying that interventions should, to the extent possible, fit with where the patient is. The research in this volume describes a variety of self-help interventions which have been successful. Many nursing interventions in the self-help category are in response to the cognitive, social, and emotional aspects of chronic illness—dealing with such issues as uncertainty, chronic sorrow, need for information, a sense of control, a renewal of self-esteem, and much more. The investigators in this book have presented evidence supporting nursing interventions to facilitate the patient and family's management of these responses either directly or indirectly through self-help interventions.

In order to move forward in clinical practice with the very powerful kinds of interventions we have heard about, what else is required? A number of authors have indicated that if we want to know what patients and caregivers need and want—what is necessary to quality of life for *them*—we should ask. In practice, then, there is a need to move away from narrow, present-oriented assessments to more reality-based, trajectory-focused, open-ended approaches. There is a need to address *priorities* amidst the many individual responses, and to move forward in identifying target populations and testing appropriate self-help interventions to help people learn:

- where and how to get information,
- how to get questions answered,
- how to manage uncertainty and its consequences,
- how to maintain and even improve functional and general health status,

and many other aspects of the physical, functional, psychological, and social dimensions of quality of life.

Index

ACE Unit, *see* Acute Care Of Elderly (ACE) Unit
Activities of Daily Living (ADLs), 122
 in assessing functional ability, 10
 BI measure of, 214
 types of, 10
Acute care hospitals, geriatric unit in, 133
Acute Care of Elderly (ACE) Unit (ACE Unit)
 assessing cognition, 137
 continence in, 138–139
 environment of, 136
 length of stay at, 139
 maintaining cognition, 136–137
 mobility of patient, 137–138
 mood of patient, 137
 nurse in, 139–140
 nutrition in, 139
 restoring cognition, 136
 sensory needs of patient, 137
Acute exacerbations in elderly, 132–140; *see also* Acute Care of Elderly (ACE) Units
 interventions, 136–140
 method of study, 135
 restoring cognition, 136
 Unit for Acute Care of the Elderly (ACE) Model, 134f
Acutely ill, chronically ill distinguished from, 24
Acute myocardial infarction (AMI), 61, 62
Adaptation, hardiness as, 17
Adaptive functioning, 10
ADLs, *see* Activities of Daily Living
Advocating, 309
Aerobic capacity, 60
Aerobic exercise
 antihypertensive effects of, 65
 psychological effects of, 71
Affects Balance Scale, 194–195
AIDS, 48, 49
 diagnosing, 50
 uncertainty and, 53
Alcoholism, managing, 14
"Altered parenting," 282
Alzheimer's disease (AD)
 characteristics of, 112–113
 exercise and, 72
 prevalence of, 112
 treatment for behavioral dysfunction, 113
Alzheimer's Disease Assessment Scale (ADAS), 122
American Association of Homes for the Aged, 117
American College of Sports Medicine, 61, 65
American Heart Association, 63, 191, 194
American Hospital Association, 22
American Medical Association, 22
American Nurses' Association, 10
American Public Health Association, 22

American Public Welfare Association, 22
Arthritis
  exercise and, 65–66
  impact of, 152
Arthritis Foundation, 150, 154, 161, 168
The Arthritis Handbook, 151, 154
Arthritis Impact Measurement Scales (AIMS), 153–154
Arthritis self-efficacy, definition of, 152
Arthritis Self-Efficacy Scale, 153
Arthritis Self-Help Course (ASHC), 150–156, 161
  course content and process, 151–152
  description of, 150–151
  goal of, 155
  improvements due to, 152
  procedure in study, 154
  program goals, 151
  results of, 154–155
ASHC, *see* Arthritis Self-Help Course
ASHC Leader's Manual, 151
Assessment/Appraisal/Intervention Guide, 171
Asthma Attitude Survey (AAS), 323
Asthma education program, 319–328
  asthma knowledge increase, 324–325
  benefits of, 320
  class length, 327
  comparison of scores on, 325T
  curricular elements of successful program, 328
  decrease in emergency visits, 324
  descriptive data for, 325–326, 326T
  emergency health care visits, comparison of experimental and control groups, 325T
  factors contributing to improvement, 326
  instruction in, 322
  instruments, 322–323
  interventions and, 321–322
  need for self-management of asthma, 320
  nurses in development of, 328
  principles of successful programs, 328
  successful and unsuccessful programs, 320
  teacher preparation, 327
Asthma Knowledge Questionnaire (AKQ), 322–323
Atherogenesis, exercise and, 62

Balancing, 307–308
Baltimore Therapeutic Evaluation (BTE), 195
Barthel Index (BI), 214, 216
BDI, *see* Beck Depression Inventory
Beck Depression Inventory (BDI), 214, 215, **216**
BI, *see* Barthel Index
Biomedical model, 28
Bipolar illness, 12
Block Nurse Program, 33
"Body listening," 12
Boston Dispensary, 39
Breast cancer, *see also* Uncertainty management in breast cancer
  exercise and, 69
  uncertainty and, 32, 51–52, 53, 56
Bureaucratic management model, 97

CAD, *see* Coronary artery disease
Cancer, exercise and, 69; *see also* Childhood cancer
Cardiorespiratory endurance, 60
Caregiver Stress Inventory (CSI), 124
Caregiving, stress of, 41–42
Case management practice model, 96
Case manager, in SCU, 97–98
Catastrophic reactions, 126
Change in practice
  change in setting, 81–82
  readiness of research for, 82–86
Childhood cancer, 312–318
  as diagnosis, 312–313
  family themes and characteristics, 315T
  incidence of, 312
  interventions, 317

nurse and, 318
siblings and impact of, 317
"Chronic," as term, 9
Chronically critically ill patient population, 94–95
Chronically ill
acutely ill distinguished from, 24
attitudes toward, 28
home care for, 41
integrative needs of, 41
management of illness by, 24–25
problems of daily living among, 24
psychosocial factors and, 26–27
redesigning care for, 25–28
special care units, (SCUs) for, 27
Chronic disease, definition of, 22
Chronic heart disease, 26
Chronic illness
cause of, 3
characteristics of, 3
definition of, 291
impact of, 3
incidence of, 3, 202
increase in, 22
prevalence of, 290–291
Chronicity, 15
Chronic lung disease
in infants, complications of, 251–252
morbidity and mortality of, 251
Chronic obstructive pulmonary disease (COPD), 69–70
depression and, 26
exercise and, 69–70
Chronic pain, nurses' perception of, 28
Chronic sorrow
determining presence of, 233
feelings associated with, 233
as normal reaction, 235
nurse's role in, 234–235, 235–236
nursing interventions in, 236
teacher/expert's role in, 235
as term, 231
triggers to feelings of, 233–234
Circuit training, 205
Clinical implications of research, 333–337
creating fitting environments, 333–334
enhancing quality of life, 334, 335
opening up to creative ideas, 335–336
Commission on Chronic Illness, 22
Compensation, in parenting, 285, 286
Conduct and Utilization of Research (CURN), 80
Conferences on nursing research, 4, 5–6
Congressional Record, 38
Continence in ACE Units, 138–139
COPD, *see* Chronic obstructive pulmonary disease
Coronary artery disease (CAD), 61–63, 189
Cost burden of low birthweight (LBW) infants, *see* Very low birthweight (VLBW) infants
Critically ill preterm infants, survival of, 250–251

Daily living uncertainty, 55–57
Death, leading cause of, 13
Decision-driven research utilization, 80
Dependence, definition of, 160
Depression
BDI measurement of, 215
exercise and, 199, 200
FRI scales and, 217
self-help response and, 162, 163–164
Diabetes, 67–69
glucoregulatory effects of exercise and, 67–68
metabolic response to exercise in IDDM, 67
metabolic response to exercise in NIDDM, 68
Diagnosis-related group (DRG) system 108
Diagnostic uncertainty, 49–51
Discharge needs, 142–149
Discharge planning, 31
benefits of, 143
by nurse, 142

[Discharge planning]
protocol for hospitalized elderly by GCNS, 144f
studies on, 143
time devoted to, 146–148, 148–149
Dysfunctional syndrome, in hospital, 133

Education, of chronically ill patient, 26; *see also* Asthma education program
Elderly
acute care units for, 27
discharge planning and, 31
in hospitals, percentage of, 142
Emory University Health Enhancement Center, 195
Enabling skills
definition of, 160
list of, 160
measuring, 163
mediating role of, 167
reduction of, 161
Self Control Schedule (SCS) in measuring, 174
Exercise
in ACE units, 137
arthritis and, 65–66
cancer and, 69
clinical evidence of glucoregulatory effects of, 68–69
COPD and, 69–70
coronary artery disease (CAD) and, 61–63
definition of, 60
diabetes and, 67–69
hypertension and, 63–65
mental health and illness and, 70–72
potential benefits for chronic illness, 61
recommended regime, 61
as symbol of hope, 63
well-being and, 62
Exercise for frail rural elderly, 202–210
aerobic capacity, 208
bike ergometry as test, 208–210
estimated VO_2 peak, 205
function measures, 200–207
goals of intervention, 205
intervention, 205–206
maintaining exercise, 204
psychoeducational training, 205
social support and, 206
Exercise for physically disabled with CAD, 189–200
arm ergometer test echocardiogram, 193
arrythmias, 198
benefits of, 196
body composition and, 199
cholesterol and, 199
ergometer exercise test with continuous analysis of expired gases, 194f
exercise test, 191–194
exercise training protocol, 191
functional capacity and, 197–198
functional restoration questionnaire, 195, 196
hemodynamic variables, 196T
isometric training, 198
M-mode echo, 191
psychological training versus endurance training, 198
self-concept and personal well-being and, 199–200
stationary wheelchair ergometer, 192f

Family
economic status of, and VLBW infant, 273–274
employment changes, 275–277. 278
functioning of, and VLBW infant, 277, 278
head injuries and role of, 212
home care by, 41
Impact on Family Scale, 274, 277
monthly income of, and VLBW infant, 277
normalization by, 282, 284–285, 286
out-of-pocket expenses for, in dollars by categories, 275T

out-of-pocket expenses for, of VLBW infants, 274–275, 278, 279
Special Care Unit and (SCU) process, 96
Specail Care Unit (SCU) programming and, 116, 121
Family caregivers of head-injured persons (HIPs), 212–218
Barthel Index scores of HIPs, 216
BDI scores of HIPs, 217
community resources used by, 216
correlations between FRI Scales and depression and anxiety, 217T
HIP deficits and problems, 216
Moos's model for coping, 213
State Anxiety Scale scores of HIPs, 217
Family Caregiving Inventory (FCI), 221
Family Concerns Interview, 305
Family Environment Scale, 214, 216
Family Leave Bill, 279
Family Perception Tool (FPT), 123–124
Family Relationship Inventory (FRI), 214–215, 217
Family response to child's chronic illness, 290–303
case illustrations of defining clusters, 295–299
children's self-perception, 301
comparison of mothers and fathers across defining themes, 293T
defining child as normal, 294, 296–297, 300
defining child as problem, 294
defining child as tragic figure, 294
defining themes, 293–295
family assessment tools, 302
illness as hateful restriction, 294
illness as manageable condition, 294
illness as ominous situation, 294
impact of illness on family, 300–301
limited understanding of illness, 294
neither parent views child as normal, 297–298
parents' agreement on view of child, 295–296
parents' definition of illness, importance of, 302
parents' discrepant view of child, 298–299
Fathers
on FFFS, 301
in illness management, 295
parental role conflict and, 288
Feetham Family Functioning Survey (FFFS), 292, 300, 301
Fisher's Least Significant Differences method, 301
Frailty, reversing, 202
Functional ability
assessing, 10
five areas of, 122
importance of, 10
Indiana Nursing Assessment of Functioning (INAF), 10, 11T
in managing chronicity, 9–12
positive effects of emphasis on, 12
Functional Abilities Checklist (FAC), 122–123, 126
Functional capacity, exercise and, 197
Functional decline, 202

Geriatric clinical nurse specialists (GCNSs), 143
discharge planning protocol by, 144, 145T
intervention in discharge needs, 144
time spent in discharge planning, 146f, 147f
Geriatric Rating Scale, (GRS), 122, 126
Geriatric units, 133
Given's Effect Scale, 173
Global Deterioration Scale (GDS), 115–116
Global Self Worth scale, 301
Graying of population, 9
Grounded theory, 291

Hamilton Depression Scale, 72
Harter Self-Perception Profile, 292

Head injured persons (HIPs), research on, 212–213; *see also* Family caregivers of head injured persons (HIPs)
Head injuries, incidence of, 212
Health
  optimism and, 16–17
  perceived versus objective, 16–17
  and person–environment fit, 14T
Health care, cost of, 39, 40, 159
Health service, cost-effectiveness of, 158
Heinz, Senator John, 38
Hill-Burton Act, 39
Home care, 38–44
  for chronically ill, 41
  cost-effectiveness of, 43
  definition of, by WHO, 41
  family responsibility for, 41
  in history, 39–40
  informal system of, 41–42
  medical model of, 42
  need to define terms, 43
  research on, 42–43
Hospital-based home care services, 33
Hospitalized chronically ill, 21–28
  acute condition and, 23
  home-facility dichotomy, 25
  hospital as environment, 21–22
  planning interventions for, 27
  psychosocial factors and, 26–27
  self-help behavior, 25
  special care units (SCUs) and, 27
  treatment modalities for, 23
Hospitals
  cost containment and reduced reimbursement, 23–24
  costs of, 93
  discharge planning and, 31
  dysfunctional syndrome and, 133
  elderly in, percentage of, 142
  as environment for chronically ill, 21–22
  transitional units in, 33
  trends in modern care in, 23
Hypertension, exercise and, 63–65

ICUs, *see* Intensive care units
Impact on Family Scale, 274, 277
Indiana Nursing Assessment of Functioning (INAF), 10, 11T
Indiana University School of Nursing, 13
Individual Incident Record (IIR), 123, 126–127
Insurance industry, 309
Intensive care units (ICUs)
  costs of, 93
  goal of, 97
  key features of, 97
  length of stay at, 93–94, 94–95
  nurses in, 248
  parents and, 239
  SCUs compared with, 100–110
International Classification of Diseases (ICD9), 94
Interventions, evaluating, 83–85
Inventory of Adult Role Behavior (IARB), 173
Inventory of Adult Self-Care (IASC), 173
Inventory of Well-Being (IWB), 163, 173
Iowa Veterans' Home (IVH), 120, 125

Jette Functional Status Index, 181–182, 185f
Journal of the American Medical Association (JAMA), 21, 22

"Knowledge creep," 80
Knowledge-driven model of research, 80
Knowledge of Alzheimer's Test (KAT), 125

Life-threatening conditions, 283
Limitation, measuring, 162–163
Loss, chronic sorrow and, 232
Low birthweight (LBW) infants; *see also* Very low birthweight (VLBW) infants
  family functioning and, 272

long-range complications of, 271
medical costs of, 271–272
mortality and, 271
non-medical costs of, 272

Madigan, Rep. Edward R., 8–9
Managing, in parenting, 308
Managing chronicity, 8–18
chronicity as feminist issue, 15
emphasis on functional ability, 9–12
person–environment fit, 13–15
quality of life, 12–13
resurgence of case study method, 16
sustaining optimism, 16–17
Maslach Burnout Inventory (MBI), 124
Medical intensive care unit, (MICU), 94
"Medically fragile," as term, 240–241
Medically fragile infant, 239–240
Medical model, 40, 41, 42
basic premise of, 42
Medical uncertainty, 49–51
managing, 52–55
Medication, as intervention, 136
Mental health and illness, 70–72
cognitive function, 72
psychiatric symptoms, 71–72
stress reduction, 70–71
Millon Behavior Health Inventory (MBHI), 195
Minnesota Multiphasic Inventory, 313
Mishel Uncertainty in Illness Scale (MUIS), 174
Morbidity, mortality versus, 8
Mothers; *see also* Nurse–mother relationship, *and* Parental role alterations
on FFFS, 301
in illness management, 295
Multidisciplinary discharge planning teams, 33
Multiple chronic illnesses, exercise and, 72
Multiple Sclerosis, diagnosing, 50
Multiple Sclerosis Self-Help Course, 168
Muscle endurance, 60
Muscle strength, 60
Myocardial infarction (MI), exercise and, 62

National Center for Nursing Research, 8
National Health Interview Survey (NHIS), 290–291
National Institute on Aging, 117
Negative certainty, 172
Neonatal Behavior Assessment Scale, 252
Neonatal ICU (NICU), 239–240
Neonatal Morbidity Scale, 254
Nightingale, Florence, 21, 333
Normalization, in parenting, 282, 284–285, 286, 307
Nurse case manager intervention, 170–172, 174–176
Nurse–mother relationship
context of negotiation, 243–244
control issues, 246
individual patterns in maternal role negotiation, 244–246mismatched perceptions, 247
process issues, 244
role negotiation in, 242–243
Nurse–parent relationship
ambiguity in, 247–248
role negotiations in, 248
trust between, 247
Nurses; *see also* PREP nurse
in ACE unit, 137–140
in asthma education program development, 328
in asthma education program instruction, 322
caring for chronically ill, 4, 7
caring for preterm CLD infants, 255, 259–260, 265
childhood cancer and role of, 318
chronic pain as perceived by, 28
chronic sorrow and role of, 234–235, 235–236
in developing interventions, 6
discharge planning by, 142

[Nurses; *see also* PREP nurse]
enhancing family health, 310–311
facilitating quality of life for patient and family, 336–337
family caregivers of HIPs and, 218
in ICUs, 248
inservice programs for, on helping parents, 248
medically fragile infants and, 240
parenting and, 335–336
patient education by, 26
in SCUs for AD, 128
in SCUs, 97, 110
working with parents of seriously ill children, 288–289
Nursing
leadership role of, 9
metatheory of, 13
Nursing Assessment of the Child with Asthma and the Family, 322
Nursing Consortium for Research on Chronic Sorrow (NCRCS), 232–233
Nursing demonstration projects, 335
Nursing model of home care, 42
Nursing research
conferences on, 4, 5–6
dissemination and use of, 4
Nursing Satisfaction Questionnaire (NSQ), 124–125

Occupational therapy, 138
Office of Technology Assessment, 93
Omnibus Reconciliation Act (OBRA)
of 1987, 38, 40
of 1990, 113
Ontario Exercise Heart Collaborative Study, 61–62
Optimism, health and, 16–17
Osteoarthritis (OA), 65–66
Osteoarthritis (OA) of knee, 178–180; *see also* Quantitative Progressive Exercise Rehabilitation (QPER)
exercise and, 179–180
hypothetical flowchart for events in, 179f
physiological muscle function and, 178
Parental role alterations, 281–289
advocating, 285
caregiving, 286
clinical implications, 288–289
compensation, 285, 286
normalization, 282, 284–285, 286
nursing diagnosis and parental role, 287–288
nurturing, 285–286
parental presence, 287
parental role alteration stress, 286
parental role changes, 285–286
parental vigilance, 287
parenting diagnoses, 282–283
parenting styles, 284–285
protecting, 285
responsibilities, 281
Parental Role Alteration Stress Scale (PRASS), 284
Parental role conflict, (PRC), 287–288
definition of, 282
Parent diary, 323
Parenting
definition of, 281
philosophies of, 294–295
success of, 281
Parents
nurse–parent relationship, 240
parent–infant relationship, 240
Patient, sensitivity to, 82–83
Perceived social support, definition of, 152
Personal Resources Questionnaire, 153
Person–environment fit, 13–15
importance of, 14–15
Pet therapy, 136
Philadelphia Geriatric Center, 112
Philadelphia Geriatric Center Morale Scale, 206
Physical fitness, 60
Physical therapy, 138
Physiological fitness indicators, 60
Physiological muscle function, 178
Positive and Negative Affect Scales, (PANAS), 173–174

Post-discharge services, 142
"Prehab Program of Patient-Centered Care," 133–134, 135
PREP nurse, 227–230
- developing contingency plans, 228–229
- documenting frequency and timing of behavior, 228
- enriching caregiving, 229–230
- rehearsal and role-playing with caregiver, 229
- reinforcing activities caregivers do well, 228

Preterm infants with chronic lung disease (CLD), 250–267
- definition of chronic lung disease, 252–253
- demographic characteristics, 258–259
- demographic variables, 254–255
- developmental outcomes for infants, 265
- infant activities, 260–262
- infant behavior, 257, 260–261, 262–264
- infant sleep–wake states, 255–256
- mean percentage of CLD infants that exhibited infant behavior, 263T
- mean percentage of observations CLD and non-CLD infants spent in sleeping and waking states, 261T
- mean percentage of observations CLD and non-CLD infants spent in sleep organization states, 262T
- nurse behaviors, 255
- nurse contexts, 255
- nursing activities, 259–260
- nursing interventions for infants, 265
- REM variables, 256–257
- respiratory regularity, 257
- sleep organization, 260
- sleep–wake states, 260, 262–264
- stereotyping of infants, 265–266

Primary nursing practice model, definition of, 97
Progressively Lowered Stimulus Threshold (PLST) Model, 119, 121
Prospective payment system (PPS), 142
Psychosocial adjustment, definition of, 159
Purpose and meaning in life, 152
Purpose in Life Test, 153

QPER, *see* Quantitative Progressive Exercise Rehabilitation
Quality of life, 12–13
- advocating, 309
- balancing, 307–308
- chronic illness in child and demands on family, 304–305
- controlling child's chronic illness, 306–309
- definition of, 160
- dimensions of, 333
- enhancing, 334, 335
- home care for chronically ill child, 304
- importance of, 12–13
- managing, 308
- measuring, 163
- minimizing, 306–307
- reframing family health, 310
- relationships of family, 304–311
- uncertainty and, 48

Quality-cost model, 33–36
Quality Cost Model of Early Hospital Discharge and Nurse Specialist Transitional Care, 243
Quantitative Progressive Exercise Rehabilitation (QPER), 178–188
- clinical implications of, 187–188
- development of, 186–187
- exercise bench used in, 180
- four-month QPER protocol for QA of knee, 182T
- functional performance after, 185–186

[Quantitative Progressive Exercise Rehabilitation (QPER)]
functional performance evaluation, 181–182
muscle function after, 183, 184f, 185, 186
muscle function measurement, 181
QPER protocol, 182–183
quantitative assessment protocols, 181–182
quantitative measurement, 187
short-term versus long-term effectiveness of, 187

Reconstitution, 16
Research, *see* Nursing research
Research Diagnostic Criteria for Depression, 72
Research use
change in setting, 81–82
clinical implications of research, 333–337
definition of, 80–81
interventions, 83–86
readiness of research for practice, 82–86
sensitivity to patient experiences, 82–83
Restrictive philosophy, 294–295
Rheumatoid arthritis (RA), 65–66
Role acquisition in family caregivers, 219–230; *see also* PREP nurse
learning about emotional needs, 223–225
learning about handling caregiving stress, 225–226
learning about physical needs, 222–223, 223T
learning about setting up services, 226
learning and role strain, 227
measures in study of, 221
as process, 219–220
post versus pre-entry, 220
sample in study of, 220–221
sources of information for caregivers, 221–222
strategies for enhancing role acquisition, 227–230
Role theory, 219
Rosenberg's Self-Esteem Scale, 206, 208

Sanger, Margaret, 14
SCUs, *see* Special care units
Self-advocacy, 56
Self-care, definition of, 160
Self-care functioning, 10
Self-Care Inventory (SCI), 173
Self-care/self-help movement, 158
Self-care skills, 38
Self-Control Schedule (SCS), 161, 163, 174
Self-efficacy, measuring, 163
Self-help
definition of, 160
uncertainty and, 51
The Self-Help Course Manual, 156
Self-Help Intervention Project (SHIP), 165
Self-Help Model
depression and, 163–164
perceived severity of illness in, 160
uncertainty and, 160
Self-help response to chronic illness, 158–168
depression and, 162, 163–164
limitation in, 162–163
Self-Help Model, 159f, 159–160
self-worth and, 162
visual analogue (VAS) response format, 163
for women with breast cancer, 165–167
Self-management programs, enabling skills and, 161–162
Self-Perception Profile, 301
Self-worth, 162
measuring, 163
Setting, need for change in, 81–82
Shared governance management model, 96–97
Shifting philosophy, 295
Sickness Impact Profile (SIP), 207, 208

Skilled care, definition of, 41
Snow's Inventory of Functional Tests (SIFT), 206–207
Socialization, as intervention, 136
Social Security Act, 40
Special Care Units (SCUs), 93–111
  admission algorithm, 101, 102f
  admission criteria, 101, 115–116
  benefits of, 95–96
  case manager in, 97–98
  chronically critically ill patient population, 94–95
  complication outcomes, 101, 106–107T, 108
  concept of, 95–96
  cost of, 95, 117
  definitions and criteria for, 114–117
  education and adjustments required by, 98–100
  as environment, 96–97
  failure to wean, 99T
  family programming and, 118, 121
  five characteristics of, 114
  ICU compared with, 100–110
  key features of, 96
  nurse in, 97, 110
  operations, 97–100
  patient cost data, 108, 109T, 110
  patient outcomes, 101, 104T, 105
  patient progress in, 98
  physical environment in, 114–115
  research on problems of, 118
  pros and cons of, 117–118
  staff of, 97, 118–120
  staff selection and training, 114
  standard criteria for, 113
  subject characteristics, 101, 103T
Special care units (SCUs) for Alzheimer's patients, 112–129
  activity programming, 116–117
  admission criteria, 115–116, 121
  behavioral dysfunction, 125–126
  cost of care, 126–127
  falls per patient week, 127T
  functional abilities, 126–127
  growth of, 112
  housing lucid and demented residents together, 117–118
  patient measures, 122–123
  phase I and II instruments, 123T
  physical environment, 114–115
  pros and cons of, 117–118
  staff, 121–122, 127–128
  staff selection and training, 114
  use of restraints per resident, 127T
STAI, *see* State-Trait Anxiety Inventory
State-Trait Anxiety Inventory (STAI), 214, 215, 216
Surgical intensive care unit (SICU), 94
Survey of Asthma Problems and Severity (SAPS), 323
Symptom Checklist 90 Revised (SCL–90–R), 313, 314–316
  means of predeath and postdeath scores by family, 316T
Symptom uncertainty, 48–49
  managing, 52–55
Systemic Lupus Erythematosis (SLE)
  diagnosing, 50
  uncertainty and, 56, 57
Systemic Lupus Erythematosis (SLE) Self-Help Course
  amount of time of participation and amount of change, 164–165
  course description, 162
  mean changes over time in participants, 164T
  as prototype, 168

Taylor Manifest Anxiety Scale, 71
Thematic Apperception Test (TAT), 313–314, 316
Thinking, research findings and, 80
Transitional care, 30–36
  costs of, 31, 32
  current and emerging models of, 32–33
  definitions of, 30
  issues in, 31–32
  key features of, 30
  length of service, 31
  patients requiring, 32

[Transitional care]
providers of, 32
quality-cost model of, 33–36

Uncertainty, 46–57
"at-risk-role" and, 51–52
constructing normative framework, 56
daily living uncertainty, 51–52
definitions of, 47, 160, 170
focusing on positive, 56
framing illness schemas, 52–53
formulating timetables, 53–54
in illness, 47–52
incorporating, 57
lack of confidence in physicians, 50–51
maintaining hope, 54–55
managing daily living uncertainty, 55–57
managing medical uncertainty, 52–55
managing symptom uncertainty, 52–55
medical diagnostic uncertainty, 49–51
occurrence of, 46
outcome of event and, 47
positive aspect of, 48
as psychological stressor, 46–47
quality of life and, 48

rituals, 57
specifying controllable circumstances, 56–57
stressful nature of, 47
survivorship, 52
symptom uncertainty, 48–49
uncertainty stress points, 52
unpredictability management, 54
Uncertainty in illness theory, 171. *See also* Mishel.
Uncertainty management in breast cancer, 170–176
intervention goals, 172

Very low birthweight (VLBW) infants, 272–279
economic status of family of, 273–274
employment of family of, 275–277
functioning of family of, 277, 278
monthly income of family of, 277
out-of-pocket expenses of family of, 274–275, 275T, 276T, 278–279
Visiting nurses, 39
Visiting Nurse Service of New York, 39, 40
Visual analogue scale (VAS), 163, 173
VLBW, *see* Very low birthweight (VLBW) infants

Wald, Lillian, 14
Web of Causation for Frailty and Disability, 202, 203f
WHO, *see* World Health Organization
WHO Collaborating Center in Healthy Cities, 13
Wilcoxin Signed Rank Test, 314–316
Women
chronicity and, 15
endurance exercise and, 64
home care and, 41
Work capacity, 62
World Health Organization (WHO), 13, 41

Yale Physical Activity Scale, 206, 208